Fundamentals of Implant Dentistry

Fundamentals of Implant Dentistry

Gerard Byrne
BDentSc. (Dublin), MSD. (Indiana)

WILEY Blackwell

This edition first published 2014 © 2014 by John Wiley & Sons, Inc.

Editorial offices: 1606 Golden Aspen Drive, Suites 103 and 104, Ames, Iowa 50010, USA
The Atrium, Southern Gate, Chichester, West Sussex, PO19 8SQ, UK
9600 Garsington Road, Oxford, OX4 2DQ, UK

For details of our global editorial offices, for customer services and for information about how to apply for permission to reuse the copyright material in this book please see our website at www.wiley.com/wiley-blackwell.

Library of Congress Cataloging-in-Publication Data
Byrne, Gerard (Dentist), author.
   Fundamentals of implant dentistry / Gerard Byrne.
      p. ; cm.
   Includes bibliographical references and index.
   ISBN 978-1-118-27496-5 (pbk.)
   I. Title.
   [DNLM: 1. Dental Implants.   2. Dental Implantation–methods.   3. Tooth Diseases–surgery.   WU 640]
   RK667.I45
   617.6'93–dc23
                              2013050477

A catalogue record for this book is available from the British Library.

Wiley also publishes its books in a variety of electronic formats. Some content that appears in print may not be available in electronic books.

Cover design by Meaden Creative

Set in 9.5/12 pt PalatinoLTStd-Roman by Toppan Best-set Premedia Limited
Printed and bound in Singapore by Markono Print Media Pte Ltd

1   2014

Contents

Acknowledgments

I would firstly like to thank my best friend and wife, Tricia; our home became my office.

Special thanks to our children for their understanding and help: Brendan Byrne, Grinnell College, Grinnell, IA, for editing the manuscript; Heather Byrne, Pomona College, Claremont, CA, for her line drawings; and Thomas Byrne, Southwest HS, Lincoln, NE, for checking and editing the references.

I am indebted to all those who have kindly given me permission to use their photographs and other copyrighted material.

Finally, many thanks to Shelby, Nancy, and the team in Ames, IA, for making this book possible.

G.B.

About the Companion Website

This book is accompanied by a companion website:

www.wiley.com/go/byrne/implants

The website includes:

- PowerPoints of all figures and tables from the book for downloading
- Appendix 1 in PDF format

1

Introduction to Dental Implants

1.1   Introduction

Implantation involves the embedding of a native or foreign tissue or substance within body tissues. The end point of dental implantation is recovered dental function and aesthetics.

It has long been a common refrain in dental practice for patients to express the desire for a "screw-in" tooth replacement. The dream of predictable stable implant prostheses and the current concept of implant "osseointegration" became a reality through the pioneering research of Brånemark and coworkers in Sweden from the mid-1960s, and Schroeder and coworkers in Switzerland from the mid-1970s. (Brånemark et al. 1969, 1977, 1985; Albrektsson et al. 1981; Schroeder et al. 1991, 1996). From a clinical standpoint, research has shown that modern titanium (Ti) endosseous implants have an overall survival rate of 90–95%.

Beginning in 1952 Brånemark discovered, in the course of vital microscopic studies of blood rheology and bone healing, that titanium (Ti) optical chambers inserted in rabbit bone became firmly attached to the bone and were difficult to remove for reuse; the living bone had "bonded" to the Ti. Later in the 1960s, Brånemark further studied this phenomenon in dogs and, from his perspective as an orthopedic surgeon, contemplated the idea of using Ti implants for artificial joints, bone repair, and edentulism. Brånemark resolved to work primarily on the rehabilitation of edentulism. He coined the term "osseointegration" to describe the stable functional bond between the metal Ti screws and living bone. Brånemark and his team, with meticulous attention to detail, adherence to sound biological principles, and

Fundamentals of Implant Dentistry, First Edition. Gerard Byrne.
© 2014 John Wiley & Sons, Inc. Published 2014 by John Wiley & Sons, Inc.
Companion website: www.wiley.com/go/byrne/implants

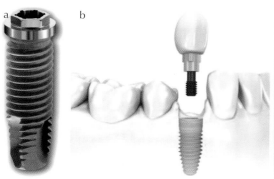
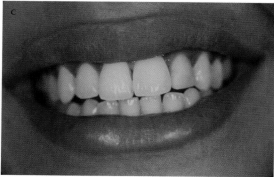

1.1. (a) Brånemark Mark III self-threading machined implant screw with Ti-Unite® surface and smooth collar (courtesy of Nobel Biocare). (b) Modern implant crown diagram comprising an implant and screw-retained combination abutment-crown (courtesy of Nobel Biocare). (c) Left central incisor implant with metal-ceramic crown.

long-term continuous study, proceeded to develop a standard set of protocols for implant rehabilitation of edentulism. Brånemark et al. (1985) postulated a two-stage surgical approach allowing the submerged implant to heal or integrate for 3–6 months before exposure to the oral environment (Fig. 1.1a,b). Schroeder et al. (1996) in later independent studies postulated a one-stage surgery, a nonsubmerged technique, with transmucosal healing and a shorter healing period of 3–4 months. Otherwise, the techniques were similar in that both used Ti, careful atraumatic site preparation, and prolonged healing.

While Brånemark's vision is now accepted and lauded, it is interesting to note that there was significant controversy and skepticism at the time in his native Sweden regarding this new implant method (Albrektsson and Sennerby 2005). In a 2005 commentary, Brånemark suggested that we need to continue to focus on the *"decisive effect of functional load on the healing process and remodeling of bone and marrow" rather than focus on the "hardware."* He further commented that: *"the mouth is a much more important part of the human body than medicine and controlling agencies recognize."*

1.2   Tooth loss

Consequences of tooth loss on alveolar bone

Bone needs functional stimulation to maintain its form and density. The alveolar bone grows with the developing and erupting teeth. Wolff's Law states that bone remodels (changes its internal and external architecture) in relation to the forces applied. The loss of a tooth and thence loss of functional bone stimulation, leads to bone atrophy and a reduction in alveolar ridge width and height (Tallgren et al. 1980). A removable prosthesis does not stimulate and maintain bone but serves to exacerbate ridge resorption. Ridge resorption of up to 22% vertically and 63% horizontally occurs within 6 months after tooth extraction in otherwise dentate patients (Tan et al. 2012). During the first year following tooth extraction, there is an average ridge width decrease of 25%, and an average 4.0 mm height reduction. Implants retain alveolar bone height, but do not completely prevent some alveolar resorption when placed immediately into tooth extraction sites.

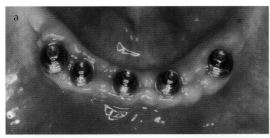

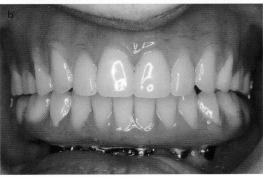

1.2. (a) Brånemark implants with attached transmucosal abutments (courtesy of Dr. E. Kim). (b) Brånemark-style reconstruction: mandibular fixed "hybrid" prosthesis supported by five implants (courtesy of Dr. E. Kim).

Demographics of tooth loss

Age is related directly to every indicator of tooth loss: caries, periodontal disease, endodontic problems, and fracture (Meskin et al. 1988; Misch 2007; Jokstad 2009). The average number of lost teeth increases with age (Müller et al. 2007; Zitzmann et al. 2007). There has been a steady increase in the global population that is over 65 years of age. Worldwide, there is a projected increase of over 65 year olds from 550 million in 2000 to 973 million in 2030. Life expectancy is increasing in economically developed countries, and was 85 years in 2001 for the United States (Kinsella 2005). Although the incidence of complete edentulism is on the decline in Europe, the United States, and other economically developed countries, as life expectancy continues to increase, and with continued immigration, the number of people requiring full dentures in the next 3–5 decades will continue to increase. The total edentulism rate in the U.S. adult population is 10.5% or approximately 18 million people. The reported rate of one and two arch edentulism is 17% or 30 million people, in the United States (Marcus et al. 1996). Global demand for complete denture prostheses is likely to continue increasing (Felton 2009) (Fig. 1.2a,b).

Partial edentulism is even more prevalent in the United States. In 45- to 54-year-old patients, 31.3% have mandibular free-end edentulism, while 13.6% have free-end maxillary edentulism. This partial edentulism rate increases to 35% (mandibular) and 18% (maxillary) in the 55- to 64-year-old age group. The number of U.S. patients with at least one quadrant of posterior teeth missing is more than 44 million (Misch 2007). Up to 70% of the adult U.S. population may be missing at least one tooth. Up until 1995, it is estimated that 1% of patients with an implant indication for tooth loss had been treated with implants. Misch (2007) estimated that a total of 74 million adults in the United States are potential candidates for dental implants. The "baby-boomer" (post-Second World War babies) population in developed countries offers significant growth potential for implant treatment due to high disposable income and longer life expectancy.

Current market research shows that the global dental implant market is expected to grow from $3.2 billion in 2010 to $4.2 billion in 2015. Europe is currently the world's largest market with a 42% market share, and a growth rate of 7%pa, followed by the United States and Japan (Market Reports 2010).

Reasons why implant treatment is increasing

- Implant success has been validated over prolonged periods.
- The population is aging; tooth loss increases with age.

- Traditional restorative dentistry procedures have a limited life span.
- Dentures deliver relatively poor function.
- Tooth loss and removable prostheses generate negative psychology for a patient.
- Dental implant treatment is viewed positively by the public.

1.3   Early dental implants

Historically, numerous attempts have been made to replace lost teeth with artificial substitutes, but with limited success (Ring 1995a, 1995b; Sullivan 2001). Dental implant therapy was initially aimed at the fully edentulous patient or dental invalid who was unable to cope with conventional dentures.

Implant classification

See NIH (1978) and Schroeder et al. (1996).
- *Subperiosteal:* A CoCr casting custom made for an edentulous bony ridge and placed subperiosteally with integral transmucosal posts for denture retention.
- *Endosseous—blade (plate), ramus frame, transosteal or staple, root form, or cylindrical:* These implants are anchored in bone and penetrate the oral mucosa to provide prosthetic anchorage. Linkow (1968) introduced the Ti blade implant. The ramus frame has a tripod of blade-like bone anchorages. Root form designs were introduced in the 1980s by Brånemark et al. (1969), Kirsch and Ackermann (1989) ("intramobil zylinder," IMZ®), Schulte (1992) (Tübingen), and Schroeder et al. (1991) ("titanium plasma sprayed screw" [TPS]/International Team for Implantology [ITI]) (Fig. 1.3a–d).

Other early implants include:

- *Submucosal implants:* A small "press-stud-like" device within the soft tissue helping to retain a denture, usually maxillary
- *Transdental fixation:* A metal implant placed through a tooth and extended into the apical bone, sometimes referred to as endodontic implants

From a practical perspective, blade, subperiosteal, ramus frame, and staple implants have enjoyed modest success. These implants enabled edentulous patients to have a stable anchored lower denture with reasonable function and comfort. Blades have been used as bridge abutments in distal edentulous areas (Kennedy Class I/II RPD cases). However, due to the surgical techniques used and immediate or early loading, there was a high incidence of chronic infection, bone loss and scar tissue envelopment of the implants. They did, however, in many cases, present the only viable alternative to mobile complete or partial dentures, albeit an invasive one.

The use of these early implants was very specialized and tended to be limited to large urban areas with little geographical spread. With the advent of predictable endosseous root-form implants, other implants have virtually disappeared from clinical practice, although they may be encountered occasionally.

Contemporary endosseous root-form implants

Modern dental implants are either cylindrical or tapered threaded screws, or unthreaded press-fit designs. The cylindrical or rotationally symmetrical implant shape allows for controlled and atraumatic osteotomy drilling or site preparation. They are manufactured from commercially pure titanium (CpTi), or titanium alloy (Ti-6Al-4V) with or without surface threads/fins and with or without surface texturing or chemical modification. Implants usually have a screw connection for prosthetic

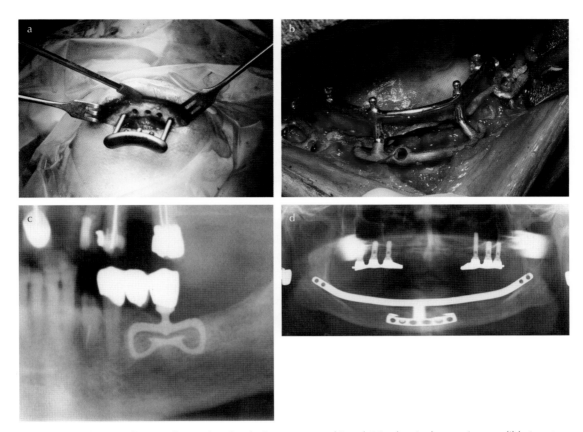

1.3. (a) External approach surgical procedure for placing a transosteal "staple" implant in the anterior mandible (courtesy of Dr. J.B. Bavitz). (b) Surgical procedure for removal of a subperiosteal implant (courtesy of Dr. J.B. Bavitz). (c) Radiograph of a blade implant (courtesy of Dr. J.B. Bavitz). (d) Ramus frame implant with a tripod of bone support.

abutments, with an anti-rotation feature. This connection enables both surgical insertion of the implant and anchorage of the prosthesis. In the past decade, implant configuration, implant surface modification, and connection design have changed and evolved. There have been repeated attempts to create more stable connections, and surfaces that favor better and more rapid osseointegration, especially in softer bone. The long-term significance of these innovations remains to be seen. Advertising relating to design enhancements is intensive and should be viewed with caution.

Implant treatment

Early implant treatment was largely geared toward complete edentulism, especially of the mandible. Implant therapy progressed to the edentulous maxilla and finally to partial edentulism. The first studies relating to single tooth implants and bridges started to appear in the early 1990s, with increasing emphasis on anchorage stability and aesthetics. The technical challenges and innovative solutions continued to grow as implant popularity spread and demand for implant crown and bridgework increased.

1.4   Pioneering implant research

The ADA Council on Scientific Affairs (ADA 2004) reported a mean survival rate of 95.4% for implants in clinical studies published since 1996. The review included 14 clinical studies covering 10,006 implants and multiple implant designs at follow-up periods of 2–16 years. An average survival rate was judged to be >90% in various clinical scenarios with single units, bridges, and overdentures.

Brånemark group

Brånemark was the pioneer of Ti root-form implants (Sullivan 2001). Beginning in 1952, studies, which have constituted the basis for permanent tissue integration of implants, were performed at the Laboratory for Vital Microscopy, Department of Anatomy, University of Lund, Sweden, also the Laboratory for Experimental Biology, University of Goteborg (since 1960), and at the Institute for Applied Biotech in Goteborg (since 1978). Early studies were vital microscopic studies of blood rheology, bone marrow, and bone healing. Early experiments in rats, rabbits, and dogs showed the phenomenon of bone condensation around the Ti implants when transcutaneous abutments were connected in jawbones. When implants were forcibly removed for examination, the bone fractured but was still adherent to the Ti surfaces. Further work in the development of clinical procedures for the rehabilitation of edentulism was undertaken in dogs. Posterior bridges were made on Ti screw implants 10.0 mm long and 4.0 mm diameter with a 10-year follow-up showing no significant problems; oral hygiene was provided once or twice per year. On the basis of these animal experiments, which showed stable osseointegration and a favorable interface with mucosal epithelium, human trials began from 1965 onwards. Edentulous subjects were treated with mandibular fixed prostheses supported by four to six screw-type implants. We now know these prostheses as "hybrid" or "fixed detachable" screw-retained fixed prostheses (FDPs). More than 4000 implants were placed in humans over approximately 10 years. Failed implants were trephined out and studied radiographically, histologically, and with scanning electron microscopy (SEM) and transmission electron microscopy (TEM). Forced mechanical failure was cohesive within bone and not adhesive between bone and the Ti implant surface. An implant survival rate of 96–99% was achieved. A summation of the group's experimentation with animal and clinical trials was presented at the Toronto Conference on Osseointegration in 1982 along with the eponymous Brånemark implant system (Zarb 1983; Brånemark et al. 1985).

Up to 50 different implant screw designs were tried before settling on the original Brånemark two-stage screw implant, marketed by Nobel Industries circa 1980. The final Brånemark implant or "fixture" for clinical use, after 30 years of laboratory and 20 years of clinical research, was a threaded commercially pure titanium (CPTi) cylindrical screw 3.75 mm diameter, 7.0 to 18.0 mm long, with a slightly wider collar (neck), and a hole and thread-formers at the apical end. The wider collar was designed to engage the cortical bone of the ridge crest for initial stability, and the apical perforation allowed bone in-growth to resist rotational forces. A transmucosal cylinder or healing abutment was added when the implant was uncovered at second-stage surgery. The original implant design has been extensively modified over the past 30+ years and many variants are now supplied by the commercial group (Nobel Biocare) affiliated with Brånemark's work. Initially, training in the Brånemark protocol was offered only in Sweden; gradually, other research and training centers were established throughout the world.

Schroeder/ITI, Schulte, and Kirsch groups

In 1975, the International Team for Implantology (ITI), the Schroeder group, in collaboration with the Straumann Company, demonstrated osseointegration of plasma-sprayed Ti (TPS) implants in monkeys (Albrektsson et al. 1986; Laney 1993; Spiekermann 1995). These ITI implants were designed for a one-stage surgery. Their findings were published in book form in German in 1988, and in English 3 years later (Schroeder et al. 1991, 1996), enabling the affiliated Straumann implant to reach the English-speaking audience and U.S. markets. The Straumann system has become one of the best researched and most popular contemporary implant systems (Jokstad 2009). One implant variant developed by Straumann and ITI was called the "Swiss screw," which had a TPS surface and integral abutments, and was primarily geared toward overdenture treatment (Babbush et al. 1986).

Another innovative ceramic (Tübingen) implant system, was developed in Germany for immediate postextraction placement (Schulte and Heimke 1976; Schulte et al. 1992). It demonstrated good osseointegration, but had some technical difficulties in the connection of abutments to the implants. The Tübingen system later adopted Ti as the base material (Frialit® II), but maintained the stepped design that was deemed favorable for implantation into tapered tooth sockets, and added some threads (d'Hoedt and Schulte 1989).

Kirsch and Ackermann (1989) (IMZ, Germany) pioneered a cylindrical, round-ended, press-fit (no threads) implant with a plasma-sprayed Ti surface (TPS). This implant was unique for having an intramobile element to help dissipate impact forces.

All three alternative press-fit implant designs (ITI, Tübingen/Frialit II, and IMZ) and surfaces (machined CPTi, TPS, and ceramic) had documented osseointegrtion and clinical success (Albrektsson et al. 1986).

1.5 Commercial implant history

According to Jokstad (2009), there are more than 600 implant systems and at least 146 manufacturers globally. Currently, the major implant companies are Nobel Biocare, Straumann, Dentsply, and Biomet-3i.

Implant brands are often a division of major biomedical enterprises with a global reach. Consolidation of the industry seems to be occurring in the West (e.g., Dentsply), but we have yet to experience the influence of developments in Asia on the Western market. It is not unusual for implant companies to change ownership or change branding. Marketing generally seems to override research and development, and in order to select the optimal system for patients, the dental professional must look closely at the ongoing clinical research data of the implant system rather than marketing campaigns for purported benefits that are not proven clinically over the long term (Jokstad 2009). It is important that the implant be serviceable throughout the lifetime of the patient. It is a rather sobering thought for dentists and patients that a treatment with long-term medical devices may be supplied by a company that goes out of business or fails to provide support.

The practicing dentist needs to be familiar with the recent history of implants, as older variants may present in patients for management of problems. There are information websites on implant identification and third-party component suppliers for discontinued implant lines. Occasionally, dental laboratories may be familiar with several systems, and stock components and instruments. Cases involving unfamiliar implant systems should be referred to the original treating dentist or a specialist prosthodontist.

Nobel Biocare (Nobel Bofors/Nobelpharma)

Nobel Biocare is the commercial arm for Brånemark's pioneering research. In 1965, the first human subject was treated with Ti implant screws and a fixed screw-retained prosthesis for an edentulous lower jaw (Brånemark 2006).

Brånemark noted the potential for mandibular flexure and confined the fixtures to the anterior mandible supporting a fixed cantilevered denture. In 1978, the Swedish Health System approved Ti implants for clinical use. In that same year, the armaments company, Bofors of Sweden (Later, Bofors Nobelpharma, and currently Nobel Biocare) agreed to partner with Brånemark for the commercial development of the implant system. In 1982, the Food and Drug Administration (FDA) approved the use of titanium dental implants in the United States. In 1983, Mats Andersson developed the Procera® method of manufacturing crowns; this technology was acquired by Nobel-pharma in 1988.

The classic Brånemark implant was a 3.75-mm diameter, 7.0- to 18.0-mm long, machined CPTi screw with a slightly wider polished collar and an "apical" thread-former. There was an external hex that allowed for surgical placement, to be followed by a screw-retained transmucosal abutment or extension cylinder. The hex became the anti-rotation device for single crowns. Historically, this is the most commonly placed implant, and many other implant companies have used a similar design. The Brånemark implant is the implant with the greatest body of clinical research (Fig. 1.4a,b).

Straumann (ITI/Bonefit®)

The Straumann Biomedical company, a pioneer in orthopedic implants, started work on dental implants in 1974 under the guidance of Dr. F. Straumann, and Professor A. Schroeder of the University of Berne, Switzerland. The early hollow-basket design evolved through various hollow cylinder, solid, press-fit, and screw designs to the current solid screw design. Implants were originally made from Ti, with no threads, a hollow perforated body, and a plasma-sprayed textured Ti surface (TPS). The early one-piece implants were designed

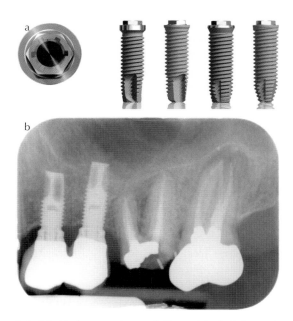

1.4. (a) Modern versions of the original Brånemark implant screw (courtesy of Nobel Biocare). (b) Radiograph of Brånemark implants with joined crowns.

with an integral transmucosal abutment (also seen with blade implants). The later two-piece implants have a flared, beveled and polished, transmucosal collar. This design pioneered the one-stage surgical technique, and favored a more natural emergence profile of crowns. Straumann introduced an internal morse taper (internal connection) for frictional retention and stability of abutments, and later modified it with an internal octagon. In 1980, under the aegis of Dr. Straumann and Professor Schroeder, the International Team for Implantology (ITI) was founded. ITI has become one of the largest independent academic organizations in implant dentistry and the related field of guided tissue regeneration. For more than 30 years, ITI has partnered with Straumann in the development of Straumann implant products (Fig. 1.5a–e) (Buser et al. 1988, 1997; Sutter et al. 1988).

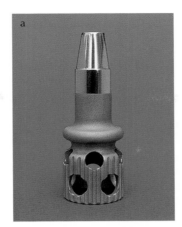

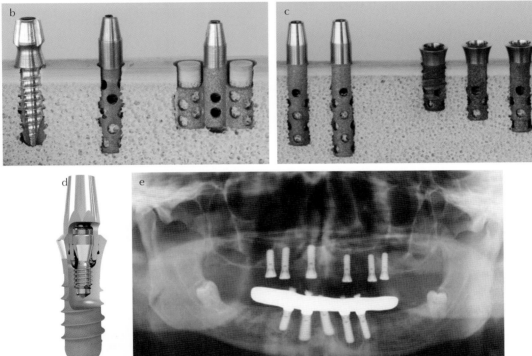

1.5. (a) Straumann implant prototype from 1974 showing hollow basket design and integral transmucosal abutment (courtesy of Straumann). (b, c) Early ITI one-piece and two-piece implants: solid (machined) and hollow (TPS-coated) (courtesy of Straumann). (d) Current solid ITI implant with abutment for a cemented crown (courtesy of Straumann). (e) Radiograph of modern, solid, flared-collar ITI implants (courtesy of Dr. T. Taylor).

Tübingen (Frialit/Friadent-Dentsply)

In 1974, Dr. W. Schulte developed a ceramic implant (Al_2O_3) at the University of Tübingen, Germany. The Tübingen implant was a tapered, stepped, root-form, press-fit design. It was designed for placement into extraction sockets and used a cemented abutment. It was the forerunner of the current Frialit implants, introduced in 1980, which have a similar stepped shape but are made from CpTi and have external threads for initial stability (Dentsply Friadent) (Schulte et al. 1992; Gomez-Roman et al. 1997). The switch to Ti and screw connections overcame the inflexibility of the original design. The Tübingen implant proved the potential of ceramic as a viable implant material (Fig. 1.6).

IMZ (Interpore/Dentsply)

A German-designed "intramobil zylinder" (IMZ) implant by Dr. A. Kirsch gained clinical popularity in the 1980s and 1990s (Kirsch and Ackermann 1989). The IMZ was a cylindrical press-fit design made from CpTi, with a plasma-sprayed Ti surface (TPS). It had a polished collar, and introduced the concept of a shock absorber or plastic "intramobile element" to mitigate functional stress. This intramobile element was later discontinued and an external hex adopted, to accommodate single crowns. Currently, an internal "spline" design is used. To date, over one million IMZ implants have been placed worldwide (Dentsply–Friadent) (Fig. 1.7a,b). More recently, Dr. Kirsch is associated with Camlog implants founded in 1999.

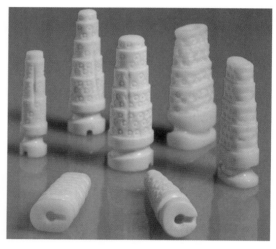

1.6. Tübingen stepped, press-fit ceramic implants (courtesy of Dentsply Implants).

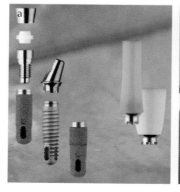
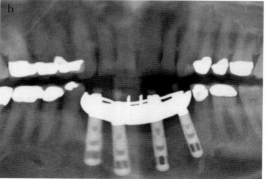

1.7. (a) Modern IMZ implants and components including the nylon intramobile element (courtesy of Dentsply Implants). (b) IMZ implants supporting a screw-retained prosthesis.

Core-Vent (Paragon/Dentsply/Sulzer/Centerpulse/Zimmer/Implant-Direct-Sybron)

The Core-Vent Corporation in North America was founded by Dr. G. Niznick (Niznick 1985). Core-Vent produced an array of implant designs and obtained numerous design patents. The original Core-Vent implant was a "hollow basket/cylinder" design. It had three threads, a patented internal hex connection, and was made from Ti alloy with a textured, grit-blasted surface (Fig. 1.8a,b). Other designs included a Swede-Vent™ implant in CpTi, similar to Brånemark's design, and a variant with a patented internal hex connection and peripheral bevel (1983) (Drago and Peterson 2007). A later modification, in 1994, tapered the internal hex walls by 1.5° to give enhanced connection stability and prevent screw loosening, especially for single crowns. Further implant designs featured press-fit with plasma-sprayed hydroxyapatite (HA) coating. Core-Vent (Paragon) implant designs were acquired first by Sulzer Medica (Centerpulse) in 2000, and later by Zimmer in 2003. Zimmer currently market Core-Vent and Sulzer designs (Fig. 1.9).

In 2006 the Niznick Company, Implant Direct, started to produce a line of implants marketed and sold over the Internet. Implant Direct merged with Sybron Implant Solutions in 2011 to form a new company—Implant Direct Sybron International. Sybron had marketed several implant designs, including "Endopore."

Calcitek (Integral/Omniloc/Sulzer)

Calcitek Integral and Omniloc implants were cylindrical, press-fit implants with a plasma-sprayed hydroxylapatite (HA) coating and several connection designs. Calcitek was a division of Sulzer Medica Inc. (Finger and Guerra 1989, 1992). Calcitek seems to be synonymous with HA coatings within the United States,

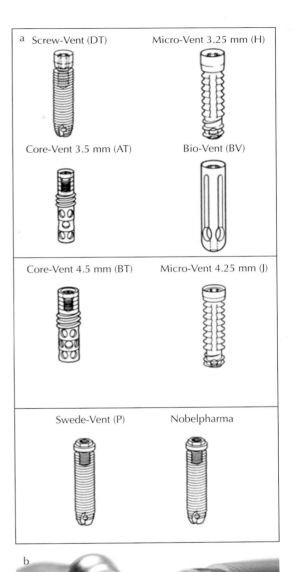

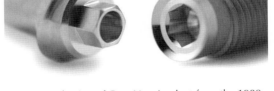

1.8. (a) A selection of Core-Vent implant from the 1980s. (b) Proprietary internal hex connection with lead-in bevel in Zimmer Screw Vent implants (courtesy of Zimmer Dental).

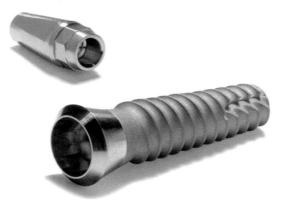

1.9. Zimmer Swissplus implant and abutment (courtesy of Zimmer Dental).

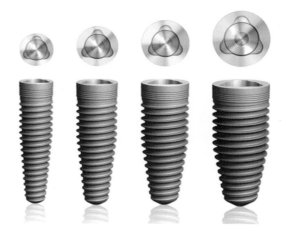

1.10. Tri-channel connection design (courtesy of /Nobel Biocare) and Replace™ Tapered Groovy implants (courtesy of Nobel Biocare).

although other companies used the same technology around the same time (Lifecore, Core-Vent, 3i, and Steri-Oss). HA surface coatings were utilized in an attempt to enhance osseointegration speed. There were some problems with the loss of the HA coating (separation of the coating from the Ti substructure) and saucerizing bone loss. This may have had more to do with the HA coating process than the HA material itself. The Albrektsson (1998) review showed unacceptable bone loss with Calcitek HA implants and this led to their withdrawal from the market (Biesbrock and Edgerton 1995; Watson et al. 1999). Ong and Chan (2000) have discussed the risk of HA dissolution. The HA surface process has largely been supplanted by other Ti-textured surface technologies that reportedly enhance osseointegration.

Steri-Oss (Nobel Biocare)

Steri-Oss implants appeared circa 1985 as straight or tapered Ti screws, with an external hex and four color-coded diameters. Surface finishes included acid etching, HA coating and TPS. A second identical line of implants (Replace Select™) had an innovative internal tri-channel internal connection. This latter design has become the most widely used and favored connection for the restorative dentist due to its simplicity and positive, intuitive clinical handling. Nobel Biocare acquired the system in 1998 and Steri-Oss products were subsumed into the Nobel Biocare implant system (Fig. 1.10).

Implant Innovations International (3i/Biomet-3i)

In 1985, Implant Innovations Inc. (3i) began manufacturing prosthetic components for implants. Later, 3i introduced its own implant, which was similar to the Brånemark design, and gradually produced a complete system of implants. In 1991, the company introduced wide-platform or wide-body implants (5.1 mm, 6.0 mm) with the same-size hex connection as for the standard 4.1 mm implant. It was discovered that when wide-platform implants were restored with narrower diameter abutments, they showed less bone loss than traditional

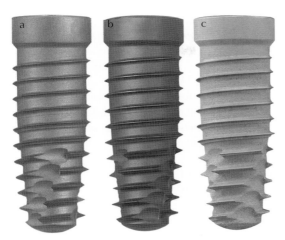

1.11. (a) Biomet 3i implant with OsseoTite® surface. (b) Biomet 3i implant with NanoTite™ surface. (c) Biomet 3i T3® implant with a combination of coarse and fine surface roughness (courtesy of Biomet 3i).

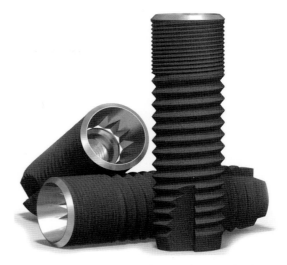

1.12. Astra Tech implants with internal connection (courtesy of Dentsply Implants).

matched implants and abutments (Lazzara and Porter 2006). This led to the concept of "platform-switching," which has been incorporated into many modern implant designs. 3i has a unique laser-coded marking system for healing abutments that simplifies data transfer for CAD/CAM laboratory work. 3i are now part of Biomet Inc. (Fig. 1.11a–c).

Astra Tech (Astra-Zeneca/Dentsply Implants)

Astra Tech has produced implants since 1985. They have focused on implants with a proprietary surface coating (TiOBlast™) and a platform-switched design with an internal tapered connection (Al-Nawas et al. 2012). Astra Tech pioneered the use of micro-threads (Hansson 1999) on the collar of their implants with a view to optimizing stress transfer in the crestal bone in order to minimize bone loss. This innovation now appears on many implant brands. Dentsply acquired Astra Tech in 2011 (Fig. 1.12).

Bicon

Bicon implants have been available since 1985 (Jokstad 2009). The design is press-fit, with fins rather than smooth walls. Bicon claims the first modern acid-etched surface, a revolutionary tapered locking connection (i.e., retaining screw) system and a reverse bevel collar design. Another significant feature of Bicon implants is their very short implant designs, as little as 5.0 mm long (Fig. 1.13).

Endopore (Sybron)

Endopore produced a unique implant that was a truncated cone, press-fit design geared toward posterior jaw locations (Jokstad 2009). These implants had a unique porous Ti surface that allowed for bone in-growth. The surface was produced with a sintered Ti alloy powder coating. It was claimed that the in-growth of bone into the Ti structure allows for optimum handling of lateral tensile loading forces, as compared with other machined and textured implant surfaces (Fig. 1.14a,b). Endopore

BICON'S 1.5° LOCKING TAPER
▸ Time-tested stable connection
▸ Proven bacterial seal

BICON'S SLOPING SHOULDER
▸ Space for bone over the implant
▸ Distributes occlusal stresses
▸ Preserves crestal bone

BICON'S PLATEAU DESIGN
▸ 30% more surface area
▸ No splinting necessary
▸ Callus bone formation
▸ Cortical-like Haversian bone between the fins

1.13. Bicon implant and friction-fit abutment (courtesy of Bicon Dental Implants).

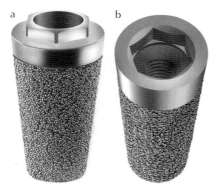

1.14. Endopore implants with (a) external hex and (b) internal hex connections and sintered Ti surfaces (courtesy of Sybron Implant Direct).

implants have been discontinued at the time of writing.

1.6   Notable implant "milestones"

NIH Harvard Conference, 1978

The U.S. National Institutes of Health (NIH) sponsored a consensus conference to review the status of oral implantology (Schnitman and Shulman 1980). The foremost experts in the field from around the United States presented the state of the art and science of oral implantology at this meeting. A consensus report was published giving clinical guidelines for the use of the various implant modalities including subperiosteal, blade, staple, and vitreous carbon. Root-form Ti endosseous implants were not on the meeting schedule, as European implant research was not represented.

Toronto Conference on Osseointegration, 1982

George A. Zarb, at the University of Toronto, recognized the potential of Brånemark's work with Ti screw implants and was instrumental in organizing the first North American Conference on Osseointegration in May 1982 (Zarb 1983). Brånemark presented the results of his group's research to a North American dental audience for the first time. He and his colleagues presented the biology of the implant–tissue interface and the results of 15 years of controlled clinical implant trials on edentulous subjects (Adell et al. 1981). This conference produced a paradigm shift in implant dentistry and the treatment of edentulism. Zarb and his colleagues was the first research group outside of Sweden to replicate and verify the clinical results obtained by the Brånemark group (Zarb and Schmitt 1990).

NIH Conference, 1988

The U.S. National Institute of Dental Research (NIDR), the U.S. NIH, and U.S. Food and Drug Administration (FDA), convened the conference to assess the rapid growth and advances in implantology in the early 1980s in the United States, Europe, and Japan (NIH 1988). The conference aimed to deal with gaps in knowledge and tried to resolve some existing controversies. The conference report emphasized the need for a multidisciplinary approach due to the complexity of the surgical and restorative procedures. The report noted the need for more controlled animal studies and clinical research, that is, randomized controlled trials (RCTs). The report also noted that it was not possible to make a definitive statement on long-term efficacy of dental implants. It was recognized that a large proportion of endosseous, subperiosteal, and transosteal implants had remained in place for more than 10 years.

1.7 Criteria for implant success

Ultimately, a long-term, functional, and stable aesthetic restoration on a stable integrated implant is the desirable outcome for both patient and dentist. Clinical implant cases may be considered a failure when the implant is failing or has failed, or when the prosthesis has aesthetic or persistent mechanical problems. The main predictors for implant survival are the quantity and quality of bone, age of patient, certain systemic health factors, smoking, the dentist's experience, loading conditions, implant length, and oral hygiene (Porter and von Fraunhofer 2005).

Implant success and survival

Albrektsson et al. (1986) designated success criteria as follows:

- The individual implant should be *clinically immobile.*
- There should be *no radiographic radiolucency.*
- There should be an *absence of persistent pain, infections, neuropathies, and paresthesia.*
- There should be *85% implant survival at the end of a 5-year period* of observation and *80% at the end of a 10-year* observation period.
- There should be *less than 0.2 mm of bone loss annually* following the implant's first year of loading.

Roos et al. (1997) proposed an update to these criteria to reflect that, as implant design evolved, early bone loss could be further minimized. The new criteria suggested a figure of <1.8 mm bone loss for the first 5 years.

- Less than 1.0 mm bone loss in the first year
- Less than 0.2 mm bone loss annually after the first year
- Functional survival of 90% after 5 years and 85% after 10 years.

Implant and prosthetic success

Implant success is predicated on the usefulness of the implant. Implant position should allow the fabrication of a successful prosthesis. Similarly, the prosthesis must be conducive to implant hygiene and transmit physiologic forces to the peri-implant bone. Criteria for success in implant dentistry have been reviewed by Papaspyridakos et al. (2012) and include:

- *Patient satisfaction:* comfort, function, aesthetics, and general satisfaction
- *Peri-implant bone health:* absence of bone loss, mobility, infection, and pain
- *Peri-implant soft tissue health:* healthy probing depth; absence of suppuration, bleeding on probing, edema, hyperplasia, swelling, and recession
- *Prosthetic success:* good function and aesthetics, with no or minor complications.

Outcome criteria vary from study to study, which makes it difficult to compare studies even about the same implants. Of the success criteria used, the most frequent is *implant survival* over the fixed time span of a study. Using this criterion, an implant may be considered a statistical survival success even if there is progressive bone loss or the implant prosthesis fails. Many studies cover a very limited timespan in terms of number of years or even months.

Another factor to be borne in mind when evaluating research or attending continuing education courses, is whether there is a research bias, or whether researchers have a conflict of interest, that is, whether their research is supported by an implant company. (Popelut et al. 2010).

1.8 Clinical studies, implant validation

Numerous clinical studies have documented the successful use of implants for tooth replacement in fully and partially edentulous patients. Expert clinical teams, in controlled conditions and with careful case selection, have conducted the vast majority of studies. PubMed, the Cochrane Library, and the ADA Evidence Based Dentistry website are good sources for systematic reviews of implant research topics.

Today, a single tooth implant replacement has the expectation of a 95% success rate (Sullivan 2001; ADA 2004; Jokstad 2009). In one of the earliest longitudinal clinical trials, Adell et al. (1981) reported implant survival of 81% (maxilla) to 91% (mandible), and a fixed full-arch prosthesis survival rate of 89–100%; peri-implant bone loss was 1.5 mm after 1 year and did not exceed 0.1 mm/year thereafter. Buser et al. (1997) wrote that the success of dental implants is well documented and an implant survival rate greater than 90% should be achievable. Esposito et al. (2003) found no differences in bone levels and failure rates for six different implant systems.

Many other studies have validated the success of implants (Albrektsson et al. 1988; Jemt et al. 1989; Adell et al. 1990; Zarb and Schmitt 1993; Lekholm et al. 1999). Authors (Berglundh et al. 2002; Lang et al. 2004) have reported 5-year survival rates of 97.5% for single crowns, 95.4% for FDPs, 94% for overdentures and a 10-year survival rate of 92.8% for FDPs. Berglundh et al. (2002), examining 10 implant systems, reported the loss of 2.5%

implants before functional loading. Implant loss during function ranged from 2% to 3% for fixed prostheses, and 5% for overdentures over a 5-year period. Implant loss for augmented ridges was significantly higher, 11.3% after 5 years. Single-implant crowns had the lowest rate of implant loss in function, 2.2%.

1.9 Implant regulation

Since 1985, the ADA had a program for Approval and, later, Acceptance for Dental Implants (ADA 2004). This Seal program was terminated in 2007. The United States and European Union have medical device regulatory guidelines (EU Standards 1993; U.S. FDA Regulations 2004).

In 1998, the FDA reclassified Ti dental implants from Class III to Class II medical devices. Class II devices need laboratory and animal testing, but not clinical human testing. Since the reclassification by the FDA of implants, there has been a proliferation of new implant systems. The vast majority of implant brands on the market today have zero clinical documentation (Jokstad 2009).

In 2003, the World Dental Federation (also known as the FDI as it was begun in France as the Fédération Dentaire Internationale) studied the issue of proliferating implant systems (Jokstadt et al. 2003) and identified 225 implant brands from 78 manufacturers. Of these, only 10 systems had more than four clinical trials, and 11 had less than four clinical trials of good methodological quality. 28 manufacturers sold implant systems without any published clinical documentation. The FDI suggested that the dental profession use implant systems that are supported by sound clinical research documentation and which conform to good manufacturing practice in compliance with International Organization for Standardization (ISO) standards, or FDA, or other regulatory standards. More than 50% of all trials reported have been on implants manufactured

Table 1.1 Clinical trials published since 2003 ($n = 530$) sorted according to implant brand

Implant brand	No. of studies	%
Nobel Biocare: Branemark/Replace/Nobeldirect/Nobelperfect/SteriOss, etc.	176	33
Straumann/ITI	101	19
Dentsply: Frialit/Frialit2/Frialit+/Friadent/Frialoc/Frios/Xive/Ankylos	53	10
Biomet 3i: Osseotite/Nanotite	41	8
Astra	23	4
Zimmer: Calcitek/Integral/Omniloc/ScrewVent/Spline/SwissPlus, etc.	22	4
IMZ	16	3
Camlog	7	1
Biohorizons/Maestro	6	1
Southern Implants	5	1
Bicon	5	1
Defcon	4	1
Sweden & Martina	4	1
Other or not stated	67	13

Source: Adapted from Jokstad (2009).

by Nobel Biocare and Straumann, and 80% of all clinical trials were limited to clinical reports conducted on implants from the first six manufacturers in Table 1.1. Bhatavadekar (2010) reviewed the literature for randomized controlled clinical implant trials and corroborated Jokstad's findings.

The onus is on the clinician to make an informed choice of the most suitable implant system for the patient's long-term benefit. This should be based on the clinical evidence, the track record, and service offered by the implant company.

1.10 Research and development

Dental implant treatments have come a long way in a short period of time. The ingenuity of implant companies and dental professionals to reinvent and tweak the designs and applications is remarkable. We still do not have scientific rationale for implant length, size, and number relative to load, nor the precise mechanics of functional loading. Destructive peak loads may be a problem, as we tend to think in terms of average occlusal forces on natural teeth that can move in function. We need a better understanding of bone response to *functional forces* and *overload*. There is still much work to be done in terms of answering fundamental questions of biology, and day-to-day treatment planning of implant supported tooth replacement. Surgical techniques continue to evolve with guided surgery, and bone augmentation solutions. Currently, there are some key areas of interest in implantology:

- Surface modification: optimizing implant design to enhance the rate of osseointegration and percentage of implant bone contact.
- Peri-implant infection (bone loss) and its management. There is controversy as to whether bone loss can be attributed to adverse biomechanical loading or whether it is simply analogous to periodontal breakdown around natural teeth.
- Ridge augmentation and guided bone regeneration
- Computer guided implant placement
- Early loading protocols and bone healing

1.11   Summary

Some of the original prostheses placed in the 1960s on Brånemark implants are still functioning today (Brånemark 2006). It is a testament to the remarkable work of Brånemark and other researchers that the original placement protocol remains essentially unchanged, and that the original implant design is still a reference and widely copied. As word spread in the dental community about osseointegration, there was a certain amount of skepticism because of the radical nature of this development. As acceptance grew so also did the input of the working dentists, bringing innovation and modification of the early Brånemark protocol and implant design. At present, certain restorative treatments have become accepted as routine procedures for general dentists namely single crowns, small multi-unit fixed prostheses, and mandibular overdentures supported by two implants.

The ADA dental education accreditation guidelines (ADA 2013) mandate competency in implant treatment. European dental education and Australian dental education have embraced implantology by producing undergraduate educational guidelines (Hicklin et al. 2009; Mattheos et al. 2009; Mattheos et al. 2010).

Evolution of surgical techniques and component design has resolved many of the early problems with implants, and today we have many excellent implant systems of high quality and utility. The technology has expanded in line with the demand for usage by the public and dentists, and finances may now be the only limitation to their universal use.

Finally, this author would highly recommend Froum's (2010) textbook on complications as a reference when embarking on implant practice.

References

ADA. (2003). Accreditation standards for dental education programs 2013. Commission on Dental Accreditation. American Dental Association, Chicago, IL. http://www.ada.org/sections/educationAndCareers/pdfs/predoc_2013.pdf (last accessed January 8, 2014).

ADA Council on Scientific Affairs. (2004) Dental endosseous implants: an update. *J Am Dent Assoc.* 135(1):92–7.

Adell R, Lekholm U, Rockler B, Brånemark P-I. (1981) A 15-year study of osseointegrated implants in the treatment of the edentulous jaw. *Int J Oral Surg.* 10(6):387–416.

Adell R, Eriksson B, Lekholm U, Brånemark P-I, Jemt T. (1990) Long-term follow-up study of osseointegrated implants in the treatment of totally edentulous jaws. *Int J Oral Maxillofac Implants.* 5(4):347–59.

Al-Nawas B, Kämmerer PW, Morbach T, Ladwein C, Wegener J, Wagner W. (2012) Ten-year retrospective follow-up study of the TiOblast dental implant. *Clin Implant Dent Relat Res.* 14(1):127–34.

Albrektsson T. (1998) Hydroxyapatite-coated implants: a case against their use. *J Oral Maxillofac Surg.* 56(11):1312–26.

Albrektsson T, Sennerby A. (2005) The impact of oral implants: past and future. *J Can Dent Assoc.* 71(5):327.

Albrektsson T, Brånemark P-I, Hansson HA, Lindström J. (1981) Osseointegrated titanium implants. Requirements for ensuring a long-lasting, direct bone-to-implant anchorage in man. *Acta Orthop Scand.* 52(2):155–70.

Albrektsson T, Zarb G, Worthington P, Eriksson AR. (1986) The long-term efficacy of currently used dental implants: a review and proposed criteria of success. *Int J Oral Maxillofac Implants.* 1(1):11–25.

Albrektsson T, Dahl E, Enbom L, Engevall S, Engquist B, Eriksson AR, Feldmann G, Freiberg N, Glantz PO, Kjellman O, Kristersson L, Kvint S, Köndell PÅ, Palmquist J, Werndahl L, Åstrand P. (1988) Osseointegrated oral implants. A Swedish multicenter study of 8139 consecutively inserted Nobelpharma implants. *J Periodontol.* 59(5):287–96.

Babbush CA, Kent JN, Misiek DJ. (1986) Titanium plasma-sprayed (TPS) screw implants for the reconstruction of the edentulous mandible. *J Oral Maxillofac Surg.* 44(4):274–82.

Berglundh T, Persson L, Klinge B. (2002) A systematic review of the incidence of biological and technical complications in implant dentistry reported in prospective longitudinal studies of at least 5 years. *J Clin Periodontol.* 29:197–212.

Bhatavadekar N. (2010) Helping the clinician make evidence-based implant selections. A systematic review and qualitative analysis ofdental implant studies over a 20 year period. *Int Dent J.* 60(5): 359–69.

Biesbrock AR, Edgerton M. (1995) Evaluation of the clinical predictability of hydroxyapatite-coated endosseous dental implants: a review of the literature. *Int J Oral Maxillofac Implants.* 10(6):712–20.

Brånemark P-I. (2006) *The Osseointegration Book: From Calvarium to Calcaneus.* Quintessence, Chicago.

Brånemark P-I, Adell R, Breine U, Hansson BO, Lindström J, Ohlsson A. (1969) Intra-osseous anchorage of dental prostheses. I. Experimental studies. *Scand J Plast Reconstr Surg.* 3(2):81–100.

Brånemark P-I, Hansson BO, Adell R, Breine U, Lindström J, Hallén O, Ohman A. (1977) Osseointegrated implants in the treatment of the edentulous jaw. Experience from a 10-year period. *Scand J Plast Reconstr Surg Suppl.* 16:1–132.

Brånemark P-I, Zarb G, Albrektsson T. (1985) *Tissue-Integrated Prostheses: Osseointegration in Clinical Dentistry.* Quintessence, Chicago.

Buser D, Mericske-Stern R, Bernard JP, Behneke A, Behneke N, Hirt HP, Belser UC, Lang NP. (1997) Long-term evaluation of non-submerged ITI implants. Part 1: 8-year life table analysis of a prospective multi-center study with 2359 implants. *Clin Oral Implants Res.* 8(3):161–72.

Buser DA, Schroeder A, Sutter F, Lang NP. (1988) The new concept of ITI hollow-cylinder and hollow-screw implants: part 2. Clinical aspects, indications, and early clinical results. *Int J Oral Maxillofac Implants.* 3(3):173–81.

d'Hoedt B, Schulte W. (1989) A comparative study of results with various endosseous implant systems. *Int J Oral Maxillofac Implants.* 4(2):95–105.

Drago C, Peterson T. (2007) *Implant Restorations: A Step-by-Step Guide,* 2nd ed. Blackwell Munksgaard, Ames.

Esposito M, Coulthard P, Worthington HV, Jokstad A, Wennerberg A. (2003) Interventions for replacing missing teeth: different types of dental implants. *Cochrane Database Syst Rev.* (3): CD003815.

EU Standards. (1993) European Commission. Harmonised Standards. Medical Devices. Council Directive 93/42/EEC of June 14, 1993 concerning medical devices OJ L 169 of July 12, 1993. http://ec.europa.eu/enterprise/policies/european-standards/harmonised-standards/medical-devices/ (last accessed December 16, 2013).

Felton DA. (2009) Edentulism and co-morbid factors. *J Prosthodont.* 18(2):88–96. Review.

Finger IM, Guerra LR. (1989) Integral implant-prosthodontic considerations. *Dent Clin North Am.* 33(4):793–819. Review.

Finger IM, Guerra LR. (1992) The Integral Implant System: prosthetic considerations. *Dent Clin North Am.* 36(1):189–206.

Froum SJ. (2010) *Dental Implant Complications: Etiology, Prevention, and Treatment.* Wiley-Blackwell, Ames.

Gomez-Roman G, Schulte W, d'Hoedt B, Axman-Krcmar D. (1997) The Tübingen Frialit-2 implant system: five-year clinical experience in single-tooth and immediately postextraction applications. *Int J Oral Maxillofac Implants.* 12(3): 299–309.

Hansson S. (1999) The implant neck: smooth or provided with retention elements. A biomechanical approach. *Clin Oral Implants Res.* 10(5):394–405.

Hicklin SP, Albrektsson T, Hämmerle CH. (2009) Theoretical knowledge in implant dentistry for undergraduate students. 1st European Consensus Workshop in Implant Dentistry University Education. *Eur J Dent Educ.* 13 Suppl 1:25–35.

Jemt T, Lekholm U, Adell R. (1989) Osseointegrated implants in the treatment of partially edentulous patients: a preliminary study on 876 consecutively placed fixtures. *Int J Oral Maxillofac Implants.* 4(3):211–7.

Jokstad A. (2009) *Osseointegration and Dental Implants.* Wiley-Blackwell, Ames.

Jokstadt A, Braegger U, Brunski JB, Carr AB, Naert I, Wennerberg A. (2003) Quality of dental implants. *Int Dent J.* 53(6 Suppl 2):409–43.

Kinsella KG. (2005) Future longevity-demographic concerns and consequences. *J Am Geriatr Soc.* 53(9 Suppl):S299–303.

Kirsch A, Ackermann KL. (1989) The IMZ osseointegrated implant system. *Dent Clin North Am.* 33(4):733–91.

Laney WR. (1993) In recognition of an implant pioneer: professor Dr. André Schroeder. *Int J Oral Maxillofac Implants.* 8(2):135–6.

Lang NP, Berglundh T, Heitz-Mayfield LJ, Pjetursson BE, Salvi GE, Sanz M. (2004) Consensus statements and recommended clinical procedures regarding implant survival and complications. *Int J Oral Maxillofac Implants.* 19 Suppl:150–4.

Lazzara RJ, Porter SS. (2006) Platform-switching: a new concept in implant dentistry for controlling postrestorative crestal bone levels. *Int J Periodontics Restorative Dent.* 26(1):9–17.

Lekholm U, Gunne J, Henry P, Higuchi K, Lindén U, Bergström C, van Steenberghe D. (1999) Survival of the Brånemark implant in partially edentulous jaws: a 10-year prospective multicenter study. *Int J Oral Maxillofac Implants.* 14(5):639–45.

Linkow LI. (1968) The blade vent—a new dimension in endosseous implantology. *Dental Concepts.* 11(2):3–12.

Marcus SE, Drury TF, Brown LJ, Zion GR. (1996) Tooth retention and tooth loss in the permanent dentition of adults: United States 1988-1991. *J Dent Res.* 75 Spec No:684–5.

Market Reports. (2010) Global Dental Implants Market. http://www.marketsandmarkets.com/Market-Reports/Dental-Implants-Market-241.html (last accessed December 16, 2013).

Mattheos N, Albrektsson T, Buser D, De Bruyn H, Donos N, Hjørting Hansen E, Lang NP, Sanz M, Nattestad A; 1st European Consensus Workshop in Implant Dentistry University Education. (2009) Teaching and assessment of implant dentistry in undergraduate and postgraduate education: a European consensus. *Eur J Dent Educ.* 13 Suppl 1: 11–7.

Mattheos N, Ivanovski S, Heitz-Mayfield L, Klineberg I, Sambrook P, Scholz S. (2010) University teaching of implant dentistry: guidelines for education of dental undergraduate students and general dental practitioners. An Australian consensus document. *Aust Dent J.* 55(3):329–32.

Meskin LH, Brown LJ, Brunelle JA. (1988) Pattern of tooth loss and accuracy of prosthodontics treatment potential in US employed and seniors. *Gerodontics.* 4:126–35.

Misch CE. (2007) *Contemporary Implant Dentistry*, 3rd ed. Mosby, St. Louis.

Müller F, Naharro M, Carlsson GE. (2007) What are the prevalence and incidence of tooth loss in the adult and elderly population in Europe? *Clin Oral Implants Res.* 18 Suppl 3:2–14.

Niznick GA. (1985) Implant prosthodontics using the Core-Vent system. *J Oral Implantol.* 12(1): 45–67.

NIH. (1978) National Institute of Health Consensus Statement Online. (1978) Dental Implants. Benefit and Risk. http://consensus.nih.gov/1978/1978DentalImplants003html.htm (last accessed December 16, 2013).

NIH. (1988) National Institute of Health Consensus Statement Online (1988) Dental Implants. http://consensus.nih.gov/1988/1988DentalImplants069html.htm (last accessed December 16, 2013).

Ong JL, Chan DC. (2000) Hydroxyapatite and their use as coatings in dental implants: a review. *Crit Rev Biomed Eng.* 28(5–6):667–707.

Papaspyridakos P, Chen CJ, Singh M, Weber H-P, Gallucci GO. (2012) Success criteria in implant dentistry: a systematic review. *J Dent Res.* 91(3): 242–8.

Popelut A, Valet F, Fromentin O, Thomas A, Bouchard P. (2010) Relationship between sponsorship and failure rate of dental implants: a systematic approach. *PLoS ONE.* 5(4):e10274. doi: 10.1371/journal.pone.0010274.

Porter JA, von Fraunhofer JA. (2005) Success or failure of dental implants? A literature review with treatment considerations. *Gen Dent.* 53(6):423–32.

Ring ME. (1995a) A thousand years of dental implants: a definitive history: part 1. *Compend Contin Educ Dent.* 16(10):1060–9.

Ring ME. (1995b) A thousand years of dental implants: a definitive history: part 2. *Compend Contin Educ Dent.* 16(11):1132–42.

Roos J, Sennerby L, Lekholm U, Jemt T, Gröndahl K, Albrektsson T. (1997) A qualitative and quantitative method for evaluating implant success: a 5-year retrospective analysis of the Brånemark implant. *Int J Oral Maxillofac Implants.* 12(4): 504–14.

Schnitman PA, Shulman LB. (1980) Dental implants: benefits and risks. Proceedings of an NIH-Harvard Consensus Development Conference, U.S. Department of Health and Human Services, Publication No. 81-1531.

Schroeder A, Sutter F, Krekeler G. (1991) *Oral Implantology: Basics - ITI Hollow Cylinder.* Thieme, New York.

Schroeder A, Sutter F, Buser D, Krekeler G. (1996) *Oral Implantology: Basics - ITI Hollow Cylinder.* Thieme, New York.

Schulte W, Heimke G. (1976) The Tübingen immediate implant. *Quintessenz.* 27(6):17–23. [in German]

Schulte W, d'Hoedt B, Axmann-Krcmar D, Gomez-Roman G. (1992) 15 years of the Tübingen Implant and its development for Frialit-2-System. *Z Zahnärztl Implantol.* 8:77–96. [in German]

Spiekermann H. (1995) *Color Atlas of Dental Medicine: Implantology.* Thieme, New York.

Sullivan RM. (2001) Implant dentistry and the concept of osseointegration: a historical perspective. *J Calif Dent Assoc.* 29(11):737–45.

Sutter F, Schroeder A, Buser DA. (1988) The new concept of ITI hollow-cylinder and hollow-screw implants: part 1. Engineering and design. *Int J Oral Maxillofac Implants.* 3(3):161–72.

Tallgren A, Lang BR, Walker GF, Ash MM Jr. (1980) Roentgen cephalometric analysis of ridge resorption and changes in jaw and occlusal relationships in immediate complete denture wearers. *J Oral Rehabil.* 7(1):77–94.

Tan WL, Wong TL, Wong MC, Lang NP. (2012) A systematic review of post-extractional alveolar hard and soft tissue dimensional changes in humans. *Clin Oral Implants Res.* 23 Suppl 5: 1–21.

U.S. FDA Regulations. (2004) Guidance for Industry and FDA Staff: Class II special controls guidance document: Root-form Endosseous dental implants and endosseous dental abutments. Document issued on: May 12, 2004. The draft of this document was issued on May 14, 2002. http://www .fda.gov/medicaldevices/deviceregulationand guidance/guidancedocuments/ucm072424.htm (last accessed January 8, 2014).

Watson CJ, Tinsley D, Ogden AR, Russell JL, Mulay S, Davison EM. (1999) A 3 to 4 year study of single tooth hydroxylapatite coated endosseous dental implants. *Br Dent J.* 187(2):90–4.

Zarb GA. (1983) *Proceedings of the Toronto Conference on Osseointegration in Clinical Dentistry.* Reprinted from the *J Prosthet Dent.* 49 and 50. Mosby, St. Louis, pp. 1–84.

Zarb GA, Schmitt A. (1990) The longitudinal clinical effectiveness of osseointegrated dental implants: the Toronto Study. Part II: the prosthetic results. *J Prosthet Dent.* 64(1):53–61.

Zarb GA, Schmitt A. (1993) The longitudinal clinical effectiveness of osseointegrated dental implants in posterior partially edentulous patients. *Int J Prosthodont.* 6(2):189–96.

Zitzmann NU, Hagmann E, Weiger R. (2007) What is the prevalence of various types of prosthetic dental restorations in Europe? *Clin Oral Implants Res.* 18(3):20–33.

2 Implant–Tissue Interface Biology

2.1	Concept of osseointegration	2.5	Soft tissue–implant interface
2.2	Implant surface chemistry	2.6	Peri-implant infection
2.3	Biology of osseointegration	2.7	Implant surface modifications
2.4	Bone healing biology		

2.1 Concept of osseointegration

An understanding of the integration between the implant and the bone and soft tissue will ensure a considered approach to implant surgery, functional loading, and maintenance of implants. Brånemark et al. (1977, 1985) coined the term osseointegration to describe a direct structural and functional connection between ordered living bone and the surface of a load-bearing implant. Brånemark's description was pivotal in that it distinguished osseointegration from other contemporary dental implants where a layer of connective tissue and downgrowth of oral epithelium (pseudo-periodontal ligament) gradually separated the implant from the bone. Schroeder et al. (1991, 1996) referred to the integration phenomenon as a functional ankylosis or osteointegration. A biomechanically oriented definition of osseointegration has been suggested by Albrektsson and Zarb (1993): "a process whereby clinically asymptomatic rigid fixation is achieved and maintained in bone during functional loading."

The Brånemark team also observed a positive healing response in skin and mucosa penetrated by Ti implants (Albrektsson et al. 1981; Brånemark et al. 1985; Adell et al. 1986). When the implant penetrates the integument, the epithelium proliferates to cover exposed connective tissue and forms an epithelial seal around the implant preventing ingress of microbiota. A junctional epithelium (JE), analogous to that of a natural tooth, forms at the surface of the exposed implant, and is attached to the implant surface via hemidesmosomes in the basal layer cells. This overlies a thin band of closely adapted connective tissue, which lies above the integrated bone (Fig. 2.1).

2.2 Implant surface chemistry

Brånemark recognized the significance of the osseointegration between bone and

Fundamentals of Implant Dentistry, First Edition. Gerard Byrne.
© 2014 John Wiley & Sons, Inc. Published 2014 by John Wiley & Sons, Inc.
Companion website: www.wiley.com/go/byrne/implants

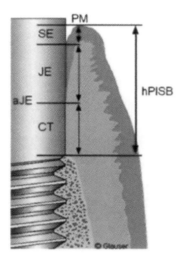

2.1. Implant osseointegration: soft-tissue and bone. Schematic diagram illustrating the histometric measurements. aJE, apical termination of junctional epithelium; CT, supracrestal connective tissue; hPISB, height of the peri-implant soft tissue barrier; JE = junctional epithelium; PM, peri-implant mucosal margin; SE, sulcular epithelium. (courtesy of Glauser R. *Clin Implant Dent Relat Res.* 7(I), 2005; Wiley-Blackwell).

commercially pure Ti (CPTi) and saw that this unique material had the biocompatibility and strength to work for clinical support of oral rehabilitation. Kasemo and Lausmaa (1985) have stated that the requirements for implanted materials are biocompatibility, adequate mechanical strength and machinability. Materials for implantation are generally polycrystalline metals and ceramics. Ceramics (metal oxides) are biocompatible and hard, but also brittle and difficult to machine. Metals are more easily machined, ductile, elastic, and chemically reactive, but are usually covered with a less reactive surface oxide (ceramic) layer that interfaces with tissue. Metals that form very stable surface oxides, Ti (TiO_2), Al (Al_2O_3), and Ta (Ta_2O_5), are very biocompatible and suitable for implantation. Ti is one of the bio-inert implant materials (Schroeder et al. 1996). Its biocompatibility has been known for some time, and repeatedly confirmed in the literature. Freshly machined Ti

immediately adsorbs oxygen molecules forming an oxide layer 20–34 Å thick within seconds. Body tissues contact only this oxide layer. The oxide layer imparts biocompatibility, while the bulk of the implant material imparts mechanical properties. Ti, or commercially pure Ti (CPTi Grades 1–4), is currently the material of choice for dental implants. It is biocompatible, easy to machine, and of adequate strength for clinical use.

The chemical properties of metal implants are governed by their surface oxide chemical composition. Various chemical processes occur at the tissue-implant interface: corrosion, selective adsorption of biomolecules, tendency of proteins to denature, and catalytic activity. Chemical reactivity, catalytic activity, and a high dielectric constant may be significant in the osteoconduction process during osseointegration. Surface contamination of Ti must be avoided during manufacture, storage, and surgery, as it could lead to unpredictable changes in surface chemistry. Theoretically, surface impurities from manufacturing or handling may lead to surface corrosion changes and osseointegration problems, which may not manifest clinically for years (Brånemark et al. 1985). Brånemark's surgical protocol was very rigid on the careful handling of implants to avoid contamination of the surface. Modification of the machined (turned) Ti surface has become popular and may enhance bio-compatibility, osteoconduction, and ultimately the quality and quantity of osseointegration.

In addition to TiO_2, other materials that are biocompatible and permit osseointegration include Al_2O_3, Ti alloys (e.g., Ti6Al4V) and other transition metals namely tantalum (Ta), zirconium (Zr), and niobium (Nb). The recently released Straumann Roxolid® implant uses an alloy of Ti and Zr; the Zimmer® Trabecular Metal™ implant uses Ta. Vitallium® alloy and stainless steel are reactive and corrosive in the body environment and may not be sufficiently biocompatible for dental implantation.

2.3   Biology of osseointegration

The concept of osseointegration was postulated by Brånemark and coworkers in 1969 and demonstrated histologically by Schroeder and coworkers in 1976. Several research teams produced exhaustive histologic findings on osseointegration between Ti and bone (Brånemark et al. 1985; Kirsch 1986; Schroeder et al. 1996; Korn et al. 1997). A further feature of functional osseointegration is the ability of the oral tissues to heal around the implant when it is exposed to the bacteria-laden oral environment, forming a peri-implant soft tissue cuff and epithelial seal. The peri-implant tissue seal is considered analogous to periodontal soft tissues in resisting bacterial infection.

The fundamental difference between an implant-supported restoration and a natural tooth is that a tooth has a periodontal ligament. The periodontal ligament is a specialized resilient organ that provides shock absorption, sensory feedback, nocioceptive reflex, and regulation of osteogenesis. It generally does not ossify, and prevents tooth resorption, which frequently occurs when an avulsed tooth is replanted, losing its ligament in the process. It accomodates physiologic tooth movement in all directions and leads to socket remodeling in response to appropriate forces.

An implant has no such support organ or mechanism and is essentially ankylosed or fixed to the bone. The only movement possible is bone flexion in response to force, the extent of which depends on bone density and volume. An implant placed in the jawbone of a growing child will be "left behind," that is, submerged relative to adjacent alveolar development, just as an ankylosed primary molar submerges (see Chapter 5, Fig. 5.2).

Implant sensory perception appears to come primarily from the sensory supply of opposing natural dentition, when present, or secondarily from contiguous soft tissues, TM joints, and masticatory muscles. Sensory innervation in bone, and proprioception and nocioception with implant restorations is poorly understood. As such, an implant crown is theoretically biomechanically more favorably opposed by a natural tooth or a denture than by another implant restoration. The latter circumstance is more likely to lead to biomechanical problems, due to lack of proprioception and risk of excessive forces.

2.4   Bone healing biology

The biology of bone healing (Jokstad 2009; Schwarz and Becker 2010) is fairly well understood, whereas the underlying metabolic and biomechanical aspects are less so (Misch 2007). The frictional heat of atraumatic bone osteotomy preparation generates a small region of bone necrosis at the edge of the osteotomy site (Schroeder et al. 1996). Following osteotomy preparation and placement of the implant in close contact with cortical and trabecular bone, a blood clot forms in the space between the two surfaces, and an osteogenic response results from the release of biochemical compounds, such as bone growth factors, from damaged cells. This is similar to the response that occurs when bone ends are immobilized in apposition after any long bone fracture. At the histological level, osseointegration is a complex process of clot organization, granulation tissue formation, and osteoid formation, followed by mineralization (Albrektsson and Jacobsson 1987; Davies 1998; Albrektsson and Johansson 2001). Ultrastructural TEM and SEM studies of fractured and recovered implant–bone specimens show a proteoglycan layer 20 Å thick between mature woven bone and the Ti surface. These studies prove the compatibility of Ti with bone (Hansson et al. 1983; Linder et al. 1983). Schroeder et al. (1996) described intimate contact between collagen, bone matrix, and the implant surface. The bone grows in a manner that seems to ignore the presence of a foreign body (Ti implant), and in fact, a textured suface proves to be osteoconductive.

The prerequisites for implant osseointegration include:

- Immobilization
  - Minimal micro-movement of the implant
- Adequate cells
  - Mesenchymal cells differentiate into pre-osteoblasts and osteoblasts.
  - Osteoclasts arise from blood monocytes.
- Adequate nutrition of cells
  - Diffusion of nutrients occurs locally until microcirculation is reestablished.
- Adequate stimulus for bone repair
  - Trauma and the subsequent inflammatory response triggers healing. Growth factors, for example, bone morphogenetic proteins (BMPs), are released by the damaged bone tissue.

Implant immobilization

Bone healing requires immobilization of the implant relative to the host bone. The literature indicates that osseointegration is favored by initial implant stability and hindered by excessive movement (Brånemark et al. 1977; Szmukler-Moncler et al. 1998). *Immobility of* the implant following surgery is considered essential to enable osteogenesis and avoid fibrous encapsulation of the implant. Initial stability or lack of mobility is afforded by the intimate fit of the implant in the osteotomy site usually aided by self-threading during insertion. Initial stability is easier to achieve in dense cortical bone and with a threaded implant, but healing may be faster in softer cancellous bone due to the latter's superior vascularity (Fig. 2.2).

Immobility of an inserted implant may be a relative term in the light of recent experience with early loading protocols. Research on immediate loading has focused attention on the amount of micro-motion that might be permissible when an implant is healing. Immediate loading relies purely on mechanical interlocking between the inserted implant and the bone. Researchers have asked the question as to how much micro-motion is permissible, and what might be a threshold for fibrous encapsulation rather than osseointegration (Szmukler-Moncler et al. 1998; Jokstad 2009). It has been suggested that a level of up to 150 µm micro-motion may be acceptable. It is also accepted that controlled loading may have a positive effect on the initial bone formation.

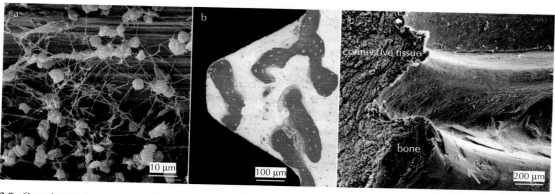

2.2. Osseointegration status quo circa 1982: (a) The fibrin meshwork *(red arrows)* of the peri-implant blood clot detached from a machined surface. (b) In trabecular bone healing, bone formation was by distance osteogenesis. (c) The smooth interfaces between bone and connective tissue and the implant surface indicated an approximation of the tissues to the surface, rather than intimate cell/surface interactions (courtesy of Davies JE, Shupbach P, Cooper L. in Jokstad 2009)

Osteogenesis and the implant surface

Terminology is used to describe the process of bone healing around an implant: (Albrektsson, Johansson 2001; Jokstad 2009):

- *Osteoinduction:* The process whereby undifferentiated and pluripotent cells are stimulated to develop into bone forming cells.
- *Osteoconduction:* The process in which an osteoconductive surface permits bone growth along the surface and into its channels and pores.
- *Contact osteogenesis:* The process whereby bone initially forms in contact with the implant if the conditions are favorable. Textured implant surfaces are more favorable than smooth machined surfaces. The textured implant surface promotes adherence of the fibrin network that acts as a scaffold for cell migration and osteoid formation directly on the implant surface. A smooth machined implant surface does not excite the same process (Davies et al. 2009) (Fig. 2.3).
- *Distance osteogenesis:* When a significant gap is present between implant and bone, or when a machined implant surface is presented, *distance osteogenesis* occurs away from the implant at the bone surface. Distance osteogenesis involves "cutting cones" of new blood vessels and osteoclastic activity. Traumatized lamellar bone is resorbed, while concentric new bone formation occurs around the new blood vessels.

Description of the three phases of bone healing

Phase 1: Inflammatory response

Within the first 48 hours after surgery, there is chemotaxis of mesenchymal cells and phagocytosis of tissue debris (Misch 2007; Jokstad 2009). Blood clotting occurs next to the implant resulting in activation of platelets and leukocytes in the hematoma, and the formation of a fibrin network attached to the implant surface. Attachment is better to textured surfaces than to smooth surfaces. Osteogenic cells migrate to the implant surface and form osteoid followed by bone, directly on the implant surface. The biochemical signaling pathways for this process are currently being elucidated.

Phase 2: Regeneration

Angiogenesis occurs within 48–72 hours, followed by granulation, which takes up to 3 weeks. Angiogenesis proceeds at a rate of 50 µm/day, taking about 10 days to restore microcirculation (Misch 2007). Osteogenesis occurs over 4–6 weeks and is stimulated by released inductive agents such as bone-morphogenetic protein (BMP). Immature *woven bone* is formed within 7 days, and this is gradually replaced by dense *lamellar bone*, which forms and matures more slowly. With textured surface implants, bone forms directly on the implant surface (contact osteogenesis), and also forms at the bone side, with gradual coalescence. With wider spaces, or with smooth, machined implants, the bone grows only from the tissue side (distance osteogenesis) toward the implant.

Phase 3: Remodeling

At 4 weeks et. seq., woven bone is gradually replaced by lamellar bone, with maximum bone deposition being achieved at 3–4 months. Radiographs have been used to demonstrate increased bone density around functioning implants. The remodeling continues in response to functional loading and reaches a "steady state" at approximately 18 months (Brånemark et al. 1985). Low interfacial strain stimulates bone regeneration, whereas high interfacial strain prevents bone regeneration at the implant bone interface. The strain threshold is unknown at this time (Brunski 1999).

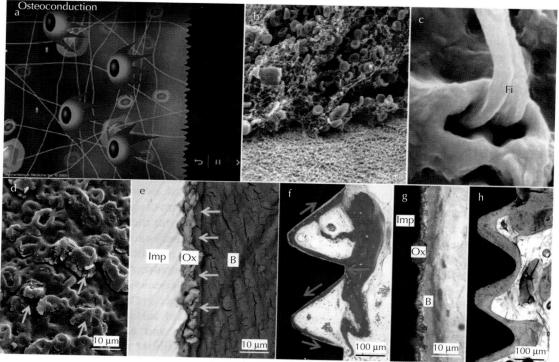

2.3. Osseointegration status quo circa 2008: (a) Osteoconduction is the recruitment and migration of osteogenic cells to the implant surface. The mechanisms are explained in this animation, which is available at http://www.ecf.utoronto.ca/~bonehead/. (b) SEM micrograph of a blood clot on an implant surface. The clot (above) can be seen to contain many red blood cells within a rich fibrin matrix that is anchored to the implant surface (below). (c) Competitive cellular activity at the implant surface can lead to osteogenic cells that come in contact with the implant surface, as can be seen in this SEM micrograph of a filopodium (Fi) anchored in an open pore of the oxidized surface. (d) Apatite deposits in the pores *(red arrows)* or around the volcano-like elevations of the anodically roughened surface *(yellow arrows)*. (e) Cement line *(yellow arrows)* interposed between the oxidized implant surface (Ox) and the body of the implant (Imp). (f) Osteoconductive bone formation outgoing from a contact point between a bone trabeculum and the implant and following the implant surface *(red arrows)*. (g) Initially formed woven bone on the crystalline oxidized layer. (h) Lamellar bone following in a wallpaper-like configuration the contour of the threads (courtesy of Davies JE, Shupbach P, Cooper L. in Jokstad 2009).

According to Misch (2007), maturation of bone surrounding the implant is expected to take a further 8 months from the time of restoration and is influenced by functional loading (size and direction of load). It is believed that cortical bone in the jaws remodels at a rate of 30–40%/year and that the bone closest to an implant remodels at a rate of 500%/year in order to mitigate the functional stresses at the implant–bone interface.

Bone loss after abutment connection

Implants are generally placed at or slightly below the ridge crest. Early crestal bone loss (2.0–3.0 mm) occurs in the first year after abutment connection (second-stage surgery) (Adell et al. 1981, 1986; Misch 2007) (Fig. 2.4). The amount of bone lost thereafter is negligible (0.1 mm p/a). For an implant placed at bone level, the bone loss or recession seems to be related to the micro-gap at the implant-abutment junction (IAJ). The microflora at the IAJ, and perhaps micro-motion of an abutment in function, especially those on an external implant connection, may determine the position of the junctional epithelial attachment on the implant and thus the fibrous tissue and bone level. Berglundh et al. (1991) observed the *biological width* between the depth of the sulcus around the implant and the bone to be approximately 2.0 mm. They also observed bone loss of 0.5 mm below IAJ within 2 weeks of abutment connection. The biological width above bone may explain the early bone recession around implants when a contaminated IAJ space is introduced (Misch 2007). For one-stage implants, such as Straumann's, with an integral smooth transmucosal collar, there is no such micro-gap introduced near the bone level, and therefore bone loss should be minimized (Cochran 2000).

Platform-switching and bone preservation

The *platform-switching* concept refers to the use of a smaller diameter abutment on a larger diameter implant platform (Fig. 2.5). This type of connection differs from original implant designs, which used abutments that were the same diameter as the implant platform (*platform-matching*). The smaller diameter abutment shifts the perimeter of the IAJ inward toward the center of the implant, and away from the bone. As a consequence, the crestal bone loss seen at second-stage surgery after abutment connection may be virtually eliminated. Lazzara and Porter (2006) theorized that the inward movement of the IAJ in this manner shifts the inflammatory cell infiltrate inward and away from the adjacent crestal bone. This minimizes crestal bone loss, and may enhance soft tissue contour, and thus aesthetics. Early

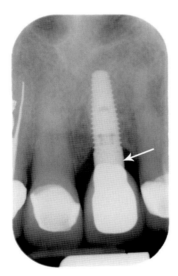

2.4. Bone loss around platform-matched implant extends from the platform to the first thread following abutment connection. Arrow indicates implant–abutment junction.

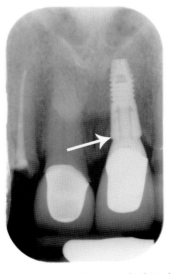

2.5. Bone loss around platform-switched implant crown extends no further than the implant platform *(arrow).*

reports on the platform-switching phenomenon relate to 3i implants. Astra Tech was also an early proponent of the design, and currently all the major implant companies produce platform-switching implants. Studies have shown a slight improvement in crestal bone height with platform-switching, but the long-term clinical significance has not been shown to date (Atieh et al. 2010; Bateli et al. 2011).

It is possible that the precise fit of the internal connection minimizes both abutment micro-motion and space for bacterial colonization of the implant–abutment junction (IAJ). This may influence peri-implant bone levels.

Implant failure or loss of osseointegration

There are several factors which prevent or cause breakdown of osseointegration:

- *Overheating bone during surgery:* Excessive surgical bone damage leads to bone sequestra, infection, connective tissue scarring, and lack of integration *(early failure).*
- *Implant movement during healing:* Early loading causing significant micro-motion and interfacial stress increases the risk of nonintegration and fibrous tissue scarring.
- *Peri-implantitis:* Bone loss during function is related to peri-implantitis and functional overload *(late failure).* Peri-implantitis is considered analogous to periodontal disease; it is the immune response to microbiota on the implant surface next to the soft tissue cuff.
- *Functional overload:* Bone loss may also be caused by overload when a negative balance between osteogenesis and osteoclasis is generated by nonphysiologic loading.

2.5 Soft tissue–implant interface

Peri-implant soft tissue cuff

A soft tissue cuff surrounds the transmucosal portion of the implant and acts as

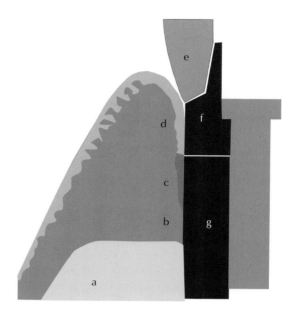

2.6. Diagram of bone and soft tissue interface/cuff with an implant and cemented crown. (a) bone; (b) connective tissue (1.0 mm); (c) junctional epithelium (1.0 mm); (d) sulcular epithelium/sulcus (1.0–2.0 mm); (e) restoration; (f) abutment; (g) implant (courtesy of H. Byrne).

an immunologic peripheral defense system (Berglundh et al. 1991; Rompen et al. 2006) (Fig. 2.6). Unlike orthopedic implants, which are "closed," dental implants must penetrate the oral mucosa and are "open" to the external bacteria-laden environment. An epithelial seal develops around the transmucosal abutment in a manner analogous to the dento-gingival junction. A junctional epithelium (JE) develops with hemidesmosomal attachment to the implant at the base of a peri-implant sulcus. The junctional epithelium provides an active biological seal against the ingress of microbiota and toxins. A band of connective tissue between the JE and bone is attached to the alveolar bone and closely adapted to the implant surface. It provides stability to the peri-implant tissue cuff and resistance to functional abrasive forces of mastication.

Junctional epithelium (JE)

Upon abutment connection and suturing of gingival tissue flaps, the epithelium proliferates to cover exposed connective tissue and forms an epithelial seal around the implant (Albrektsson et al. 1981). The junctional epithelium (JE) is a product of the basal epithelial cells; the cells have the ability to adhere to tooth structure and Ti. A similar JE forms on the surface of the exposed titanium implant, attaching in the same way via hemidesmosomes (Bosshardt and Lang 2005) (Fig. 2.7 and Fig. 2.8). Berglundh and Lindhe (1996) reported that the JE extends up to 2.0 mm along the implant surface, and is 40 μm in width. The JE extends to within 1.0 mm of the crestal bone. According to Schwarz and Becker (2010), biologic width is the distance from the most coronal extension of the JE to the alveolar bone. It comprises the JE (approx.

1.0 mm) and the CT attachment (approx. 1.0 mm).

Connective tissue

The architecture of the underlying connective tissue is somewhat uncertain. There is approximately 1.0 mm of connective tissue between bone and junctional epithelium. This connective tissue is closely adapted to the implant, with collagen bundles organized in a circular pattern parallel to, and in intimate contact with, the implant. It appears to limit the apical proliferation of the JE. Schroeder et al. (1996) and Schüpbach and Glauser (2007) have demonstrated collagen fibres running perpendicular (functionally oriented) to rough implant surfaces and parallel to smooth implant surfaces. Glauser et al. (2005) have measured a biologic

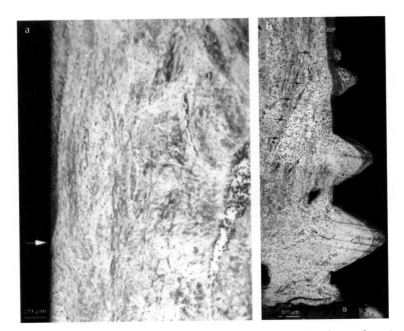

2.7. (a) Apical end of the junctional epithelium *(arrow)* as observed with textured implant surfaces (courtesy of Glauser R; *Clin Implant Dent Relat Res*. 7(I), 2005; Wiley-Blackwell). (b) Downgrowth of the junctional epithelium toward the alveolar bone crest, as observed with machined surfaces. aJEP, apical termination of the junctional epithelium; CT, connective tissue; B, bone (courtesy of Glauser R, *Clin Implant Dent Relat Res*. 7(I), 2005; Wiley-Blackwell).

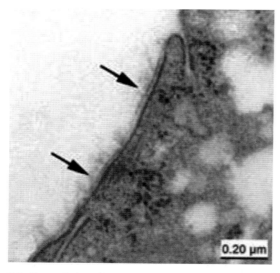

2.8. Transmission electron micrograph of surface of cell directly in contact with implant. Note presence of basal lamina and hemidesmosomes *(arrows)* (bar = 0.2 μm) (courtesy of Schupbach P, Glauser R. 2007, reprinted from *J Prosthet Dent.,* 2007; Elsevier-Mosby).

width of approximately 4.0 mm for machined, etched and oxidized implant surfaces. The JE was longer (3.4 mm) for smooth machined surfaces as compared with rough surfaces (1.8 mm). The height of the connective tissue seal was >2.0 mm for rough surfaces and 0.6 mm for machined surfaces. Schwarz and Becker (2010) noted the same phenomenon (Fig. 2.9a,b).

The implant–abutment junction (IAJ)

The type of implant–abutment connection (switching or matching), micro-movement, and the presence of micro-flora in the gap between implant and abutment influence the level of crestal bone and position of junctional epithelium. The following approximate values have been suggested for the implant-gingival junction: gingival sulcus of

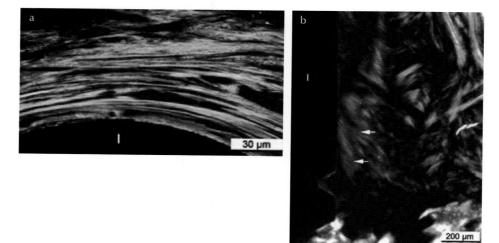

2.9. (a) Horizontal section through connective tissue around implant viewed in polarized light. Note bundles of circumferentially oriented collagen fiber bundles following parallel to implant surface in horizontal plane (bar = 30 μm) (courtesy of Schupbach P, Glauser R. 2007, reprinted from *J Prosthet Dent.,* Elsevier-Mosby). (b) Longitudinal section through human implant with oxidized surface showing functionally oriented collagen fibrils in apical portion of peri-implant connective tissue (bar = 200 μm) (courtesy of Schupbach P, Glauser R. 2007, reprinted from *J Prosthet Dent.,* Elsevier-Mosby).

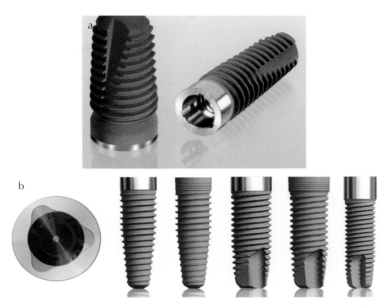

2.10. (a) Implant collar variations (courtesy of Camlog). (b) Implant collar variations (courtesy of Nobel Biocare).

1.0 mm, a junctional epithelium of 1.0 mm, and a connective tissue attachment of 1.0 mm (Berglundh and Lindhe 1996). It is unclear whether junctional epithelium attaches either side of the IAJ.

The implant collar

It is widely accepted that the transmucosal portion of an implant should have a smooth polished surface to facilitate plaque control. However, textured implant surfaces promote osseointegration, and may even favor adhesion of soft tissue cells (epithelial cells and fibroblasts) and functional orientation of connective tissue. A balance must be achieved between texture and machined surfaces on the collar of the implant (Quirynen and Bollen 1995) (Fig. 2.10a,b). Glauser et al. (2005) and Schwarz and Becker (2010) have drawn attention to a tendency for further apical migration of the junctional epithelium, and greater marginal bone

loss for smooth as compared with textured implant collars.

2.6 Peri-implant infection

Bacterial plaque biofilms are considered etiologic for both mucositis and peri-implantitis. Schwarz and Becker (2010) have discussed the histopathology and treatment of peri-implant disease at length. The accumulation of bacterial biofilms may lead to an inflammatory response in peri-implant tissues (Lindquist et al. 1996). Soft tissue inflammation around implants is referred to as *mucositis*. *Peri-implantitis* is a combination of soft tissue inflammation and bone loss (Fig. 2.11).

Factors that facilitate peri-implant bone loss

- History of chronic or aggressive periodontal disease (Heitz-Mayfield 2008)

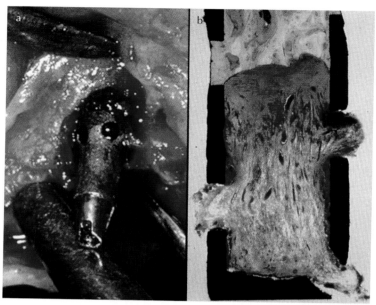

2.11. Implant peri-implantitis: (a) Hollow cylinder implant with peri-implantitis and bone loss. The lesion has reached the inner compartment of the implant body. (b) Histology of the removed implant showing osseointegration still present at the apical portion of the implant (courtesy of Lang NP, Tonetti MS. in Froum 2010; Wiley-Blackwell).

- Cigarette smoking (Strietzel et al. 2007)
- Systemic disease, for example, poorly controlled diabetes
- Occlusal overload: Isidor (1996, 1997) observed in monkeys that occlusal overload had a greater influence on the loss of osseointegration of implants than plaque accumulation. Researchers have noted different patterns for bacterial- and nonbacterial-caused peri-implant bone resorption (Rosenberg et al. 1991; Sanz et al. 1991)
- Inadequate band of keratinized mucosa
- Gingival inflammatory conditions, for example, lichen planus
- Exposed threads or textured surfaces of implants
- Plaque control limited by poorly fitting and designed prostheses (Klinge 2012).

Clinical signs and symptoms of peri-implant disease

- Bleeding on probing
- Redness, edema, pain
- Suppuration
- Pocket formation
- Bone resorption
- Gingival recession
- Implant mobility.

Ligature induced peri-implantitis model

Pontoriero et al. (1994) showed that plaque accumulation around implants follows a similar pattern to that of natural teeth and leads to an increase in the gingival index and clinical pocket probing depths. The development of inflammatory infiltrate is comparable with that of natural teeth. An experimental peri-implantitis model has shown that lack of plaque control leads to rapid breakdown of peri-implant soft and hard tissues (Lang et al. 1993; Lang and Tonetti 2010), similar to periodontal disease, but with extension of inflammatory infiltrate directly into bone marrow spaces. Such extension into bone does not occur in periodontitis. Incomplete seating of abutments can lead to significant plaque accumulation and inflammatory complications, such as fistula formation. It is not clear how important the size of the micro-gap between abutment and implant is, or the influence of micro-motion.

Progression of peri-implant infections (mucositis and peri-implantitis)

Schwarz and Becker (2010) provide an account of the pathogenesis of peri-implant disease.

- *Healthy peri-implant mucosa:* junctional epithelium and adjacent connective tissue have a small number of random polymorphonuclear leukocytes.
- *Early mucositis:* increased polymorph infiltrate, thickening of junctional epithelium, and damage to collagen fibers.
- *Established mucositis:* increase in polymorphs and collagen breakdown, increased lymphocytes and plasma cells, and activation of osteoclasts
- *Advanced mucositis:* formation of a "true" pocket, ulcerated pocket epithelium, and initial bone resorption.
- *Peri-implantitis:* persistence of "true" pocket, dominance of plasma cells, activation of osteoclasts, and resorption of bone.

2.7 Implant surface modifications

The original Brånemark implant had a threaded machined surface. The threads enabled excellent implant stability in the prepared osteotomy, and also increased the surface area of the implant significantly. Other early implants, including ITI and IMZ, utilized a press-fit (no threads) design that had a textured surface (titanium plasma sprayed [TPS]). Esposito et al. (2002) reported that there were no differences in survival rates between the different types of implant systems.

Currently, there is a significant shift away from Brånemark-style machined surfaces toward textured Ti surfaces of proprietary manufacture that have little long-term data (Froum 2010). Most implant companies offer surface textured implants that claim *osseoconductive* properties, with superior speed and quality of osseointegration or bone–implant contact (BIC) over traditional machined-surface implants (Fig. 2.12). The machined screws work best in high-density bone, whereas textured implants are shown to be superior in clinical situations with softer bone or bone grafts (Becktor et al. 2004). Gotfredsen et al. (1992) showed that textured surfaces have superior biomechanical properties.

Research has shown that textured surfaces can be osteoconductive and lead to more rapid and complete osseointegration with successful loading being feasible within 6–8 weeks (Bornstein et al. 2005; Cochran 1999, 2000; Testori et al. 2002; Albouy et al. 2008; Lambert et al. 2009). It is not clear whether this effect is due to surface texture or to changes in surface chemistry (Junker et al. 2009). There is continued research and development to chemically engineer surfaces in order to enhance bioactivity (Kasemo and Gold 1999; Variola et al. 2011).

A variety of textured surfaces are shown in Fig. 2.12. Textured surfaces:

- Increase the surface area for bone contact (Wennerberg et al. 1996).
- Accelerate osseointegration (Larsson et al. 1996; Schüpbach et al. 2005).
- Increase the percentage of bone-implant contact (BIC).

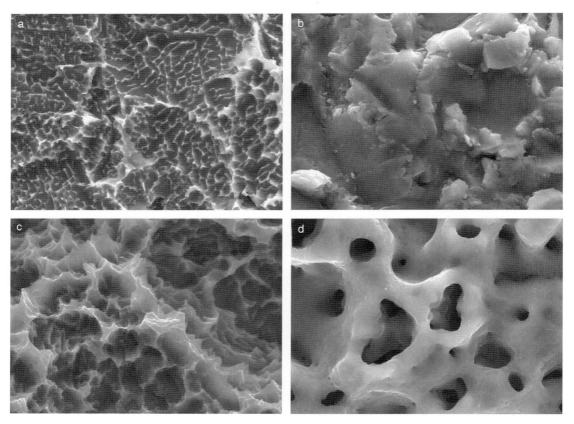

2.12. Different implant surface textures: (a) SEM of Osseotite™ surface (original magnification × 5000); (b) SEM of TiOblast™ surface (original magnification × 5000); (c) SEM of SLA™ surface (original magnification × 5000); (d) SEM of TiUnite® surface (original magnification × 5000) (courtesy of Gottlow J. in Jokstad 2010; Wiley-Blackwell).

- May limit downgrowth of junctional epithelium (Glauser et al. 2005; Schüpbach and Glauser 2007).

Davies (2003) proposed that textured surfaces promote blood clot adhesion and bone formation directly on the implant surface *(contact osteogenesis)*. In contrast, a clot shrinks away from a smooth machined surface creating a micro-gap. The osteogenic cells cannot reach the implant surface and new bone will start forming away from the implant *(distance osteogenesis)*. Thus osseointegration is faster for textured surfaces (Glauser et al. 2005; Schüpbach

et al. 2005; Cochran et al. 2007). A beneficial bone response from surface modifications with growth factors has yet to be validated (Junker et al. 2009).

Currently, there are many proprietary surface texture modifications available. They are created by a number of etching, sintering, anodizing, blasting, or other chemical processes. Each manufacturer markets unique features for their products, as can be seen on their websites.

(1) *Nobel Biocare TiUnite®*
   TiUnite is produced by anodic oxidation of the implant surface. It is a highly

crystalline phosphate enriched TiO$_2$ porous surface. Nobel Biocare has received FDA clearance to claim more rapid bone formation and greater amount of bone in contact with the surface during healing. The TiUnite implant surface has been shown to give an enhanced bone response when compared with machined surfaces with immediate placement (Rocci et al. 2003; Schüpbach et al. 2005).

(2) *Straumann TPS, SLA®, and SLActive®*
The Straumann SLA surface is produced by sandblasting followed by acid etching. The SLA surface is characterized as hydrophobic, while the newer SLActive surface has hydrophilic properties produced by storage in isotonic saline solution. The SLA implant reduces osseointegration time in half (6–8 weeks) over Ti plasma-sprayed implants (TPS). According to Straumann literature, SLActive surfaces further reduce osseointegration time in half, from 6–8 weeks to 3–4 weeks when compared with SLA (Buser et al. 2004).

(3) *Astra Tech TiOblast™, OsseoSpeed™*
The TiOblast surface is produced by blasting the implant surface with particles of TiO$_2$ (Rasmusson et al. 2005). It was launched in 1990 and is the precursor of the newer OsseoSpeed™ surface. TiOblast was the first moderately textured implant surface with long-term (10-year) follow-up reported in the literature (Al-Nawas et al. 2012). OsseoSpeed, a fluoride "bio-active" modification of TiOblast, was launched in 2004 (Rocci et al. 2008).

(4) *Biomet-3i Osseotite®, Nanotite™*
Osseotite is created by a dual acid-etching process. Nanotite is a modification of osseotite with a crystalline deposition of calcium phosphate. Animal studies have demonstrated an increase in rate and extent of osseointegration for the newer surface (Lazzara et al. 1999).

(5) *Neoss Bimodal surface*
The Bimodal surface is a hydrophilic surface created by multi-stage blasting with ZrO$_2$ and Ti particles, etching, cleaning, and chemical treatment.

(6) *Dentsply Friadent® Plus surface*
The Friadent Plus surface is grit-blasted then etched. It claims hydrophilic properties.

(7) *Zimmer MTX™ (micro-rough), MP1® HA coating, Trabecular Metal Technology™*
Zimmer's MTX surface is produced by grit-blasting with HA particles, followed by washing with nonetching acid. Trabecular Metal Technology is an engineered porous layer rather than a surface texture. It is created from Ta deposition and allows for bone in-growth to the surface of the implant. The surface is used in Zimmer's orthopedic implants (Fig. 2.13a,b).

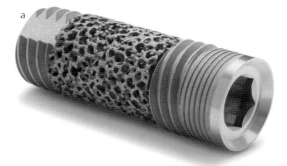

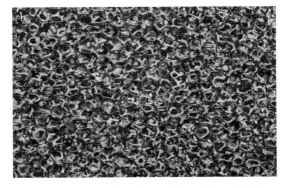

2.13. (a) Zimmer® trabecular metal™ surface. (b) Micrograph of trabecular metal™ surface texture (courtesy of Zimmer Dental)

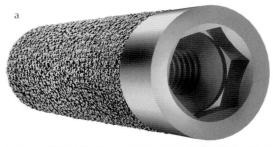

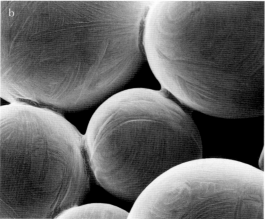

2.14. (a) Endopore implant with sintered Ti particle surface. (b) Micrograph of endopore sintered surface (courtesy Sybron Implant Direct)

(8) *Endopore sintered porous surface.*
    The Endopore porous surface is created by sintering a 0.3 mm layer of Ti6Al4V particles onto the implant surface. The porous surface allows bone growth into the pores, and was claimed to be biomechanically favorable (Jokstad 2009) (Fig. 2.14a,b).

(9) *Camlog Promote® surface.*
    The Camlog Promote surface is produced by abrasive blasting followed by acid etching.

With the discovery of more rapid and more complete osseointegration of implants with textured surfaces, implant manufacturers' focus has shifted to enhancing implant surfaces for use in problem areas with softer bone and for cases that require early or immediate loading. The experimentation with osseoconductive surfaces is likely to continue for some time and offers tangible benefits for dental implantology.

References

Adell R, Lekholm U, Rockler B, Brånemark P-I. (1981) A 15-year study of osseointegrated implants in the treatment of the edentulous jaw. *Int J Oral Surg.* 10(6):387–416.

Adell R, Lekholm U, Rockler B, Brånemark P-I, Lindhe J, Eriksson B, Sbordone L. (1986) Marginal tissue reactions at osseointegrated titanium fixtures (I). A 3-year longitudinal prospective study. *Int J Oral Maxillofac Surg.* 15(1):39–52.

Albouy JP, Abrahamsson I, Persson LG, Berglundh T. (2008) Spontaneous progression of peri-implantitis at different types of implants. An experimental study in dogs. I: clinical and radiographic observations. *Clin Oral Implants Res.* 19(10):997–1002.

Albrektsson T, Jacobsson M. (1987) Bone-metal interface in osseointegration. *J Prosthet Dent.* 57(5): 597–607.

Albrektsson T, Johansson C. (2001) Osteoinduction, osteoconduction and osseointegration. *Eur Spine J.* 10(2 Suppl):S96–101.

Albrektsson T, Zarb GA. (1993) Current interpretations of the osseointegrated response: clinical significance. *Int J Prosthodont.* 6(2):95–105.

Albrektsson T, Brånemark P-I, Hansson HA, Lindström J. (1981) Osseointegrated titanium implants. Requirements for ensuring a long-lasting, direct bone-to-implant anchorage in man. *Acta Orthop Scand.* 52(2):155–70.

Al-Nawas B, Kämmerer PW, Morbach T, Ladwein C, Wegener J, Wagner W. (2012) Ten-year retrospective follow-up study of the TiOblast dental implant. *Clin Implant Dent Relat Res.* 14(1):127–34.

Atieh MA, Ibrahim HM, Atieh AH. (2010) Platform-switching for marginal bone preservation around dental implants: a systematic review and meta-analysis. *J Periodontol.* 81(10):1350–66.

Bateli M, Att W, Strub JR. (2011) Implant neck configurations for preservation of marginal bone level: a systematic review. *Int J Oral Maxillofac Implants.* 26(2):290–303.

Becktor JP, Isaksson S, Sennerby L. (2004) Survival analysis of endosseous implants in grafted and nongrafted edentulous maxillae. *Int J Oral Maxillofac Implants.* 19(1):107–15.

Berglundh T, Lindhe J. (1996) Dimension of the peri-implant mucosa. Biological width revisited. *J Clin Periodontol.* 23(10):971–3.

Berglundh T, Lindhe J, Ericsson I, Marinello CP, Liljenberg B, Thomsen P. (1991) The soft tissue barrier at implants and teeth. *Clin Oral Implants Res.* 2(2):81–90.

Bornstein MM, Schmid B, Belser UC, Lussi A, Buser D. (2005) Early loading of non-submerged titanium implants with a sandblasted and acid-etched surface. 5-year results of a prospective study in partially edentulous patients. *Clin Oral Implants Res.* 16(6):631–638.

Bosshardt DD, Lang NP. (2005) The junctional epithelium: from health to disease. *J Dent Res.* 84(1): 9–20.

Brånemark P-I, Hansson BO, Adell R, Breine U, Lindström J, Hallén O, Ohman A. (1977) Osseointegrated implants in the treatment of the edentulous jaw. Experience from a 10-year period. *Scand J Plast Reconstr Surg Suppl.* 16:1–132.

Brånemark PI, Zarb GA, Albrektsson T. (eds.) (1985) *Tissue-Integrated Prostheses: Osseointegration in Clinical Dentistry.* Quintessence, Chicago.

Brunski JB. (1999) In vivo bone response to biomechanical loading at the bone/dental-implant interface. *Adv Dent Res.* 13:99–119.

Buser D, Broggini N, Wieland M, Schenk RK, Denzer AJ, Cochran DL, Hoffmann B, Lussi A, Steinemann SG. (2004) Enhanced bone apposition to a chemically modified SLA titanium surface. *J Dent Res.* 83(7):529–33.

Cochran D, Oates T, Morton D, Jones A, Buser D, Peters F. (2007) Clinical field trial examining an implant with a sand-blasted, acid-etched surface. *J Periodontol.* 78(6):974–82.

Cochran DL. (1999) A comparison of endosseous dental implant surfaces. *J Periodontol.* 70(12): 1523–39.

Cochran DL. (2000) The scientific basis for and clinical experiences with Straumann implants including the ITI Dental Implant System: a consensus report. *Clin Oral Implants Res.* 11 Suppl 1:33–58.

Davies JE. (1998) Mechanisms of endosseous integration. *Int J Prosthodont.* 11(5):391–401.

Davies JE. (2003) Understanding peri-implant endosseous healing. *J Dent Educ.* 67(8):932–49.

Davies JE, Schüpbach P, Cooper L. (2009) The implant surface and biological response: the changing interface. In: A Jokstad (ed.), *Osseointegration and Dental Implants.* Wiley-Blackwell, Ames, pp. 213–23.

Esposito M, Coulthard P, Worthington HV, Jokstad A, Wennerberg A. (2002) Interventions for replacing missing teeth: different types of dental implants. *Cochrane Database Syst Rev.* (4):CD003815.

Froum SJ. (2010) *Dental Implant Complications: Etiology, Prevention, and Treatment.* Wiley-Blackwell, Ames.

Glauser R, Schüpbach P, Gottlow J, Hämmerle CH. (2005) Peri-implant soft tissue barrier at experimental one-piece mini-implants with different surface topography in humans: a light-microscopic overview and histometric analysis. *Clin Implant Dent Relat Res.* 7 Suppl 1:S44–51.

Gotfredsen K, Nimb L, Hjörting-Hansen E, Jensen JS, Holmén A. (1992) Histomorphometric and removal torque analysis for TiO2-blasted titanium implants. An experimental study on dogs. *Clin Oral Implants Res.* 3(2):77–84.

Hansson HA, Albrektsson T, Brånemark P-I. (1983) Structural aspects of the interface between tissue and titanium implants. *J Prosthet Dent.* 50(1): 108–13.

Heitz-Mayfield LJ. (2008) Peri-implant diseases: diagnosis and risk indicators. *J Clin Periodontol.* 35(8 Suppl):292–304.

Isidor F. (1996) Loss of osseointegration caused by occlusal load of oral implants. A clinical and radiographic study in monkeys. *Clin Oral Implants Res.* 7(2):143–52.

Isidor F. (1997) Histological evaluation of peri-implant bone at implants subjected to occlusal overload or plaque accumulation. *Clin Oral Implants Res.* 8(1):1–9.

Jokstad A. (2009) *Osseointegration and Dental Implants.* Wiley-Blackwell, Ames.

Junker R, Dimakis A, Thoneick M, Jansen JA. (2009) Effects of implant surface coatings and composition on bone integration: a systematic review. *Clin Oral Implants Res.* 20 Suppl 4:185–206.

Kasemo B, Gold J. (1999) Implant surfaces and interface processes. *Adv Dent Res.* 13:8–20.

Kasemo B, Lausmaa J. (1985) Metal Selection and Surface Characteristics. In: P-I Brånemark, GA Zarb, T Albrektsson (eds.), *Tissue-Integrated Prostheses: Osseointegration in Clinical Dentistry.* Quintessence, Chicago, pp. 99–116.

Kirsch A. (1986) Plasma-sprayed titanium-I.M.Z. implant. *J Oral Implantol.* 12(3):494–7.

Klinge B. (2012) Peri-implant marginal bone loss: an academic controversy or a clinical challenge? *Eur J Oral Implantol.* 5 Suppl:S13–9.

Korn D, Soyez G, Elssner G, Petzow G, Brès EF, d'Hoedt B, Schulte W. (1997) Study of interface phenomena between bone and titanium and alumina surfaces in the case of monolithic and composite dental implants. *J Mater Sci Mater Med*. 8(10):613–20.

Lambert FE, Weber HP, Susarla SM, Belser UC, Gallucci GO. (2009) Descriptive analysis of implant and prosthodontic survival rates with fixed implant-supported rehabilitations in the edentulous maxilla. *J Periodontol*. 80(8):1220–30.

Lang NP, Tonetti MS. (2010) Peri-implantitis: etiology, pathogenesis, prevention, and therapy. In: SJ Froum (ed.), *Dental Implant Complications: Etiology, Prevention, and Treatment*. Wiley-Blackwell, Ames, pp. 119–33.

Lang NP, Brägger U, Walther D, Beamer B, Kornman KS. (1993) Ligature-induced peri-implant infection in cynomolgus monkeys. I. Clinical and radiographic findings. *Clin Oral Implants Res*. 4(1):2–11.

Larsson C, Thomsen P, Aronsson BO, Rodahl M, Lausmaa J, Kasemo B, Ericson LE. (1996) Bone response to surface-modified titanium implants: studies on the early tissue response to machined and electropolished implants with different oxide thicknesses. *Biomaterials*. 17(6):605–16.

Lazzara RJ, Porter SS. (2006) Platform-switching: a new concept in implant dentistry for controlling post-restorative crestal bone levels. *Int J Periodontics Restorative Dent*. 26(1):9–17.

Lazzara RJ, Testori T, Trisi P, Porter SS, Weinstein RL. (1999) A human histologic analysis of osseotite and machined surfaces using implants with 2 opposing surfaces. *Int J Periodontics Restorative Dent*. 19(2):117–29.

Linder L, Albrektsson T, Brånemark P-I, Hansson HA, Ivarsson B, Jönsson U, Lundström I. (1983) Electron microscopic analysis of the bone-titanium interface. *Acta Orthop Scand*. 54(1):45–52.

Lindquist LW, Carlsson GE, Jemt T. (1996) A prospective 15-year follow-up study of mandibular fixed prostheses supported by osseointegrated implants. Clinical results and marginal bone. *Clin Oral Implants Res*. 7(4):329–36.

Misch CE. (2007) *Contemporary Implant Dentistry*, 3rd ed. Mosby-Elsevier, St. Louis.

Pontoriero R, Tonelli MP, Carnevale G, Mombelli A, Nyman SR, Lang NP. (1994) Experimentally induced peri-implant mucositis. A clinical study in humans. *Clin Oral Implants Res*. 5(4):254–9.

Quirynen M, Bollen CM. (1995) The influence of surface roughness and surface-free energy on supra- and subgingival plaque formation in man. A review of the literature. *J Clin Periodontol*. 22(1):1–14.

Rasmusson L, Roos J, Bystedt H. (2005) A 10-year follow-up study of titanium dioxide-blasted implants. *Clin Implant Dent Relat Res*. 7(1):36–42.

Rocci A, Martignoni M, Gottlow J. (2003) Immediate loading of Brånemark System TiUnite and machined-surface implants in the posterior mandible: a randomized open-ended clinical trial. *Clin Implant Dent Relat Res*. 5 Suppl 1:57–63.

Rocci M, Rocci A, Martignoni M, Albrektsson T, Barlattani A, Gargari M. (2008) Comparing the TiOblast and Osseospeed surfaces. Histomorphometric and histological analysis in humans. *Oral Implantol (Rome)*. 1(1):34–42.

Rompen E, Domken O, Degidi M, Pontes AE, Piattelli A. (2006) The effect of material characteristics, of surface topography and of implant components and connections on soft tissue integration: a literature review. *Clin Oral Implants Res*. 17 Suppl 2:55–67.

Rosenberg ES, Torosian JP, Slots J. (1991) Microbial differences in 2 clinically distinct types of failures of osseointegrated implants. *Clin Oral Implants Res*. 2(3):135–44.

Sanz M, Alandez J, Lazaro P, Calvo JL, Quirynen M, van Steenberghe D. (1991) Histo-pathologic characteristics of peri-implant soft tissues in Brånemark implants with 2 distinct clinical and radiological patterns. *Clin Oral Implants Res*. 2(3):128–34.

Schroeder A, Sutter F, Krekeller G. (1991) *Oral Implantology: Basics-ITI Hollow Cylinder*. Thieme, New York.

Schroeder A, Sutter F, Krekeller G. (1996) *Oral Implantology: Basics, ITI Hollow Cylinder*. Thieme, New York.

Schüpbach P, Glauser R. (2007) The defense architecture of the human peri-implant mucosa: a histological study. *J Prosthet Dent*. 97(6 Suppl):S15–25.

Schüpbach P, Glauser R, Rocci A, Martignoni M, Sennerby L, Lundgren A, Gottlow J. (2005) The human bone-oxidized titanium implant interface: a light microscopic, scanning electron microscopic, back-scatter scanning electron microscopic, and energy-dispersive x-ray study of clinically retrieved dental implants. *Clin Implant Dent Relat Res*. 7 Suppl 1:S36–43.

Schwarz F, Becker J. (2010) *Peri-Implant Infection: Etiology, Diagnosis and Treatment*. Quintessenz, Berlin.

Strietzel FP, Reichart PA, Kale A, Kulkarni M, Wegner B, Küchler I. (2007) Smoking interferes with the prognosis of dental implant treatment: a systematic review and meta-analysis. *J Clin Periodontol*. 34(6):523–44.

Szmukler-Moncler S, Salama H, Reingewirtz Y, Dubruille JH. (1998) Timing of loading and effect of micro-motion on bone-dental implant interface: review of experimental literature. *J Biomed Mater Res*. 43(2):192–203.

Testori T, Del Fabbro M, Feldman S, Vincenzi G, Sullivan D, Rossi R Jr, Anitua E, Bianchi F, Francetti L, Weinstein RL. (2002) A multicenter prospective evaluation of 2-months loaded Osseotite implants placed in the posterior jaws: 3-year follow-up results. *Clin Oral Implants Res*. 16(6):631–8.

Variola F, Brunski JB, Orsini G, Tambasco de Oliveira P, Wazen R, Nanci A. (2011) Nanoscale surface modifications of medically relevant metals: state-of-the art and perspectives. *Nanoscale*. 3(2):335–53.

Wennerberg A, Albrektsson T, Johansson C, Andersson B. (1996) Experimental study of turned and grit-blasted screw-shaped implants with special emphasis on effects of blasting material and surface topography. *Biomaterials*. 17(1):15–22.

3

Implant Biomechanics

3.1 Introduction

Implant therapy is a relatively new modality, and treatment plans are based on empirical, traditional prosthetic treatments. We must always be mindful of the difficult oral environment in which our prostheses must function. Overloading implant restorations may contribute to peri-implant bone loss and implant failure or cause mechanical complications with the prosthesis. Biomechanical research data are fragmented and incomplete, and opinions are diverse. The relative influence of overload, as distinct from the host immune response to plaque deposits, on peri-implantitis bone loss, has not been elucidated satisfactorily.

Biomechanics

Biomechanics is the study of the mechanics of a living body, especially of the forces exerted by muscles on the skeletal structure. It involves engineering concepts applied to biological situations. In implantology, one is concerned with the dynamics of masticatory loading, and the response of bone to loading stresses at the implant–bone interface. Implant biomechanics is a function of masticatory forces, osseointegration, bone density, and the integrity of implant-abutment connection.

Force has magnitude, direction, frequency, and duration, and is expressed in Newtons (N). The stress (force/unit area) created at the implant–bone interface is a combination of the force and the direction of the force. Compressive, tensile, and shear forces act on bone at the implant–bone interface.

Implant proprioception and nocioception

Natural teeth have a supporting periodontal ligament, which acts as a shock absorber and

Fundamentals of Implant Dentistry, First Edition. Gerard Byrne.
© 2014 John Wiley & Sons, Inc. Published 2014 by John Wiley & Sons, Inc.
Companion website: www.wiley.com/go/byrne/implants

provides sensory feedback during function to limit trauma. Implants are effectively anky-losed to bone and without proprioceptive or nocioceptive mechanisms (Tokmakidis et al. 2009) (Fig. 3.1). From the outset, researchers have been concerned that overloading implants could result in bone loss and implant loss. Proprioception for implant prostheses may be supplied by the periodontium of opposing teeth, muscle and joint receptors, and oral soft tissues. Early studies on implant-supported prostheses (hybrid) concluded that the functional capacity of these patients was similar to that of dentate subjects (Lundqvist and Haraldson 1984; Lundgren et al. 1987; Carlsson 2009). It was considered that the lack of periodontal receptors could lead to impaired fine motor control of the mandible, risking overload. This concern led to the use of resin occlusal surfaces rather than porcelain ones in order to mitigate forces (Brånemark et al. 1985). The IMZ implant system produced an "intramobile" nylon spacer between implant and abutment to act as a stress-breaker or shock absorber for occlusal force (Babbush et al. 1987). Currently, implant-borne metal-porcelain or ceramic restorations are used routinely, both in full and partial arch fixed prostheses, without apparent ill effects.

Functional bone remodeling

The masticatory muscles act on implant restorations in function and parafunction generating occlusal forces. The biological reaction in bone to normal, subnormal, or excessive forces determines whether productive bone remodeling or destructive bone loss occurs. With natural teeth, forces are dissipated by a combination of the periodontal ligament, bone deformation, and reflex jaw opening. With implants, only bone deformation or strain can occur and the nocioceptive reflex may be negated. Strain can have a positive effect whereby bone remodels and gets denser (Brånemark et al. 1985), or can have a negative effect whereby bone could be

damaged and susceptible to resorption and replacement by less specialized connective tissue. Bone density and bone volume may be major factors in determining the bone response to functional forces. In a well-designed clinical case, there should be a positive bone remodeling response to functional loading.

Peri-implant bone loss related to overload

It is accepted that excessive force on a natural tooth may cause some bone resorption and increased mobility. Although a cause–effect relationship has not been established between bruxism and implant failure, it is accepted that implant overload may lead to marginal bone loss or mechanical problems (Isidor 1997, 2006). Naert et al. (2002) suggested that short implants, a low number of implants per prosthesis, and bone grafting were linked to increased risk for implant failure, and that prosthesis splinting may be advantageous. Implant survival has also been found to be lower in less dense bone, and with shorter implants, which may implicate overload in bone loss and failure (Friberg et al. 1991; Sennerby and Roos 1998; Weber and Cochran 1998; Telleman et al. 2011).

Peri-implant infection and bone loss

It is widely accepted that bone loss around implants can be caused by the host immune response to microbiota and their toxins. Bacterial plaque, as a causative factor in peri-implant disease and bone loss, has been put forward by periodontics researchers, as the primary cause of bone loss after osseointegration (Schwarz and Becker 2010). This disease process is analogous to periodontitis (Lang et al. 1993; Froum 2010).

In a long-term study of mandibular implant-supported fixed prostheses, factors associated with occlusal loading, such as bite force, clenching, and cantilever length were of less importance for peri-implant bone loss than smoking and poor oral hygiene (Lindquist et al. 1996).

Mechanical failure

Overload may lead to mechanical failure of the implant, implant screw, or the prosthesis. Adverse loading conditions must be anticipated and managed at the treatment planning stage in order to reduce the risk of prosthesis failure.

3.2 Natural tooth: functional response

Natural tooth support is provided by the periodontium (Fig. 3.1). The tooth root and alveolar bone are joined by the periodontal ligament (a syndesmosis). Fibers of the periodontal ligament (PDL) attach directly to the tooth via cementum and to the alveolar bone. Proprioceptors in the PDL monitor the forces when

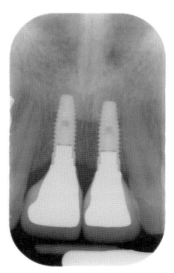

3.1. Radiograph showing two maxillary central incisor implant crowns. Note the periodontal ligaments (syndesmosis) of adjacent natural teeth and macroscopic bone-implant contact (ankylosis).

biting and chewing. The gingival attachment consists of a fibrous attachment to cementum, and a junctional epithelium, which attaches to the tooth surface via hemidesmosomes. The gingival attachment forms a physical and immunologic barrier to oral microbiota. The periodontal ligament is highly vascular, innervated, and forms a resilient suspensory and force dissipating system for the tooth and has several key features (Brånemark et al. 1985):

(1) *Shock absorption:* Oblique, relaxed collagen fiber groups and periodontal vascularity are responsible for a dampening effect or viscoelastic property of the periodontal ligament. This counters functional forces and effectively dissipates force. Natural teeth can move rapidly vertically, horizontally, and rotationally in response to loading (Giargia and Lindhe 1997). The longer the tooth root, the lower the load distribution to the crestal bone. Teeth, both anterior and posterior, move vertically approximately 28 μm and between 56 and 108 μm bucco-lingually under light forces (Parfitt 1960). Heavier or progressive force on a tooth causes bone flexion with secondary tooth movement of up to 40 μm depending on bone density and volume (Mühlemann 1967). Given tooth and bone configurations, there is significant variability of tooth movement in different directions.

(2) *Proprioception:* The periodontal ligament is well innervated, and mechanoreceptors reflexly protect against excessive force. Sensory regulation of the masticatory process takes place through mechanoreceptors in the PDL, the temporomandibular joints (TMJs), the masticatory muscles and the oral mucous membrane. Mandibular movements are coordinated with significant input from these receptors. Thus, tooth movement and reflex jaw opening accommodate heavy or sudden impact forces (Okeson 2013).

(3) *Control of osteogenesis and accommodation of tooth movement:* It is believed that the periodontal ligament regulates osteogenesis as a consequence of external forces that bring about tooth movement. Normally, there is constant remodeling of the alveolus to accommodate external forces and reestablish equilibrium, as seen with supereruption and drifting, or in orthodontic movement. When the periodontal ligament is lost, as with a replanted tooth, the tooth becomes ankylosed and osteoclasts attack and resorb the root.

3.3 Implant: functional response

Unlike a natural tooth, an implant is fixed to bone and has been called a functional ankylosis (Schroeder et al. 1996). Bone is elastic and undergoes elastic deformation in response to force, but the speed and magnitude of the deformation is not equivalent to that of the PDL.

Osseointegration

Clinically, the integrated implant is immobile with no discernible movement, and maintains its position even as teeth can move relative to it (Fig. 3.2). The osseointegration concept implies direct bone contact with the implant surface. As with a natural tooth, there is alveolar bone distortion/deformation under loading, especially with progressive or sustained loading. Implant mobility has been measured at between 2 and 3 μm vertically and between 12 and 66 μm horizontally. Occlusal loads are transmitted directly to the bone at the implant–bone interface. The loads are not distributed uniformly and the crestal bone bears the greatest load, especially when forces are off-axis as with cantilevers and bruxism. Under small transient occlusal loads, there is no implant

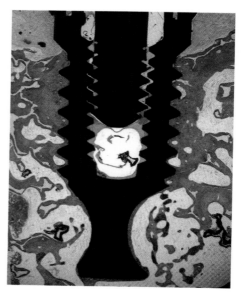

3.2. Microphotograph of an immediately loaded implant after 9 months in function. The histological evaluation showed a bone-to-implant contact of 93% and a densification of the surrounding bone. The marginal bone level is coronal to the first implant thread (courtesy of Gottlow J. in Jokstad 2010; Wiley-Blackwell).

movement; under heavy or prolonged force, there is a small amount of elastic bone deformation.

Implant–bone interface

The macro- and microscopic configuration of the implant surface, the percentage of bone-to-implant contact (BIC), and the bone density and volume determine the biomechanics of force transference. Microscopically, there is intimate contact between bone and the oxide layer of the implant surface. Bone fills implant surface irregularities at macroscopic, microscopic (Angstrom), and molecular levels. According to Skalak (1985), this intimate contact allows the direct transfer of force from the implant to the bone without any *relative movement* between implant and bone. The potential movement of the implant, or slippage, is resisted by the implant surface roughness and the intimate interfacial contact. Excessive force may disrupt this interface or cause direct damage to the bone, as the modulus of elasticity (Young's modulus) is much higher for Ti than for bone.

Bone response to load: remodeling or loss

Bone resists compressive forces best and resists tensile and shear/sliding forces worst (Misch 2007). A shear or sliding force may be visualized as a machine screw implant resisting rotational or unscrewing force. The physical response to functional force is strain and deformation of bone at the implant–bone interface. Movement of the opposing dentiton or movement of the abutment at the IAJ may also dissipate some of the force. Bone will deform elastically under the biting force, but may be damaged (plastic deformation) when an unknown threshold force is exceeded.

Physiologic forces lead to remodeling as in the rest of the human skeleton, and an increase in bone density around the implant (Brånemark et al. 1985) (Fig. 3.3). It is theorized that overload leads to micro-strain and micro-fractures, which stimulate a cellular response by means of changes in fluid dynamics or electromagnetic stimuli. The mechanobiology of bone response to strain has been discussed at length by Henneman et al. (2008) and Krishnan and Davidovitch (2009). Bone adjacent to an implant is 60% mineralized at 4 months, and 100% mineralized at 1 year (Misch 2007). Remodeling under physiologic loads will lead to an increase in bone–implant surface contact, and an increase in bone density.

Bone resistance to elastic or plastic deformation is a function of its density and volume. Dense cortical bone (Type I) has a higher elastic modulus (10-fold) than spongy cancellous bone (Type IV), and hence Type I bone is more resistant to stress-induced elastic or plastic deformation. It has been shown that implants in

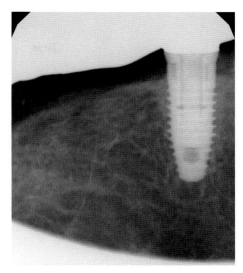

3.3. Radiograph of functional bone densification around a long-standing implant.

dense bone can resist greater forces and have a higher survival rate (Lin et al. 2008; Jokstad 2009).

Loading sequelae

Bone adapts to functional forces and can increasingly withstand greater force as it remodels in line with these physiologic forces. Excessive force has been implicated in bone loss, although a causative relationship has not been proven clinically (Quirynen et al. 1992; Isidor 1997, 2006; van Steenberghe et al. 1999; Misch et al. 2005). If an *unknown loading threshold* is exceeded, there are several possible sequelae for an implant restoration:

- The restoration may fracture
- The connection screw may loosen or fracture
- The implant may fracture
- There may be progressive marginal bone damage/loss (secondary failure), with bone being replaced by fibrous connective tissue.

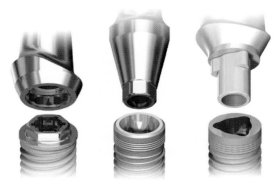

3.4. Three implant-abutment connections: external hex, internal hex with platform-switching, and tri-lobe connection (courtesy of Nobel Biocare).

The implant–abutment connection

It is not clear whether the type of abutment connection makes a difference in force transmission to bone (Fig. 3.4). It has been suggested that external connections may lead to peak strain in crestal bone and hence the risk of bone stress and damage in this area (Tokmakidis et al. 2009). With external connections, all the occlusal force and strain is transmitted to the bolt-like abutment retaining screw, risking screw loosening and fracture, but in the process, relieving some of the strain in bone. With a precisely fitting internal connection, more stress is directed apically along the implant body and away from the bony crest (Hansson 2003). Thus, internal connections may lead to more even loading of bone over the entire surface of the implant. Internal connections also place less strain on abutment screws, but introduce the risk of implant collar "hoop" fracture due to the precise fit and force transfer in this area.

3.4 Functional and nonfunctional forces

Sir Isaac Newton's second law of motion states that the acceleration of a body is inversely proportional to its mass and directly proportional to the force that caused the acceleration. Mass is measured in kilograms (kg). Acceleration is measured in meters per second squared (m/s^2).

Thus, force (F) = the product of mass and acceleration kg·m/s^2.

A force of 1 kg·m/s^2 is 1 newton (N).

In dental literature, bite force is sometimes expressed as kilograms (kg), and in older literature, force may be expressed as pounds (lb). Forces are represented by vectors; they have magnitude and direction. Forces on teeth and implants vary in magnitude, direction, frequency, and duration. Bite force has been estimated at between 40 and 90 kg on the first molar and between 13 and 23 kg on the central incisor and greater in bruxism (Okeson 2013). Maximum bite force measured on different teeth ranges from 150 to 710 N (Misch 2005). Males generally have larger maximum bite forces than females. Dolichofacial patients (Class II division 1) tend to have less force-generating potential than brachiofacial patients (Class II division 2) (Fig. 3.5). These latter patients may have hypertrophy of the masticatory musculature and bruxing habits. The osseointegrated implant must be able to resist normal masticatory forces that may have axial and nonaxial (horizontal, twisting, and rotational) components. The resolution of the force and its effect on living bone at the implant bone interface is complex and the outcome is unpredictable.

Functional occlusal force

Functional force arises from mastication and swallowing actions. It is predominantly vertical in the tooth long-axis or perpendicular to the occlusal plane, with a varying lateral component depending on arch location. In the natural dentition, horizontal forces tend to be in a mesial direction, with a facial component in the maxilla and a lingual component in the mandible. Occlusal forces are directed through a food bolus or by direct contact in maximum

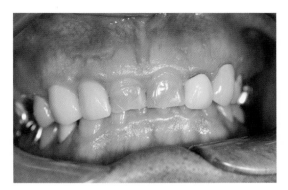

3.5. Class II division 2 occlusion with increased vertical overlap and bruxism wear.

intercuspation or eccentric contact positions. Force gradually increases, peaks, and suddenly declines. Conscious effort can greatly magnify the normal masticatory force. Bruxing and clenching can create massive directional loads of prolonged duration. Force can also be a sudden impact force, such as when a hard object is encountered during chewing, or when the mandible receives an external blow.

Nonfunctional (secondary) force

Force on implants also occurs indirectly through mandibular distortion or flexion (during opening, protrusion, or chewing) and may have implications for long rigid prostheses that cross the midline in the mandible. It has been estimated that the mandible can expand up to 800 μm in the cross-arch dimension measured at the first molars during opening (Misch 2007). The clinical significance of mandibular flexure on implant survival is not known (Law et al. 2012). Ill-fitting multi-unit "splinted" implant prostheses that are screw-retained can create stress at the abutment connection that is transmitted to the implant–bone interface. Although it has been suggested that misfit does not lead to bone loss (Jemt et al. 2000), it would

seem clinically prudent that an implant restoration system should be strain-free at rest, and should not resist natural mandibular flexion (Monteiro et al. 2010).

3.5   Dissipation functional forces

Force is transmitted directly and without mitigation through relatively rigid ceramics, plastics, and metals of a dental prosthesis to the implant–bone interface. Ultimately, force transmission to the implant–bone interface results in strain with elastic or plastic deformation of the bone, which dissipates the force. Strain within the bone may cause remodeling or bone damage and resorption. Force transmission and bone deformation is influenced by factors such as bone volume and density, the quality of bone-implant contact (BIC), and the mechanical interlocking configuration of the implant with the bone. Physiologic functional forces must be planned in order to promote a healthy remodeling bone response.

Bone–implant contact

The amount of *bone contact* with the implant surface (BIC) varies greatly and is lower in fine cancellous bone than in dense cortical bone. This has implications for load bearing capacity. Albrektsson et al. (1993) demonstrated a BIC of 80% in retrieved Brånemark machined implants from anterior mandible bone. The amount of bone in contact with the implant will depend on the conditions for osseointegration and whether the implant has a machined or textured surface. BIC can be expected to be greater at an earlier stage with textured surfaces, and to increase over time. Significant improvement in implant–bone contact has been demonstrated with newer textured implant surfaces (Khang et al. 2001; Stach and Kohles 2003). Rocci et al. (2003) demonstrated a BIC >80% for TiUnite surfaces in the posterior mandible. The

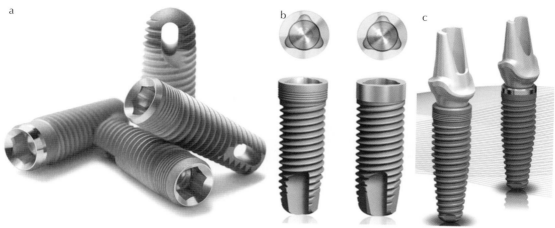

3.6. (a) Zimmer Tapered Screw-Vent® (TSV) implants with various surface features: threads, micro-grooves, machined collar, textured collar, thread formers, internal hex connection, and textured surfaces (MTX™ and HA surface) (courtesy of Zimmer Dental). (b) Nobel Replace™ implant configurations (courtesy of Nobel Biocare). (c) Nobel Replace™ implant variations with platform switching connection (courtesy of Nobel Biocare)

phenomenon of contact osteogenesis is considered to be significant in improving osseointegration, especially in lower density bone (Jokstad 2009). Bone loss may be related to low BIC percentage, immature bone, low bone density, or excessive forces leading to osteoclasis or a net negative bone turnover.

Implant body surface configuration

Threads and surface texture greatly increase the surface area for potential implant contact with bone. This is positive for force transmission and dissipation. Threads are usually rounded to avoid stress concentrations, but also in order to present a favorable configuration for vertical compression loading (Brånemark et al. 1985). This same effect can be expected with surface microscopic texture, as there is intimate implant–bone contact at this level. The interlocking of bone and Ti asperites can transmit shear stresses in a manner similar to screw threads. Macroscopic and microscopic textures create a substantial increase in bone contact area, and thus the capacity of the implant to

dissipate forces in contiguous bone. Much has been written relative to biomechanics of screw implants in bone. However, nonthreaded, textured-surface implants have been used equally successfully, implying that force is transferred successfully to bone by many implant designs. Machined surface implants have good long-term outcomes in dense bone but show increased failure rate due to crestal bone loss in soft or grafted bone (Jokstad 2009; Van de Velde et al. 2010). Histomorphometric analyses of BIC have confirmed higher values for textured surface implants compared with machined surfaces (Trisi et al. 2002; Schwartz et al. 2005; Wennerberg and Albrektsson 2009). Finite element analysis (FEA) and photoelastic analysis have been used to rationalize implant shape and thread designs by evaluating stress concentration (Brunski et al. 2009) (Fig. 3.6a–c).

Implant collar configuration

The role of overload in peri-implant crestal bone damage or loss is not well understood. At the outset of osseointegration and implant therapy, it was believed that bone loss would be a direct consequence of occlusal overload. Misch (2007) has suggested that forces on the implant lead to stress concentration on bone in the collar region, and to bone resorption. The implication of this is that overload may account for bone loss around the collars of implants (Isidor 1997; Misch et al. 2005). It has been suggested that micro-threaded or textured collar designs may lead to bone preservation around the implant collar by giving more favorable force transmission to bone (Hansson 1999). However, Bateli et al. (2011) found no connection between collar configuration and marginal bone loss. It is thought that implants with smooth machined collars may lose bone by a phenomenon known as *stress shielding*, whereby functional forces are not well dissipated by the smooth implant–bone junction in an area of high stress. This phenomenon is similar to disuse atrophy. A smooth polished 4.0 mm collar has been associated with more crestal bone loss than a 2.0 mm smooth polished one (Misch 2007). Schwarz and Becker (2010) noted more epithelial downgrowth on smooth than on rough collars.

Implant length (crown-to-implant length ratio)

Biomechanically, short implants have less bone contact, but also may have a poor clinical crown-to-implant ratio (C/I). The significance of a high C/I is not known. Implant restorations with C/I ratios of up to 2/1 may be acceptable clinically, and might be considered as an alternative to procedures that require more advanced surgery aimed to increase bone volume and decrease the C/I ratio in atrophic ridges (Sanz and Naert 2009) (Fig. 3.7).

According to Misch (1999) and Misch et al. (2006), implant length may not be as important in stress mitigation as the implant diameter and number. Some reports show that short implants

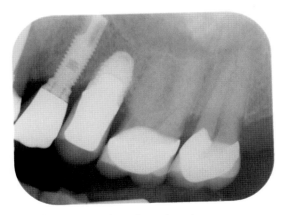

3.7. Clinical examples of good and poor crown-to-implant ratios.

are at a higher risk of failure, especially in less dense bone (Friberg et al. 1991; Hobkirk et al. 2006). However, Annibali et al. (2012) in a systematic review of short implants (5.0–8.0 mm), found that surgical technique, implant location, and type of edentulism and prosthetic restoration did not affect short-implant survival. Short-term success rates were high (99.1%); textured surface implants had a slightly higher success rate than machined surfaces.

3.6 Bite force mechanics and implant prostheses

Stress and strain

The stress (force/unit area) created at the implant–bone interface is a function of the force and the area of implant–bone contact (BIC). The strain induced may be compressive, tensile or shear. The strain may lead to elastic or plastic bone deformation. Bone resists compressive stress better than tensile or shear stress, although the clinical significance of this is unknown (Carlsson 2009). Off-axis forces represent a 50–200% increase in compressive stress as compared with axial loading, while tensile and shear stress may increase 10-fold (Misch 2007).

Moment forces

Occlusal force can have a *moment* or torsional (twisting) and bending action on an implant if the force acts along a lever arm, such as a cantilevered pontic. The moment of a force is the product of the force and the distance (moment arm) to the point of action of the force from the axis of rotation or fulcrum (class I lever arm). The greater the distance of the force along the lever arm, the greater the *moment force*. From a clinical standpoint, the fulcrum point may be considered the abutment screw. An axial force of 30 N on the implant does not induce a moment load. However, a 30 N force offset by 1 cm gives a horizontal bending force, and/or a torsional (unscrewing) moment force of 30 Ncm (abutment screws are often tightened/torqued to approximately 30 Ncm). A longer lever arm or cantilever increases the moment force, and hence greatly magnifies the force at abutment screw, and ultimately, at the implant–bone interface (Fig. 3.8a,b).

Clinical cantilevers or moment forces

A moment force can occur in the following clinical conditions:

- On a portion of the crown outside the diameter of the implant (a small diameter implant with a large crown)
- Off-axis loading of an implant crown (common with poorly angled implants or anterior implant crowns)
- On a cantilevered pontic.

Cantilever action can be visualized as lateral force (off-axis force) on a maxillary canine implant crown, or on a cantilevered pontic. In many cantilever scenarios, there will not only be a bending moment but also a torquing moment, which tends to stress the implant-abutment connection, or the implant itself around its long axis. A single cantilevered

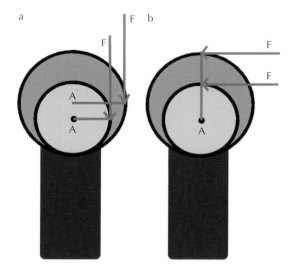

3.8. Increasing crown size in (a) width or (b) height increases axial and horizontal cantilevers and moment forces (F) around imaginary axes (A) (courtesy of H. Byrne).

pontic from a single implant is a greater risk than a single cantilevered pontic in an FDP with two or more implants (Romeo and Storelli 2012).

The mechanics are considerably more complex for a restoration involving several implants and pontics, in that forces will be resolved based on the location of several fulcrum points and lever arms. It is suggested that implants be evenly spaced for optimum force distribution. Skalak (1985) considers the geometry of curved constructions too complex to be easily quantified mathematically. The implant positioning, the complex forces of occlusion, and deformation of the prosthesis, screws, and jawbone must all be taken into account (Fig. 3.9a,b).

Impact forces

An additional force that affects implants is impact or sudden force. Impact forces also have

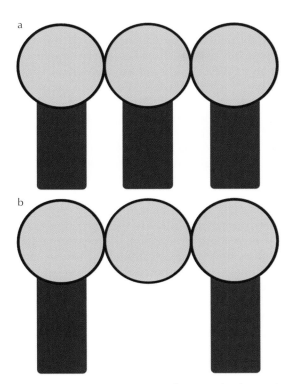

3.9. (a) Ideal implant support configuration for three-unit FDP. (b) Acceptable implant support configuration for a three-unit FDP (courtesy of H. Byrne).

magnitude, duration, and direction. In the natural dentition, these forces are resisted hydrodynamically by the periodontal ligament and reflexly by jaw opening. If severe, impact forces may result in tooth fracture or fracture of restorative components. Unlike a tooth, when an impact force is applied to an implant, the force is transmitted directly to bone without any hydrodynamic mitigation.

Fatigue failure

Occlusal forces are repetitive. These forces may be very large during bruxing and clenching. Such repetitive forces over a long duration could to lead to *fatigue failure* of the implant or more likely restorative components. Screw loosening and fracture is a common outcome. Fatigue failure is a function of the materials, the loading geometry, and the loading frequency (Fig. 3.10a,b).

Lack of implant proprioception

It has been claimed (Misch 2005) that rigidly fixed implants generate more strain in bone (up

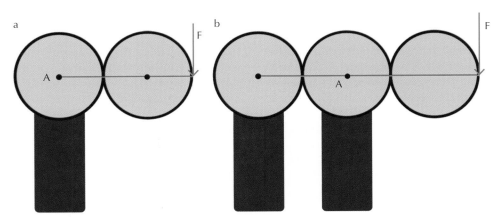

3.10. (a) Implant FDP configuration that is rarely acceptable due to moment forces. (b) Implant FDP configuration may be acceptable depending on the available bone volume and implant size. The moment force (F) is counteracted by the rigid splinting of the implants (courtesy of H. Byrne).

to fourfold) than natural teeth. This is partly due to the relative lack of proprioception from an implant. There is no PDL to act as a limiting factor (van Steenberghe and de Vries 1978). Excessive force may lead to ceramic fractures, component fracture, screw loosening, and interfacial bone damage. Bone damage has not been quantified in relation to force magnitude thus far. It is not clear to what extent the proprioception system works for implants, especially with opposing implant restorations. Hämmerle et al. (1995) showed that the tactile sensitivity threshold of implants is less by a factor of $9\times$ compared with natural teeth. As a consequence, the loads on implant restorations are often three times higher on removable implant-borne prostheses and nine times higher on fixed single-tooth implant-borne restorations than on the natural dentition (Tokmakidis et al. 2009).

3.7 Quality of osseointegration

Ultimately, the survival of an implant will be determined by the magnitude of force, the quality of the surrounding bone, and the quality of the interface between implant and bone or osseointegration. The bone–implant interface has been intensively studied, bone densities have been classified, and attempts have been made to determine the quality of osseointegration in terms of bone–implant contact (BIC) with various diagnostic tools, such as Periotest® and Osstell™ resonance frequency analysis (RFA). Finite element analysis and photoelastic analysis have been extensively applied to implant design and strain patterns in bone.

Strain testing (Periotest and Osstell)

Techniques and instruments have been designed in an effort to quantify the quality of osseointegration in order to better predict

clinical outcome. The subject has been thoroughly reviewed by Chang et al. (2010), and Jong-Chul et al. (2011). Resonance frequency analysis (RFA) was invented by Meredith and Cauley in 1992. Osstell RFA uses a magnetic pulse which, when applied to an implant abutment, provides an implant stability quotient (ISQ) value in the range of 1 to 100; the higher the ISQ value, the higher the implant stability. Although high values indicate better osseointegration, it is not clear what parameters of osseointegration are being measured (Hobkirk et al. 2006). The Periotest consists of an instrument designed to identify the damping capacity of a tooth or implant by measuring the contact time of an electronically driven and monitored rod after percussing the test surface. A Periotest value (PTV) ranges from -8 (low mobility) to $+50$ (high mobility). A Periotest value (PTV) of -8 to -6 indicates excellent implant stability.

Both Periotest and Osstell RFA measurements are influenced by variables such as bone density, bone volume, and implant diameter and length (above and within bone) (Cranin et al. 1998; Meredith 1998). Data suggest that high ISQ values and low Periotest values indicate successfully integrated implants, and that low or decreasing ISQ values and high or increasing Periotest values may be signs of ongoing disintegration and/or marginal bone loss (Aparicio et al. 2006).

Currently, these devices are not sufficiently validated clinically as prognostic biomechanical indicators. They are, however, useful research tools and are becoming more clinically relevant with the increase in immediate implant loading.

Photoelastic and finite element analysis (FEA)

Laboratory photo-elastic and finite element models have been used to simulate the effect of forces at the implant–bone interface, showing peak strains around the implant collar (Brunski 1992; Schroeder et al. 1996; Misch 2005; Brunski et al. 2009). These models show that lateral forces tend to be transmitted to crestal bone in dense bone situations, whereas the same forces are transmitted more apically in softer cancellous bone. External connections tend to create peak stresses in crestal bone, whereas internal connections move the stress more apically. While these simulations may seem impressive, and may be useful in implant design, the clinical relevance of these laboratory models is not validated (Assunção et al. 2009).

3.8 Clinical force management

Overload may lead to bone loss or mechanical component failure. A goal of treatment planning is to design a treatment, which minimizes adverse forces and evenly distributes mechanical stress in the implant system and contiguous bone (Tokmakidis et al. 2009). Occlusal forces vary depending on the nature of the opposing arch, whether a denture, implant overdenture, natural teeth, or implant crowns, and the proportion of residual functional occlusion present. The more natural teeth that remain, the more favorable the loading situation will be due to natural proprioception.

Force on an implant restoration is mitigated by:

- Movement of the opposing tooth or denture with negative sensory feedback
- Movement of the abutment relative to the implant at the connection (external connections allow more movement than internal conical connections)
- Micro-motion of the implant via elastic bone deformation.

Theoretical means of mitigating force include:

Increasing implant surface area

- *Increased implant number:* the logical choice when feasible
- *Increased implant length:* increase of bone contact area
- *Increased implant diameter:* changing from the smallest to largest may increase surface area by 25–50% (Fig. 3.11a,b)
- *Use of macroscopic features:* threads and fins
- Microscopic texture.

Reducing adverse loads

- Facilitate axial loading of implants
- Avoid cantilevers: offset forces result in larger moment forces
- Use longer implants to give a favorable crown/implant ratio (Fig. 3.12)
- Employ accurate harmonious adjustment for static and dynamic occlusion
- Splint implants with rigid frameworks to distribute load
- Use protective rigid orthotic bruxism devices.

Prevention of screw loosening by preloading the abutment connection

It is current practice to *preload* abutment screws by torquing them into place at predetermined torque values to prevent abutment screw loosening. Torque value is a measurable means of developing tension in a screw joint (Drago 2007). Preloading elastically deforms the screw thread. The strain thus created, called the preload, keeps the implant and abutment clamped together. Preload must be overcome before the screw can come loose. This is a standard engineering technique and requires the use of calibrated *torque drivers*. Implant

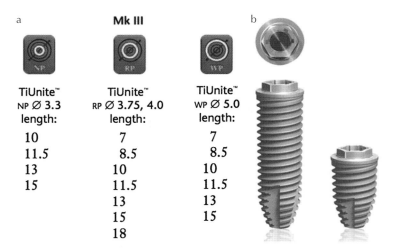

3.11. (a) Implant platform diameter and length variations for Brånemark Mark III implants (courtesy of Nobel Biocare). (b) Implant length; NobelSpeedy™ Groovy and Shorty™ (courtesy of Nobel Biocare).

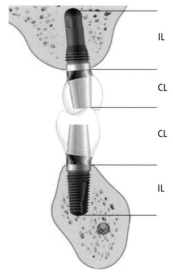

3.12. Diagram of optimal axial loading showing crown (CL)/implant (IL) ratios. The maxillary implant has a more favorable C : I ratio (courtesy of CAMLOG).

companies have used various surface treatments on screws (e.g. Nobel TorqTite®) in order to reduce friction and increase preloading. Each implant system will have its own torque driver

and specific recommended preload value. Functional stress on an abutment screw may, over time, lead to lessening of preload and loosening of screws. Screw loosening may indicate inadequate preload or excessive forces. External implant connections place virtually all the strain on the abutment screw, due to the "bolt" type retention design. Well-fitting, cone-shaped internal connections reduce the strain on the abutment screw, because load is transferred directly to the implant body, and a lesser preload is needed.

3.9 Biomechanical treatment planning

Mechanical complications with implant restorations are often traced back to unfavorable loading. There are no evidence-based guidelines for designing implant support. While there is no demonstrated cause-and-effect relationship between bruxing and implant failure, a precautionary approach is recommended in treatment planning (Manfredini et al. 2011). Misch (2007) has given guidelines regarding implant positioning, or key implant locations for support of fixed bridgework. He advocates more implants when adverse force factors are present by, for example, using one implant per tooth as a baseline, with longer and wider implants when feasible. The clinician who is contemplating more complex cases is advised to refer to other more advanced implant textbooks.

Recommendations for implant diameter, number, and length

- A 3.0 to 3.5 mm (small diameter) implant for mandibular incisors and maxillary lateral incisors
- A 4.0 to 4.5 mm (regular/medium diameter) implant for premolars, canines, occasionally first molars
- A 5.0 to 6.0 mm (wide/large diameter) implant for molars
- Two implants for two adjacent teeth and two or three implants for three adjacent teeth (not including first molars and canines as pontics)
- A generally accepted reference length is 10.0 mm. Implant lengths range from approximately 6.0–18.0 mm.

Some general guiding principles

- If in doubt, use one implant per tooth.
- Canine and first molars are "key" locations for multi-unit fixed restorations (Misch 2005)
- Splinting a natural tooth to an implant, or implants, via a fixed prosthesis creates a cantilever force situation and should be avoided because the implant moves less than the natural tooth.
- Two or more rigidly splinted implants may allow for better load distribution than individual implants
- Implants should be spaced evenly for multi-unit prostheses

- Avoid cantilevers or moment arms especially in cases of parafunction; use terminal implant abutments. Small cantilevers may be acceptable, as with a canine implant supporting a lateral incisor pontic, provided the occlusion is favorable. Occlusion is favorable when there is adequate posterior occlusal function and minimal eccentric contact. A fixed dental prosthesis (FDP) cantilever may be considered when the alternative treatment would require advanced surgery
- Use a maximum of two pontics (premolar size) per bridge span—a long-span fixed prosthesis with end support implants may have force moments on each implant from flexure of a long pontic span. A rigid framework is paramount
- Precise internal connections may present greater risk of implant fracture (than screw fracture) than external hex designs when large forces are anticipated.
- Poorly angled implants lead to adverse off-axis moment forces. Off-axis placement and loading may be unavoidable, but incorrect implant angulation in a good site is avoidable
- Poorly fitting multi-unit restorations having direct screw retention to implants may induce resting strain within the abutment screw or at the implant–bone interface.
- Mandibular full-arch fixed prostheses should be segmented (due to mandibular flexion) when implants are to be placed both anteriorly and posteriorly
- Do not restore second molars except in ideal circumstances. They are in the highest force area and have the lowest quality bone.

Clinical scenarios

(1) *Single units*
  - A poor crown/implant ratio risks a lateral moment force
  - A cantilever or moment force occurs when a smaller diameter implant

(3.0–4.0 mm) supports a larger (e.g., molar size) crown

- A moment force occurs with poor angulation of implant relative to the crown

(2) *Multi-unit implant prostheses (FDPs)*
- Avoid cantilevered pontics.
- Use one implant per tooth.
- Central incisor, canine, and first molars are important implant support positions
- Two-stage screw retained restorations are desirable in patients with bruxism
- Adjacent single units may be splinted in order to spread the load over both implants.

(3) *Multi-unit prostheses with implants and natural teeth.*

If an implant is combined with a natural tooth to support a three-unit FDP, greater movement of the natural tooth relative to the implant can occur, especially with lateral forces (Fig. 3.13) (Hoffmann and Zafiropoulos 2012). This effectively results in an implant FDP supporting two cantilevered pontics (Boldt et al. 2012). It is a practice that cannot be justified biomechanically, except perhaps in cases with elderly patients where the natural abutment is a canine or molar and is relatively immobile. A systematic review by Pjetursson et al. (2007) found that the practice of joining natural teeth to implants had a lower success rate than either tooth supported or implant supported FDPs.

(4) *Fixed full-arch FDP (hybrid denture)*

With fixed full-arch prostheses, it is generally accepted that distal cantilevers should not exceed the anterior–posterior spread of the implants (Rangert et al. 1989; Sanz et al. 2009) (Fig. 3.14a,b). When parafunction is present or when there is an opposing natural dentition or implants, cantilevers should be minimal. V-shaped arches allow a more favorable anterior–posterior distribution of implants.

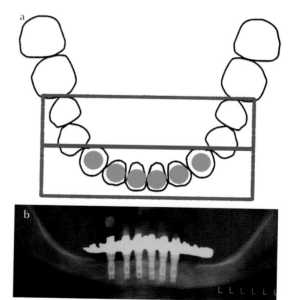

3.14. (a) Diagram of implant positions (green dots) for a fixed full-arch hybrid FDP with distal cantilevers. It is accepted practice to limit distal cantilevers to the distance between the most anterior and posterior implant (courtesy of H. Byrne). (b) Radiograph showing hybrid cantilever extensions.

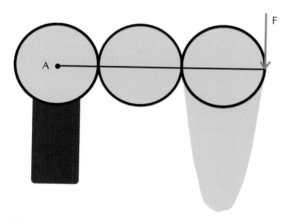

3.13. Diagram of implant-natural tooth combination FDP. Due to the greater relative motion of a natural tooth in function, this configuration is equivalent to a two-unit implant cantilever FDP (courtesy of H. Byrne).

(5) *Overdentures*

From a biomechanical standpoint, resilient clips should be used for overdentures to allow for movement of the denture base where it is supported by the residual ridge. The use of three or more implants gives more support, but presents the risk that the denture will "rock" in function. Also, joining two or more implants with a bar should give a more favorable loading scenario when compared with two individual implants, in that forces are distributed to both implants simultaneously by virtue of the rigid connection. This treatment is considered favorable in the upper jaw. Since most overdenture cases use resilient clips and are opposed by a complete denture, forces on the implants are minimal. Excessive force would likely lead to premature failure of the retentive clips or resin base.

(6) *Shortened dental arch*

It is not uncommon in prosthetic treatment to accept the loss of second or even first molars without replacement (Carlsson 2009) There is no clinical research to guide the clinician in this decision. It is ideal to have at least first molar occlusion, and when circumstances are favorable, a first molar implant crown may be planned. Occasionally, when premolars and molars are missing, replacement of the premolars only may be considered. This solution may be more desirable for the patient than a removable prosthesis or more complex implant treatment. Bruxers are not good candidates for the shortened arch implant treatment.

3.10   Adjusting occlusion

There is no evidence to date to recommend any unique method of occlusal design or occlusal adjustment for implant prostheses (Kim et al. 2005; Taylor et al. 2005; Gross 2008). Therefore, occlusion of implant-supported prostheses can be managed successfully by using the standard jaw registration methods, occlusal adjustment, and traditional occlusion concepts used for fixed and removable prostheses (Carlsson 2009; Okeson 2013). It is paramount to be focused on the management of occlusion, static and dynamic, on an implant restoration in order to harmonize occlusal forces on the implants or between natural teeth and implants.

Precise occlusal adjustment, in general, is extremely taxing due to difficulties in achieving consistent jaw positions and movements, marking contact and adjusting contact. Harmony of tooth contact in the maximum incuspation (MI) jaw position and eccentric jaw positions (test glides) is desirable. Shimstock film (5 μm thick) is a valuable tool for confirming contact or lack of contact.

In the case of a single implant crown with an opposing natural tooth, the natural tooth can move in function, thereby accommodating the relatively immobile implant crown. The occlusion may be adjusted either as a conventional crown, or so that the implant crown is out of contact in MI when checked with shimstock. The crown may be in contact in forceful biting.

When two implant restorations oppose, occlusal adjustment should leave the crowns out of contact in forceful biting (shimstock drags but does not tear). Thus, following occlusal adjustment, when the patient closes normally in MI, in light contact, the implant restorations may be out of contact.

In the course of time, the dentition will adapt to the implant fixed restoration, and an occlusal equilibrium will be reestablished.

References

Albrektsson T, Eriksson AR, Friberg B, Lekholm U, Lindahl L, Nevins M, Oikarinen V, Roos J, Sennerby L, Astrand P. (1993) Histologic investigations on 33 retrieved Nobelpharma implants. *Clin Mater.* 12(1):1–9.

Annibali S, Cristalli MP, Dell'Aquila D, Bignozzi I, La Monaca G, Pilloni A. (2012) Short dental implants: a systematic review. *J Dent Res.* 91(1): 25–32.

Aparicio C, Lang NP, Rangert B. (2006) Validity and clinical significance of biomechanical testing of implant/bone interface. *Clin Oral Implants Res.* 17 Suppl 2:2–7.

Assunção WG, Barão VA, Tabata LF, Gomes EA, Delben JA, dos Santos PH. (2009) Biomechanics studies in dentistry: bioengineering applied in oral implantology. *J Craniofac Surg.* 20(4):1173–7.

Babbush CA, Kirsch A, Mentag PJ, Hill B. (1987) Intramobile cylinder (IMZ) two-stage osteointegrated implant system with the intramobileelement (IME): part I. Its ratinale and procedure for use. *Int J Oral Maxillofac Implants.* 2(4):203–16. Review.

Bateli M, Att W, Strub JR. (2011) Implant neck configurations for preservation of marginal bone level: a systematic review. *Int J Oral Maxillofac Implants.* 26(2):290–303.

Boldt J, Knapp W, Proff P, Rottner K, Richter EJ. (2012) Measurement of tooth and implant mobility under physiological loading conditions. *Ann Anat.* 194(2):185–9.

Brånemark P-I, Zarb GA, Albrektasson T. (eds.) (1985) *Tissue-Integrated Prostheses: Osseointegration in Clinical Dentistry.* Quintessence, Chicago.

Brunski JB. (1992) Biomechanical factors affecting the bone-dental implant interface. *Clin Mater.* 10(3): 153–201.

Brunski JB, Currey JA, Helm JA, Leucht P, Nancy A, Wazen R. (2009) The healing bone-implant interface: role of micromotion and related strain levels in tissue. In: A Jokstad (ed.), *Osseointegration and Dental Implants.* Wiley-Blackwell, Ames, pp. 205–11.

Carlsson GE. (2009) Dental occlusion: modern concepts and their application in implant prosthodontics. *Odontology.* 97(1):8–17.

Chang PC, Lang NP, Giannobile WV. (2010) Evaluation of functional dynamics during osseointegration and regeneration associated with oral implants. *Clin Oral Implants Res.* 21(1):1–12.

Cranin AN, DeGrado J, Kaufman M, Baraoidan M, DiGregorio R, Batgitis G, Lee Z. (1998) Evaluation of the Periotest® as a diagnostic tool for dental implants. *J Oral Implantol.* 24(3):139–46.

Drago C. (2007) *Implant Restorations: A Step-by-Step Guide,* 2nd ed. Blackwell Munksgaard, Ames.

Friberg B, Jemt T, Lekholm U. (1991) Early failures in 4641 consecutively placed Brånemark dental implants: a study from stage 1 surgery to the connection of completed prostheses. *Int J Oral Maxillofac Implants.* 6(2):142–6.

Froum SJ. (2010) *Dental Implant Complications: Etiology, Prevention, and Treatment.* Wiley-Blackwell, Ames.

Giargia M, Lindhe J. (1997) Tooth mobility and periodontal disease. *J Clin Periodontol.* 24(11):785–95.

Gross MD. (2008) Occlusion in implant dentistry. A review of the literature of prosthetic determinants and current concepts. *Aust Dent J.* 53 Suppl 1:S60–8.

Hansson S. (1999) The implant neck: smooth or provided with retention elements. A biomechanical approach. *Clin Oral Implants Res.* 10(5):394–405.

Hansson S. (2003) A conical implant-abutment interface at the level of the marginal bone improves the distribution of stresses in the supporting bone. An axisymmetric finite element analysis. *Clin Oral Implants Res.* 14(3):286–93.

Hämmerle CH, Wagner D, Bragger U, Lussi A, Karayiannis A, Joss A, Lang NP. (1995) Threshold of tactile sensitivity perceived with dental endosseous implants and natural teeth. *Clin Oral Implants Res.* 6:83–90.

Henneman S, Von den Hoff JW, Maltha JC. (2008) Mechanobiology of tooth movement. *Eur J Orthod.* 30(3):299–306.

Hobkirk JA, Wiskott HW; Working Group 1. (2006) Biomechanical aspects of oral implants. Consensus report of Working Group 1. *Clin Oral Implants Res.* 17 Suppl 2:52–4.

Hoffmann O, Zafiropoulos GG. (2012) Tooth-implant connection: a review. *J Oral Implantol.* 38(2): 194–200.

Isidor F. (1997) Histological evaluation of peri-implant bone at implants subjected to occlusal overload or plaque accumulation. *Clin Oral Implants Res.* 8(1):1–9.

Isidor F. (2006) Influence of forces on peri-implant bone. *Clin Oral Implants Res.* 17 Suppl 2:8–18.

Jemt T, Lekholm U, Johansson CB. (2000) Bone response to implant-supported frameworks with differing degrees of misfit preload: in vivo study in rabbits. *Clin Implant Dent Relat Res.* 2(3):129–37.

Jokstad A. (2009) *Osseointegration and Dental Implants.* Wiley-Blackwell, Ames.

Jong-Chul P, Jung-Woo L, Soung-Min K, Jong-Ho L (2011) implant stability: measuring devices and randomized clinical trial for ISQ value change pattern measured from two different directions by magnetic RFA. http://cdn.intechopen.com/pdfs/18417/InTech-Implant_stability_measuring_

devices_and_randomized_clinical_trial_for_isq_ value_change_pattern_measured_from_two_ different_directions_by_magnetic_rfa.pdf (accessed December 17, 2013).

Khang W, Feldman S, Hawley CE, Gunsolley J. (2001) A multi-center study comparing dual acid-etched and machined-surfaced implants in various bone qualities. *J Periodontol.* 72(10):1384–90.

Kim Y, Oh TJ, Misch CE, Wang HL. (2005) Occlusal considerations in implant therapy: clinical guidelines with biomechanical rationale. *Clin Oral Implants Res.* 16(1):26–35.

Krishnan V, Davidovitch Z. (2009) On a path to unfolding the biological mechanisms of orthodontic tooth movement. *J Dent Res.* 88(7):597–608.

Lang NP, Brägger U, Walther D, Beamer B, Kornman KS. (1993) Ligature-induced peri-implant infection in cynomolgus monkeys. I. Clinical and radiographic findings. *Clin Oral Implants Res.* 4(1):2–11.

Law C, Bennani V, Lyons K, Swain M. (2012) Mandibular flexure and its significance on implant fixed prostheses: a review. *J Prosthodont.* 21(3):219–24.

Lin CL, Wang JC, Ramp LC, Liu PR. (2008) Biomechanical response of implant systems placed in the maxillary posterior region under various conditions of angulation, bone density, and loading. *Int J Oral Maxillofac Implants.* 23(1):57–64.

Lindquist LW, Carlsson GE, Jemt T. (1996) A prospective 15-year follow-up study of mandibular fixed prostheses supported by osseointegrated implants. Clinical results and marginal bone. *Clin Oral Implants Res.* 7(4):329–36.

Lundgren D, Laurell L, Falk H, Bergendal T. (1987) Occlusal force pattern during mastication in dentitions with mandibular fixed partial dentures supported on osseointegrated implants. *J Prosthet Dent.* 58:197–203.

Lundqvist S, Haraldson T. (1984) Occlusal perception of thickness in patients with bridges on osseointegrated oral implants. *Scand J Dent Res.* 92:88–95.

Manfredini D, Bucci MB, Sabattini VB, Lobbezoo F. (2011) Bruxism: overview of current knowledge and suggestions for dental implants planning. *Cranio.* 29(4):304–12.

Meredith N. (1998) Assessment of implant stability as a prognostic determinant. *Int J Prosthodont.* 11(5):491–501.

Misch CE. (1999) Implant design considerations for the posterior regions of the mouth. *Implant Dent.* 8(4):376–86.

Misch CE. (2005) *Dental Implant Prosthetics.* Elsevier Mosby, St. Louis.

Misch CE. (2007) *Contemporary Implant Dentistry*, 3rd ed. Elsevier Mosby, St. Louis.

Misch CE, Suzuki JB, Misch-Dietsh FM, Bidez MW. (2005) A positive correlation between occlusal trauma and peri-implant bone loss: literature support. *Implant Dent.* 14(2):108–16.

Misch CE, Steignga J, Barboza E, Misch-Dietsh F, Cianciola LJ, Kazor C. (2006) Short dental implants in posterior partial edentulism: a multicenter retrospective 6-year case series study. *J Periodontol.* 77(8):1340–7.

Monteiro DR, Goiato MC, Gennari Filho H, Pesqueira AA. (2010) Passivity in implant-supported prosthesis. *J Craniofac Surg.* 21(6):2026–9.

Mühlemann HR. (1967) Tooth mobility: a review of clinical aspects and research findings. *J Periodontol.* 38(6 Suppl):686–713.

Naert I, Koutsikakis G, Quirynen M, Duyck J, van Steenberghe D, Jacobs R. (2002) Biologic outcome of implant-supported restorations in the treatment of partial edentulism. Part 2: a longitudinal radiographic study. *Clin Oral Implants Res.* 13(4):390–5.

Okeson JP. (2013) *Management of Temporomandibular Disorders and Occlusion*, 7th ed. Elsevier Mosby, St. Louis.

Parfitt GJ. (1960) Measurement of the physiological mobility of individual teeth in an axial direction. *J Dent Res.* 39:608–18.

Pjetursson BE, Brägger U, Lang NP, Zwahlen M. (2007) Comparison of survival and complication rates of tooth-supported fixed dental prostheses (FDPs) and implant-supported FDPs and single crowns (SCs). *Clin Oral Implants Res.* 18 Suppl 3: 97–113. Review. Erratum in: Clin Oral Implants Res. (2008) 19(3):326–8.

Quirynen M, Naert I, van Steenberghe D. (1992) Fixture design and overload influence marginal bone loss and fixture success in the Brånemark system. *Clin Oral Implants Res.* 3(3): 104–11.

Rangert B, Jemt T, Jomeus L. (1989) Forces and moments on Brånemark implants. *J Oral Maxillofac Implants.* 4(3):241–7.

Rocci A, Martignoni M, Burgos P, Gottlow J, Sennerby L. (2003) Histology of retrieved immediately and early loaded oxidized implants. Light microscopic observations after 5 to 9 months of loading in the posterior mandible of 5 cases. *Clin Implant Dent Relat Res.* 12 Suppl 1:88–98.

Romeo E, Storelli S. (2012) Systematic review of the survival rate and the biological, technical, and aesthetic complications of fixed dental prostheses with cantilevers on implants reported in longitudinal studies with a mean of 5 years follow-up. *Clin Oral Implants Res.* 23 Suppl 6:39–49.

Sanz M, Naert I; Working Group 2. (2009) Biomechanics/risk management. *Clin Oral Implants Res.* 20 Suppl 4:107–11.

Schroeder A, Sutter F, Buser D, Krekeler G. (1996) *Oral Implantology: Basics: ITI Hollow Cylinder.* Thieme, New York.

Schwartz Z, Nasazky E, Boyan BD. (2005) Surface microtopography regulates osteointegration: the role of implant surface microtopography in osteointegration. *Alpha Omegan.* 98(2):9–19.

Schwarz F, Becker J. (2010) *Peri-Implant Infection: Etiology, Diagnosis and Treatment.* Quintessence, London.

Sennerby L, Roos J. (1998) Surgical determinants of clinical success of osseointegrated oral implants: a review of the literature. *Int J Prosthodont.* 11(5): 408–20.

Skalak R. (1985) Aspects of biomechanical considerations. In: P-I Brånemark, GA Zarb, T Albrektsson (eds.), *Tissue-Integrated Osseointegration in Clinical Dentistry.* Quintessence, Chicago, pp. 117–28.

Stach RM, Kohles SS. (2003) A meta-analysis examining the clinical survivability of machined-surfaced and osseotite implants in poor-quality bone. *Implant Dent.* 12(1):87–96.

van Steenberghe D, de Vries JH. (1978) The influence of local anaesthesia and occlusal surface area on the forces developed during repetitive maximal clenching efforts. *J Periodontal Res.* 13:270–4.

van Steenberghe D, Naert I, Jacobs R, Quirynen M. (1999) Influence of inflammatory reactions vs. occlusal loading on peri-implant marginal bone level. *Adv Dent Res.* 13:130–5.

Taylor TD, Wiens J, Carr A. (2005) Evidence-based considerations for removable prosthodontic and dental implant occlusion: a literature review. *J Prosthet Dent.* 94(6):555–60.

Telleman G, Raghoebar GM, Vissink A, den Hartog L, Huddleston Slater JJ, Meijer HJ. (2011) A systematic review of the prognosis of short (<10mm) dental implants placed in the partially edentulous patient. *J Clin Periodontol.* 38(7):667–76.

Tokmakidis K, Wessing B, Papoulia K, Spiekermann H. (2009) Load distribution and loading concepts on teeth and implants. *J Dent Implantol.* 25(1): 44–52.

Trisi P, Lazzara R, Rao W, Rebaudi A. (2002) Bone-implant contact and bone quality: evaluation of expected and actual bone contact on machined and osseotite implant surfaces. *Int J Periodontics Restorative Dent.* 22(6):535–45.

Van de Velde T, Collaert B, Sennerby L, De Bruyn H. (2010) Effect of implant design on preservation of marginal bone in the mandible. *Clin Implant Dent Relat Res.* 12(2):134–41.

Weber HP, Cochran DL. (1998) The soft tissue response to osseointegrated dental implants. *J Prosthet Dent.* 79(1):79–89.

Wennerberg A, Albrektsson T. (2009) Effects of titanium surface topography on bone integration: a systematic review. *Clin Oral Implants Res.* 20 Suppl 4:172–84.

4

Implant Systems

4.1 Introduction

Implants introduce to clinical dentistry a new lexicon of terminology that needs to be understood by all parties involved in implant dentistry—the clinician, the patient, and the auxiliary support personnel.

The implant, formerly referred to as a *fixture*, is the principal component of any implant system and is supplemented by a host of ancillary components. Modern implants are generally two-piece, consisting of the implant that is osseointegrated in bone, and the abutment that is attached to the implant and supports the prosthesis. Some one-piece implants, with an integral abutment are also available, for example, the Nobel Biocare NobelDirect® implant.

The Brånemark system was a two-piece implant with an external hex anti-rotation feature. ITI initially used a one-piece implant abutment combination, IMZ had a screw connection with no anti-rotation feature, and Tübingen had a proprietary post connection.

Other manufacturers involved in early implant development were Core-Vent, 3i, Astra, Bicon, and, more recently BioHorizons, Camlog, Southern Implants, and others.

From a practical standpoint, the profession needs reliable manufacturers and suppliers of comprehensive systems. Implant pioneers, such as Brånemark and Schroeder, worked in tandem with manufacturing companies to research, develop, and engineer systems that were brought to the marketplace. Development of the early systems was empirical, both clinically and biomechanically. The pioneers designed and optimized implant shapes that could osseointegrate and maintain integration, and connection systems that could support functioning restorations (Fig. 4.1a,b).

4.2 Implant materials

Most modern implants are manufactured from commercially pure titanium grade 4 (CPTi).

Fundamentals of Implant Dentistry, First Edition. Gerard Byrne.
© 2014 John Wiley & Sons, Inc. Published 2014 by John Wiley & Sons, Inc.
Companion website: www.wiley.com/go/byrne/implants

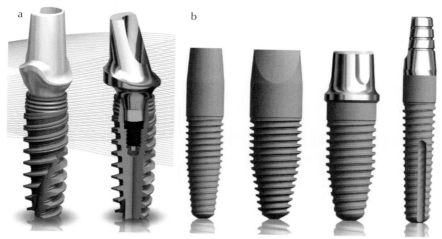

4.1. (a) A modern endosseous two-piece implant design comprising the implant and a screw-retained abutment (courtesy of Nobel Biocare). (b) Modern one-piece implant with integral abutment (courtesy of Nobel Biocare).

Yield strength and O_2 content increase from grade 1 through grade 4. Occasionally, a Ti-alloy, called aircraft-grade titanium (Ti-6/4 or Ti 6Al4V or grade 5 Ti), is used. It consists of 90% titanium, 6% aluminum, and 4% vanadium, and has many industrial applications. Other implant materials that are used include tantalum (Ta), which is used by Zimmer, and zirconium (Zr), which is used by Straumann. In the past, Tübingen implants were made from solid aluminum oxide (Al_2O_3), while other implants used plasma-sprayed surface coatings of Ti or $CaPO_4$. (Schroeder et al. 1996; Jokstad et al. 2003).

Ti oxides form a passivating layer on Ti implants, largely preventing further dissolution, while providing the chemicals that are responsible for the biochemical reaction with bone. Modern surfaces may be machined, but most have proprietary textured surfaces. Some implants with $CaPO_4$ surfaces had problems with dissolution in body tissues and breakdown in osseointegration (Spiekermann 1995). There is very little long-term clinical data for $CaPO_4$-coated implants. Wataha (1996) has comprehensively reviewed implant materials.

4.3   Evolution of implant systems

Evolution of systems

The earliest system to enter the world marketplace was Nobelpharma's Brånemark system from Sweden. This was followed by Straumann/Bonefit/ITI from Switzerland, CoreVent and Implant Innovations/3i within the United States, IMZ from Germany, and others. Over the past 30 years, convergence of implant systems has occurred, with implant companies providing a range of largely similar products with slight variation often related to details of shape, thread design, connection, abutment, and surface texture. Innovations such as internal connections, surface texturing, and platform-switching have been rapidly adopted and incorporated into all the major systems. Some companies (Dentsply) offer several implant systems. Although there are many similarities between implant systems, components and tools are not generally intercompatible. However, within systems, components and tools are often "back-compatible."

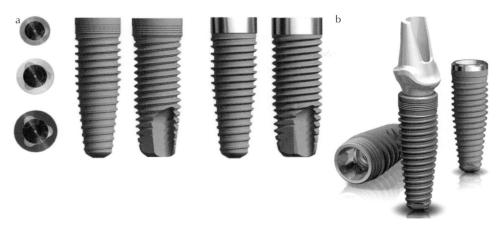

4.2. (a) Nobel Biocare Replace™ implants (three diameters) with tri-channel connections (courtesy of Nobel Biocare). (b) Nobel Biocare collar and connection variations (courtesy of Nobel Biocare)

Modern implant systems

Currently, there is an abundance of implant systems and components to satisfy most surgical and restorative situations. Modern dental implant systems comprise a comprehensive array of precision instruments, components, interactive software and techniques for creation of implant restorations. Instruments and components are generally color-coded for ease of identification and use. There are treatment planning, surgical and restorative armamentaria supplied by the implant companies, together with educational, logistical, and laboratory support networks. In addition, detailed instructions are provided for the use of each system, surgical and restorative, and pertinent literature relating to the system, it's nuances and indications.

Research

Credibility and reputation have been achieved through research and innovation, service and quality control. The Nobel Biocare system is the most researched, the most popular, and may be considered a reference system; all other systems tend to be compared to it.

Implant shape, surface, and connection

Significant changes have occurred with implant design in terms of shape, thread design surface texture, and connection design in response to demand for implant use in softer bone and prosthetic flexibility. The change to an internal connection was a significant step forward in implant evolution and clinical utility (Fig. 4.2a,b).

Implant-level impression coping and implant-level restoration (UCLA abutment)

Early Brånemark implants had used an intermediary transmucosal abutment (cylinder) attached to the implant which compromised the aesthetics of crown and bridgework and encroached on the crown height space. Implant-level impression copings and the implant-level abutments (UCLA abutment) were introduced by Lewis et al. (1988, 1992) as clinicians endeavored to produce more aesthetic fixed restorations. The implant-level impression coping allowed the reproduction of the implant position and surrounding soft tissue on a laboratory cast. This enabled a crown to be shaped so that it emerged from the implant platform and through the mucosa in a manner similar to a natural tooth. The intermediary transmucosal abutment of the Brånemark design was thus eliminated for single crowns and bridges, and the final restorative abutment or crown (incorporating the UCLA abutment) was screwed directly to the implant. The UCLA abutment was an important development, allowing great prosthetic flexibility.

Prefabricated customizable abutments

Along with the UCLA abutment, implant companies started to produce standardized prefabricated abutments of different shapes and lengths in Ti or ceramic (Al_2O_3 or ZrO_2), which could be torqued into the implant and form the equivalent of a tooth preparation for conventional crown and bridgework. Some of these were designed to be modified or customized depending on the clinical situation. The final restoration could be cemented in place.

Computer-aided design (CAD) and computer-aided manufacturing (CAM) of Ti and ceramic abutments

Gradually, abutments became available in ceramic materials to meet aesthetic demands. Eventually, abutments could be custom fabricated by CAD/CAM techniques for optimum configuration and aesthetics. We are approaching a juncture when intraoral digital scanning for CAD/CAM prosthetics will rapidly become the norm.

Interactive software, and instrumentation for computer-guided surgery and prosthetics

Many companies provide interactive treatment planning software (e.g., NobelClinician™) that utilizes computed tomography (CT) data and customized implant guides to plan and guide implant placement. Custom surgical guides can be manufactured, and special drill kits are available for guided surgery. This technology further interfaces with CAD/CAM technology for the fabrication of immediate restorations to be inserted at the time of surgery.

4.4 Surgical instrumentation

Implant companies provide high quality surgical instrument sets with instructions for use, maintenance and sterilization (Fig. 4.3a,b). Guidelines are also furnished for osteotomy preparation:

- Sterile implant vials with implant data labels
- Step-by-step instructions for osteotomy preparation
- Surgical engines and handpieces with suitable irrigation devices
- Color-coded drills with millimeter markers that correspond to the implant shape and length
- Direction indicators and depth guides with millimeter markers
- System of graded osteotomes for preparation of soft bone sites
- Unique drills as needed for accommodating specific implant collar shapes
- Tapping drills for thread creation in dense bone
- Tissue punch devices and bone mills to be used when uncovering implants at second-stage surgery.

32302 Brånemark System® Surgery Kit

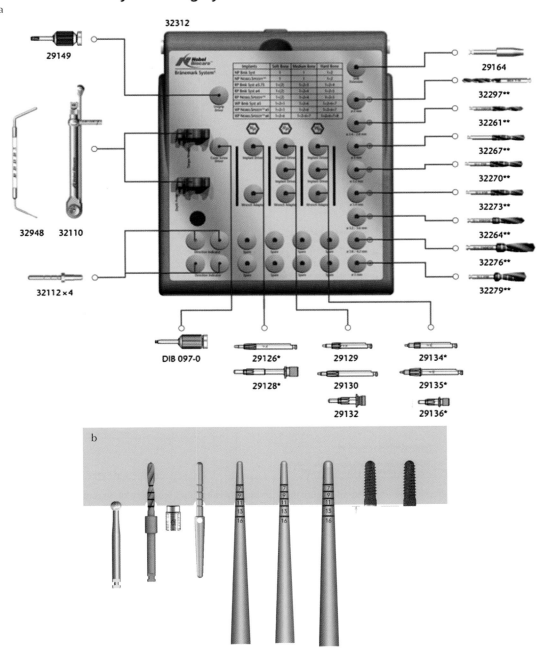

4.3. (a) Implant surgical set (courtesy of Nobel Biocare). (b) Osteotome set and implant site preparation guide for soft bone (courtesy of CAMLOG).

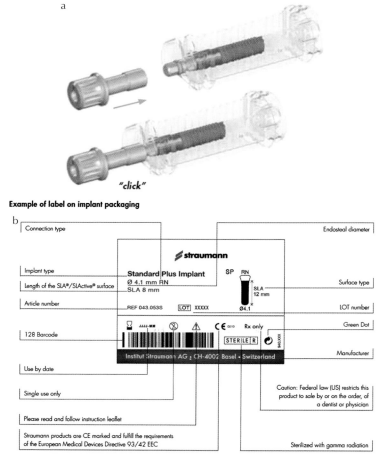

4.4. (a) Sterile implant package (courtesy of Straumann). (b) Implant data label (courtesy of Straumann).

The clinician must be aware of instrument dimensions and sharpness of drills. Dull drills, with or without excessive pressure, may cause bone damage and implant failure. Many implant companies are introducing single-use bone drills. Implants are supplied sterile in sealed vials, with custom connections for insertion drivers (motor or hand). Press-fit implants have mallet devices for tapping the implants into the prepared osteotomy (Fig. 4.4a,b).

4.5   Features of endosseous implants

Thread design

The original Brånemark implant was a cylindrical Ti self-tapping screw. It had a smooth machined surface, and the threads extended from the apical end to the *collar* and restorative *platform* (Fig. 4.5). Threads enable good primary stability and increase the effective surface area of an implant, thereby increasing the potential

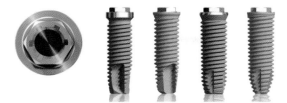

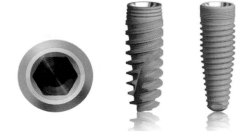

4.5. Nobel Biocare Brånemark Mark III and Mark IV implants with modifications to collar, grooves, and apical designs (from left to right) (courtesy of Nobel Biocare). The platform diameter is slightly greater than the body diameter due to machining to produce the threads (courtesy of Nobel Biocare).

4.6. Two implant variants that are tapered, with deep or shallow grooves and an internal hex platform-switched connection (courtesy of Nobel Biocare).

area for bone conact and force transmission to bone.

The collar and platform were slightly wider than the body and this created a *flange*, which engaged the cortical bone at the ridge crest, aiding initial stability. Contemporary implant designs are parallel or tapered, have modified thread design, and may have no flange. Three alternative early designs (ITI, IMZ, and Tübingen) had no threads and were called press-fit. Some press-fit designs (Frialit® and IMZ) have adopted surface threading.

Currently, most implants have surface threads, and textured surfaces produced by a variety of proprietary treatments. However, there are still some press-fit designs available. Some press-fit designs (Frialit and IMZ) have adopted surface threads. Thread shape varies with a view to giving better initial stability especially in softer bone and better biomechanical force distribution to bone (Fig. 4.6). A slight apical taper is often incorporated with or without deeper threads to ensure initial stability in softer bone. To date, the effects of thread design and taper parameters on implant success have not been validated.

Implant length

Implant length may range from 5.0 to 18.0 mm long depending on the implant company.

Longer implants are specifically available for insertion into the zygomatic bone. Many of the early cases used Brånemark implants that were only 7.0 mm long. There was a gradual trend toward using the longest implant feasible, which would engage both mandibular cortical plates for optimum stability. Currently, it seems acceptable to use an implant length of between 10.0 and 15.0 mm for 3.0 to 4.0 mm diameter implants, while accepting less length on 5.0 to 6.0 mm diameter implants. Research cannot give the clinician a definitive answer as to the optimum length of implant to use in a particular clinical circumstance. Studies have shown comparable survival rates for short (<10.0 mm long) implants (Annibali et al. 2012a), although longer implants might have a slightly better survival rate in partially dentate cases (Telleman et al. 2011). For approximate comparative purposes, an implant measuring 4.0 × 10.0 mm is equivalent to a 5.0 × 8.0 mm, or a 6.0 × 6.0 mm implant assuming the same implant and bone configuration and bone density. It is likely that the number of implants is the more important treatment planning factor. Some implant companies, for example, Bicon, promote shorter implants.

Implant body and platform diameter

Implants are often referred to in terms of body diameter and platform diameter (Fig. 4.7).

External connection

 NP Ø 3.5 mm
interface

 RP Ø 4.1 mm
interface

 WP Ø 5.1 mm
interface

Internal connection

 NP Ø 3.5 mm
interface

 RP Ø 4.3 mm
interface

 WP Ø 5.0 mm
interface

 6.0 Ø 6.0 mm
interface

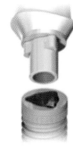

**NobelActive™ (Internal
conical connection)**

 NP Ø 3.5 mm

 RP Ø 3.9 mm

NobelDirect® Posterior

 RP Ø 4.3 mm

 WP Ø 5.0 mm

 6.0 Ø 6.0 mm

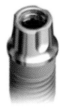

4.7. Diagram showing a range of implant (platform) diameters, and connection options; NP, narrow platform; RP, regular platform; WP, wide platform (courtesy of Nobel Biocare).

Implant *diameter* refers to the widest part of the implant body that fits within the osteotomy site. Tapered implants have a gradient of diameter, being widest toward the platform. The *platform*, onto which a prosthetic component sits, is the "top" or occlusal aspect of an implant. It is often wider than the implant body itself as with the Brånemark design and Straumann flared-neck (one-stage surgery) implants. The term platform was more relevant for external hex implants in that the platform supported the abutment, but is less relevant for many modern conical internal connection implants. Platform-switching allows abutments to attach within the tapered, conical connection channel without fully covering the implant platform.

Increasing the implant diameter increases the potential area for osseointegration and force transmission to bone. In many cases, the retaining screw diameter also increases as the implant diameter increases. Implant diameter is selected with reference to bone volume and tooth size. Typical implant diameters range from 3.0 to 6.0 mm, and implants are often termed narrow/small, regular/standard, wide, or extra-wide platform, based on the diameter of the platform or implant body at its widest section:

Narrow/small: Approximately 3.0 mm, suitable for mandibular incisors and maxillary lateral incisors
Regular/standard: Approximately 4.0 mm, suitable for all teeth except small incisors
Wide: Approximately 5.0 mm, suitable for molars
Extra-wide: Approximately 6.0 mm, also suitable for molars.

Implant collar

The collar, sometimes referred to as the neck, is the portion of the implant that lies just apical to the implant platform (Fig. 4.8). Traditional implants had a smooth machined body and transmucosal collar. The collar was placed

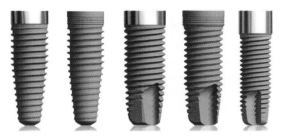

4.8. Implants with machined, or grooved and textured collar configurations (courtesy of Nobel Biocare).

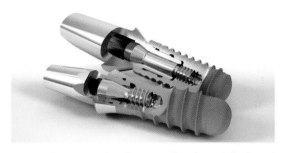

4.9. Implant examples showing "flared" (polished) and "straight" (textured) collars, and internal connections (courtesy of Straumann).

within the bony osteotomy thus making the implant platform "flush" with the bony crest. The height of the polished collar surface varies in width, and in many cases, a textured surface runs all the way to the coronal extent or platform. Polished collars are now designed to extend above the crestal bone (next to the soft tissue), whereas textured collars are placed within the bone. Collar diameter, height and surface finish vary from product to product. Many collars also now incorporate micro-threads or grooves. ITI use a smooth machined transmucosal collar for mucosal contact, for their one-stage surgery implants; the implant surface for bone contact is textured (Fig. 4.9).

It had been theorized that bone loss may occur because of excessive strain at threads in the collar area, or because the smooth machined collar does not engage bone as well as a textured surface. This led to the use of micro-threads, or textured surfaces in the collar area in contact with bone, for better force distribution to bone (Hansson 1999, 2000, 2003). It is not known yet whether collar design variations have a significant bearing on long-term implant outcomes.

Prosthetic connection and anti-rotation feature

The majority of implants require a screw retained prosthetic abutment, although one

system uses a parallel post with frictional locking (Bicon) (Taylor 2009). The abutment may be similar to a crown preparation, a combination abutment-restoration (using a customized UCLA abutment), an overdenture patrix (anchor), or a bar support. The prosthetic connection permits retention of the prosthesis and provides a convenient method of transferring the clinical implant position to the laboratory master cast through the use of precisely fitting impression copings (impression abutments). Abutment retaining screws often have greater diameter on larger diameter implants.

Modern implants have an internal or external engaging or anti-rotation feature, which is used for implant placement and is essential for single-unit crowns but not essential for multi-unit restorations.

Early CoreVent designs incorporated the first internal hex connection for use with cementable overdenture and single crown abutments (Drago 2007). Zimmer implants and others use an updated version of this patented design. Many current implants use a variant of the Brånemark external or the CoreVent internal connection.

With an internal connection, it is easier for the clinician to find a positive seat for abutments sub-gingivally (Fig. 4.9). A Nobel Biocare tri-channel internal connection is currently the most popular connection design.

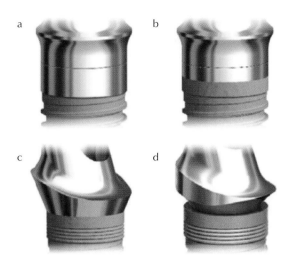

a   b

c   d

4.10. The implant-abutment junction: platform-matching (a, b, c) and platform-switching (d) designs (courtesy of Nobel Biocare).

One-piece implant

Integral abutments were a feature of subperiosteal, blade, and other implants such as early ITI implants, current NobelDirect implants, and some Zimmer implants. Integral abutments present the risk of not achieving osseointegration because of inadvertent early functional contact. On the positive side, an integral abutment cannot loosen from the implant in function.

Implant platform

Traditionally, the implant platform is the surface upon which a restorative abutment sits (Fig. 4.7). The "flat" platform is surmounted by a protruding hex with a central screw hole. With the advent of wider diameter implants, the platform increased in diameter, thereby giving more support to the abutment and restoration. Many implants are of tapered design, and the implant diameter then refers to the diameter of the implant platform. Although external hex designs are still popular, many new internal connection designs have been introduced. These may no longer have a flat supportive platform, but instead have an internal cone-shaped or tapered connection with an anti-rotation feature (Figs. 4.5,4.6,4.9).

Platform-switching design

For traditional implants, the diameter of the abutment and implant platform was the same at the connection point (Fig. 4.10). This is referred to as *platform-matching*. Lazzara and Porter (2006) showed that the connection of a smaller-diameter abutment reduced the amount of bone loss around implants after abutment connection. This concept, called *platform-switching*, has been embraced by some leading clinicians and implant companies, and such designs are now widely offered. It is most desirable to minimize bone loss around implants, and thereby possibly increase soft tissue support especially in the aesthetic zone. However, more evidence is needed to validate the clinical benefits of platform-switching (Annibali et al. 2012b; Stafford 2012).

Surface finish/texture

Brånemark popularized smooth, machined, and threaded screws. Early IMZ and ITI implants had plasma-sprayed, Ti-coated, textured surfaces (TPS). CoreVent had a threaded and sandblasted surface. Calcitek, Steri-Oss®, and IMZ used plasma-sprayed hydroxyapatite (HA) surfaces.

Currently, major implant companies offer implants with a variety of proprietary surface textures or modifications created by a number of etching, sintering, anodizing, or blasting processes. Surface texture increases the surface area for osseointegration, and creates an interlocking mechanical interface with bone.

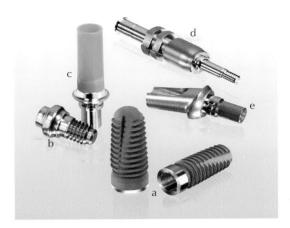

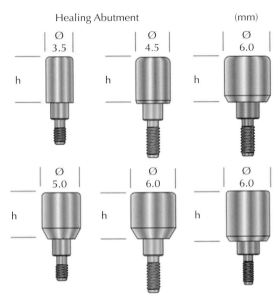

Healing Abutment   (mm)

4.11. (a) Implants with polished collars and textured threaded bodies. (b) Healing abutment. (c) UCLA abutment. (d) Impression coping for open tray. (e) Angled prefabricated abutment (courtesy of CAMLOG).

4.13. Healing abutments, color coded and available in various heights and diameters (courtesy of Nobel Biocare).

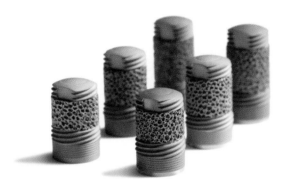

4.12. Zimmer family of Trabecular Metal® Technology (TMT) implants (courtesy of Zimmer Dental).

Textured surfaces show *osseoconductive* properties, with superior speed and area of osseointegration over traditional smooth machined surface implants (Cochran 2000) (see Chapter 2) (Fig. 4.11 and Fig. 4.12).

Cover screw, healing abutment

In *one-stage* implant placement, a cover screw is used to fill the implant screw hole to prevent ingress of debris. Alternatively, a larger healing abutment can be used to develop a soft tissue emergence profile for the future restoration. Different implant companies provide various shapes of healing abutments for this purpose.

In *two-stage* implant placement, after the implant is inserted into the osteotomy site, a cover screw is placed to minimize the risk of infection, and prevent bone growth over the implant platform. At second-stage surgery, the cover screw is replaced by a transmucosal healing abutment. The healing abutment may be parallel-sided or flared.

Healing abutments come in different shapes and sizes and their diameter may be the same or larger than the implant platform, Expanded shapes are used to help create an optimum emergence profile *(tissue shaping)* for the final restoration; this decision being made at the discretion of the restorative dentist (Fig. 4.13).

One manufacturer (Biomet 3i) produces laser coded abutments (3i Encode) to enable data transfer for CAD/CAM prosthesis fabrication.

4.6 Prosthetic components

The original Brånemark implant was placed so that the platform was flush with the bone crest. At second-stage surgery, a cylindrical *transmucosal abutment* was attached with an abutment screw. This abutment was surmounted by a secondary abutment, to which the restoration was attached by means of a smaller *prosthetic screw.* Currently, a transmucosal healing abutment is placed at second-stage surgery. This healing abutment is removed for impression taking and eventually is replaced by a *prosthetic transmucosal abutment.* This prosthetic abutment may stand alone for a cemented crown such as a prefabricated Nobel Biocare Snappy™ abutment, or be an integral part of the final restoration, such as with UCLA abutments, for example, the Nobel Biocare GoldAdapt abutment. It may also be a Zest Locator® anchor. There are many versions of stock or prefabricated and customizable abutments available. The UCLA prefabricated abutment gradually superseded the traditional Brånemark *transmucosal healing abutment* for single crowns (Lewis et al. 1988). The UCLA *prefabricated abutment* allows a custom abutment or crown to be screwed directly to the implant.

Prosthetic implant components enable the clinician and laboratory technician to produce the final clinical prosthesis. The prosthesis may be one of the following, which may be screwed or cemented in place:

- *Single units (crowns):* screw or cement
- *Multi-unit (FDPs):* one-stage (screw or cement), two-stage (screw only)
- *Full arch fixed multi-unit (FDP):* screw or cement (usually two-stage)
- *Overdentures:* resilient retentive anchors (Zest, Dalbo) or customized bars.

Screw retention is engineered to create a durable connection while balancing the strength of the screw and implant. A tapered or conical inlet to the screw-hole gives a very secure immobile abutment fit that inhibits screw loosening and limits ingress of microflora at the implant-abutment junction (IAJ). Abutments are retained by abutment screws that are torqued into the implant using a torque driver. Screw diameter and length varies.

Healing abutment/transmucosal abutment, tissue-shaping abutment

These abutments are placed at second-stage surgery and allow the soft tissue to heal against a smooth Ti surface. This leads to the formation of a junctional epithelium and a close adaptation of connective tissue around the implant and abutment. The soft tissue around the implant may be modified or shaped in order to create an optimal emergence profile for the final restoration. This can be achieved with a tapered, stock healing abutment or with a custom fabricated provisional crown. Healing abutments are tightened with finger-held screwdrivers.

Impression coping or abutment, implant analog or replica

An impression coping or abutment screws into the implant, fits the implant precisely and permits transfer of accurate implant positional information from the mouth to the laboratory master cast using a conventional dental impression (Fig. 4.14). There are two types of impression coping: pick-up and transfer copings. The pick-up coping remains in the impression, while the transfer coping stays in the implant after taking the impression. Prior to pouring the master cast, the impression coping is connected to a matching implant analog/replica. The cast will have the implant *analog* in its correct 3D position for laboratory fabrication of the prosthesis.

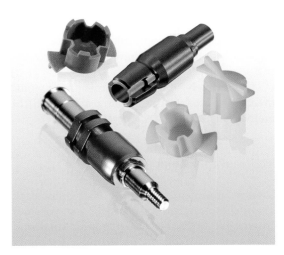

4.14. Impression copings for open and closed tray techniques (courtesy of CAMLOG).

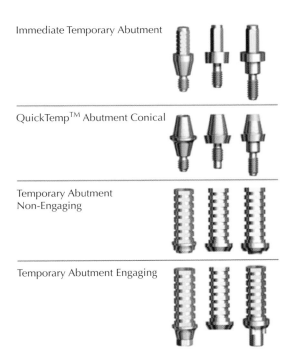

Immediate Temporary Abutment

QuickTemp™ Abutment Conical

Temporary Abutment
Non-Engaging

Temporary Abutment Engaging

4.15. A variety of provisional abutments (courtesy of Nobel Biocare).

Provisional restoration abutments

Several different types of provisional restoration abutments are available, made from Ti or resin (Fig. 4.15). Some types of abutments screw directly into the implant and can be modified to receive a cemented provisional crown. Other abutments have a textured surface for resin application, and are retained to the implant by a central abutment screw. The screw-hole access for maxillary anterior units is often on the labial side due to implant angulation, and must be filled with a suitable correction resin.

Stock/prefabricated abutments

There are many varieties of stock abutments, such as multi-unit abutments, used for two-stage screw-retained prostheses, crown preparation-shaped abutments, and overdenture abutments (Fig. 4.16a,b). The estorative abutment may have an anti-rotation connection with the implant depending on its planned usage. It will usually be retained by an abutment screw. Stock abutments are made from Ti

and a variety of ceramics or metal alloys. They may or may not be customizable in terms of angle, height, and finish-line configuration. The soft tissue height determines the subgingival collar height of such abutments, and different *subgingival collar heights* are available. Restorative abutments are torqued into place at manufacturer-determined torque. The final restoration is cemented over the abutment.

Custom restorative abutments

Custom restorative abutments are fabricated by waxing and casting directly onto a UCLA-type cylindrical abutment that has a machined implant connection and a plastic waxing sleeve (Fig. 4.16a,b). These abutments can be configured in wax with appropriate marginal and axial preparation configurations for cemented crowns/FDPs, and then "cast-to" in noble alloy. They may also be configured as the final framework for porcelain application, creating a one-piece metal-ceramic, screw-retained crown/FDP.

Alternatively, custom ceramic or Ti abutments can be fabricated using a CAD/CAM method such as NobelProcera® (Fig. 4.17).

Multi-unit abutments

Conical abutments are traditional Brånemark abutments designed for *two-stage screw-retained* crowns and FDPs. The abutments are small and have a custom "carrier" or "handle" for safety of oral placement. They may be straight or angled. They have a range of subgingival collar heights. Appropriate abutment heights are chosen by the clinician or laboratory technician based on the implant level impression. They are torqued into the implants, and the final restoration is secured using small prosthetic screws. The use of multi-unit abutments is declining.

Standard abutments

Standard abutments, also known as gold cylinders, are the traditional transmucosal abutments used in the early Brånemark "hybrid" fixed cases. They extend through the gingiva and provide the platform for the final prosthesis, which is retained by prosthetic screws. Traditionally, the cylinder could be grasped supra-gingivally with a special hemostat in order to supply counter-torque to the implant fixture while the abutment screw was tightened.

Overdenture abutments

The two most popular overdenture abutments are Zest Locator® (Zest Anchors) and Dalbo-Plus® ball (Cendres Métaux) attachments or

a
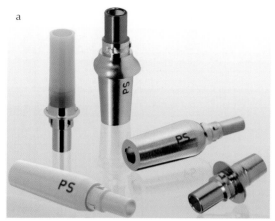

b
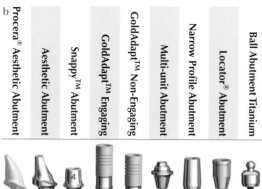

4.16. (a) A variety of pre-fabricated restorative abutments (courtesy of CAMLOG). (b) A variety of prefabricated restorative abutments (courtesy of Nobel Biocare).

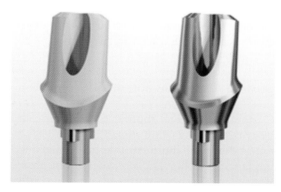

4.17. Custom milled Nobel/Procera™ abutments (ceramic and Ti) for cemented crowns (courtesy of Nobel Biocare).

anchors (see Chapter 10). Other variants include generic stock abutments to which various bars can be soldered for retention of overdentures. All these abutments are made of Ti; Zest anchors have a gold colored Ti–nitride coating. Both Zest and Dalbo attachment systems permit approximately 30° of off-axis implant alignment (Fig. 4.18a,b).

4.7   Screws, screwdrivers, and torque drivers

Screwdrivers

Screwdrivers (drivers) are designed for finger use or latch-type handpiece drill use intra-orally. There are certain popular screwdriver tips such as slotted, square, hex, and star-shaped. For each finger driver, there is usually a latch-type version for a handpiece or a hand-held torque driver. It is important to select the correct driver for the correct screw in order to avoid damaging screw heads or losing screws intraorally. Finger-held drivers usually have a hole for threading floss and making the driver captive (Fig. 4.19 and Fig. 4.20).

Abutment screws and prosthetic screws

Abutment and prosthetic screws are made from Ti, Ti alloy, or Au-based alloy. Designated screws must be used as per manufacturer's directions for optimum results. Screws for ceramic and metal abutments may be of different design. Laboratory screws are also provided for use during fabrication of prostheses. Many modern abutment screws are designed to be *prestressed* at specific tightening torques, thereby creating thread distortion and preventing screw loosening.

Surface treatments (e.g., carbon coating) have been variously used by implant companies to reduce tightening friction in order to enhance preload.

4.8   Implant marketplace and system selection

Without reliable manufacture and supply, implantology cannot progress. Without industry support for research, academic impetus, and independent implant innovation by working dentists, dental implantology will stagnate. The needs of the profession have thus far been answered by the implant industry with continuous development of new products. (Jokstad et al. 2003; Bhatavadekar 2010).

Currently, Nobel Biocare is the worldwide market leader, followed closely by Straumann and others. Nobel Biocare marketed the first Ti screw implant and this was also the first implant for dental use approved by the U.S. Food and Drug Administration (FDA). Straumann, Dentsply, Biomet 3i, BioHorizons, and Zimmer also have a large share of the implant market, and have comprehensive systems, training programs, and support.

Consistency and conservatism should guide our approach to new implant products. It is important that when using a system of implants for your patients, you should expect compatible components to be available for a period of perhaps 50 years or the lifetime of the patient.

Jokstad (2009) wrote that there were up to 600 different implant systems produced by 146 different manufacturers. He discussed the issue of FDA approval criteria and the difficulties for current and future clinicians coping with so many systems. He further noted that the vast majority of systems had no clinical research documentation. The presence in the marketplace of so many systems and aggressive marketing leaves the clinician with thoughtful decisions to make in his or her clinical practice.

Name of item	Accessory components available from*	Shape/size	Ø Thread
a			
Ball Ø 2.5 mm compatible with TSB	Nobel Biocare	Ball-shape Ø 2.5 mm	Ø 2.2 mm × 0.45
Metal Housing compatible with TSB			
Retentive Cap White compatible with TSB	Rhein 83 www.rhein83.com		
Ball Ø 2.0 mm compatible with OSO™ (Retentive caps not included, please order separately from Preat Corporation)	Nobel Biocare	Ball-shape Ø 2.0 mm	Ø 2.2 mm × 0.45
Ball Ø 2.25 mm compatible with Dalbo®-Plus	Nobel Biocare	Ball-shape Ø 2.25 mm	Ø 2.2 mm × 0.45
Dalbo®-Plus elliptic	Cendres & Métaux www.cmsa.ch		
Ball Ø 2.2 mm compatible with Bredent™ (Retentive caps not included, please order separately from Bredent™)	Nobel Biocare	Ball-shape Ø 2.2 mm	Ø 2.0 mm × 0.25
Metal Housing compact + Bredent™ Occlusal (Retentive caps not included, please order separately from Bredent™)			
b			
Attachment compatible with Anchor System M3	Nobel Biocare	Conical	Ø 3.0 mm × 0.5
Metal Housing Anchor System M3	Servo Dental www.servo-dental. de		
Rigid Retention Anchor System M3			
Zest® Anchor Bar Locator®	Zest Anchors Inc www.zestanchors.com	Conical	Ø 2.0 mm × 0.4
Zest® Anchor Bar Cap			
Gold Rider Dolder® Macro	Cendres & Métaux www.cmsa.ch	U-shape	No threaded parts needed
Gold Rider Dolder® Macro			
Gold Rider Dolder® Round Bar	Cendres & Métaux www.cmsa.ch	Round-shape	
Metal Housing Hader	Servo Dental www.servo-dental. de	Round-shape	
Hader Clip Plastic (yellow)			

4.18. (a) and (b) A variety of pre-fabricated overdenture abutments (courtesy of Nobel Biocare).

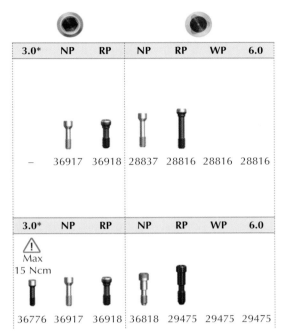

3.0*	NP	RP	NP	RP	WP	6.0
–	36917	36918	28837	28816	28816	28816

3.0*	NP	RP	NP	RP	WP	6.0
⚠ Max 15 Ncm						
36776	36917	36918	36818	29475	29475	29475

4.19. Abutment screws for Nobel Biocare internal connection implants; upper screws are for Zirconia, and lower for Ti abutments (courtesy of Nobel Biocare).

When selecting an implant company and system, the following should be considered:

- The history, reputation, and longevity of the company
- The quality of service and support from the company
- The quality and strength of the company's research
- The preferences of other members of the implant team.

The dental patient population is mobile and patients may need follow-up maintenance by other dentists. Therefore company name, support, and universality become important when choosing an implant system. The lack of compatibility between systems, and the evolution of components and tool sets may lead to problems for patients and dentists in the future, as patients move and dentists retire.

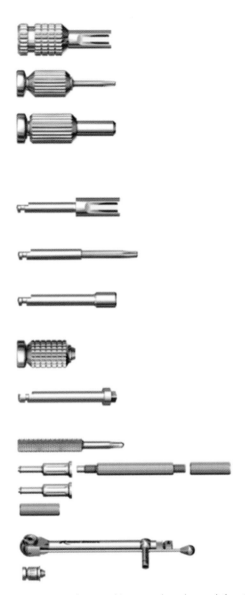

4.20. A variety of screwdrivers and tools used for the Nobel Biocare System (courtesy of Nobel Biocare).

References

Annibali S, Cristalli MP, Dell'Aquila D, Bignozzi I, La Monaca G, Pilloni A. (2012a) Short dental implants: a systematic review. *J Dent Res.* 91(1):25–32.

Annibali S, Bignozzi I, Cristalli MP, Graziani F, La Monaca G, Polimeni A. (2012b) Peri-implant marginal bone level: a systematic review and meta-analysis of studies comparing platform-switching versus conventionally restored implants. *J Clin Periodontol*. 39(11):1097–113.

Bhatavadekar N. (2010) Helping the clinician make evidence-based implant selections. A systematic review and qualitative analysis ofdental implant studies over a 20 year period. *Int Dent J*. 60(5): 359–69.

Cochran DL. (2000) The scientific basis for and clinical experiences with Straumann implants including the ITI Dental Implant System: a consensus report. *Clin Oral Implants Res*. 11 Suppl 1:33–58.

Drago C. (2007) *Implant Restorations: A Step-by-Step Guide*, 2nd ed. Wiley-Blackwell, Ames.

Hansson S. (1999) The implant neck: smooth or provided with retention elements. A biomechanical approach. *Clin Oral Implants Res*. 10(5):394–405.

Hansson S. (2000) Implant-abutment interface: biomechanical study of flat top versus conical. *Clin Implant Dent Relat Res*. 2(1):33–41.

Hansson S. (2003) A conical implant-abutment interface at the level of the marginal bone improves the distribution of stresses in the supporting bone. An axisymmetric finite element analysis. *Clin Oral Implants Res*. 14(3):286–93.

Jokstad A. (2009) How many implant systems do we have and are they documented? In: A Jokstad (ed.), *Osseointegration and Dental Implants*. Wiley-Blackwell, Ames, pp. 3–26.

Jokstad A, Braegger U, Brunski JB, Carr AB, Naert I, Wennerberg A. (2003) Quality of dental implants. *Int Dent J*. 53(6 Suppl 2):409–43.

Lazzara RJ, Porter SS. (2006) Platform switching: a new concept in implant dentistry for controlling postrestorative crestal bone levels. *Int J Periodontics Restorative Dent*. 26(1):9–17.

Lewis S, Beumer J 3rd, Hornburg W, Moy P. (1988) The "UCLA" abutment. *Int J Oral Maxillofac Implants*. 3(3):183–9.

Lewis SG, Llamas D, Avera S. (1992) The UCLA abutment: a four-year review. *J Prosthet Dent*. 67(4): 509–15.

Schroeder A, Sutter F, Buser D, Krekeler G. (1996) *Oral Implantology: Basics: ITI Hollow Cylinder*. Thieme, New York.

Spiekermann H. (1995) *Color Atlas of Dental Medicine: Implantology*. Thieme, Stuttgart.

Stafford GL. (2012) Evidence supporting platform-switching to preserve marginal bone levels not definitive. *Evid Based Dent*. 13(2):56–7.

Taylor TD. (2009) Stability of implant-abutment connections. In: A Jokstad (ed.), *Osseointegration and Dental Implants*. Wiley-Blackwell, Ames, pp. 269–73.

Telleman G, Raghoebar GM, Vissink A, den Hartog L, Huddleston Slater JJ, Meijer HJ. (2011) A systematic review of the prognosis of short (<10 mm) dental implants placed in the partially edentulous patient. *J Clin Periodontol*. 38(7):667–76.

Wataha JC. (1996) Materials for endosseous dental implants. *J Oral Rehabil*. 23(2):79–90.

5 Assessment, Diagnosis, and Treatment Planning

5.1 Introduction

Effective and complete data collection is required for diagnosis and treatment planning. Once data have been gathered, diagnoses can be made and treatment plans can be formulated and presented to the patients for their approval. It is fundamental that the dentist be comfortable with the implant proposal; if in doubt, one should consult with, or refer to, more experienced colleagues.

Diagnosis and treatment planning is a process that may require several visits and discussions to collate all the necessary information and options. The dentist of record will have joint consultations with specialist colleagues as necessary and ensure that suitable referral and laboratory support is available. Patient preferences, treatment modalities, treatment timetables and sequencing, patient education, and

financial commitments must all be addressed. The risks and benefits of all treatment options must be presented before a patient can make an informed decision.

A good working relationship within the implant team, predicated on knowledge and mutual respect, should ensure the best treatment outcomes for the patient. The general sequence of assessment, treatment planning, and treatment, may be outlined as follows:

- Presenting problem
- History: medical and dental
- Clinical examination
- Medical consultations, surgery consultation
- Diagnosis
- Consideration of treatment options; patient education
- Surgical and restorative treatment plan
- Informed consent

Fundamentals of Implant Dentistry, First Edition. Gerard Byrne.
© 2014 John Wiley & Sons, Inc. Published 2014 by John Wiley & Sons, Inc.
Companion website: www.wiley.com/go/byrne/implants

- Implant surgery
- Restorative treatment
- Maintenance.

When data collection and treatment planning are well organized, the diagnosis, treatment planning, and treatment sequence should be more efficient.

A multidisciplinary approach

The implant treatment group combines the knowledge and skills of a general dentist, hygienist, dental technician, and various specialists as needed (periodontist, oral surgeon, prosthodontist, and orthodontist). The restoring dentist is at the center of and coordinates the implant treatment group. This must be the case, as patients will return to the restorative dentist if questions or problems arise later about any aspect of treatment, whether real or perceived. The quality of the final restoration will depend on the communication within the group during the process, and the skills of the group members.

5.2 Patient interview

The potential implant patient may attend the dental practice for reasons that may have nothing to do with implants (Fig. 5.1a,b). The range of presenting problems is myriad. In due course, the topic of implants may arise, and the process of patient education will begin.

A patient may request implant treatment based on information from other dentists and/or from personal research. It is important to listen to the patient and probe for further information without prejudging.

The patent may have a space from a congenitally absent tooth, a traumatic injury, or a prior extraction, which is not an immediate problem for them, or they may have a pain from a failing restored tooth or fixed prosthesis. The patient

5.1. General appearance. (a) Patient with low smile line, bruxism tooth wear and failing restorations. (b) Neglected dentition with active caries and periodontitis in a patient who is a heavy smoker.

may be struggling to cope with dentures, or may have been thinking of having dentures remade because of chronic discomfort. The primary tool of the diagnostician is trained observation, and this should not be underestimated at the expense of technology, algorithms, and business formulae. The following observations about the patient should be noted at the initial interview:

- Demeanor: nervous, confrontational, demanding, and hyperactive
- General appearance: pallor, flushed, obese, anorexic
- Breath odor suggesting poor hygiene, smoking, diabetic ketosis
- Aesthetics of existing teeth and prostheses

- Smile line and facial asymmetry
- Extreme variations of the skeletal base
- Excessively developed masticatory musculature, possibly indicating a bruxing or clenching habit
- TMJ "popping," asymmetrical jaw movements, mandibular dyskenesia
- "Overclosed" mandible with angular cheilosis and "invisible" teeth in an edentulous patient

Additionally, one needs to gauge these factors:

- Dental IQ
- Reason for tooth loss
- Motivation, for example, embarrassment at state of dentition
- Compliance and cooperation
- Financial constraints (will impact on the plan)

If there is an immediate presenting condition, this should be addressed as needed following history and examination.

5.3   Medical history

A thorough medical history is essential, with special emphasis on medical conditions that may complicate elective surgery, compromise healing, or preclude implant treatment. The dentist should be satisfied that the patient is physically and psychologically fit for the rigor of implant procedures. Treatment may be contraindicated or suspended for reasons of ill health, drug addiction, or psychiatric problems (Froum 2010).

Certain medical conditions or medications may compromise bone healing and thus the prognosis of implants. Implant survival depends on the ability of tissues to heal following surgery, and therefore any condition that adversely affects healing increases the risk of implant failure. The referral implant surgeon

will also make an assessment of surgical risks at a later stage.

The dentist must decide, in the light of medical history and the clinical exam, whether implant treatment will bring the quality of life improvement sought by the patient, or whether there are alternative treatments that pose less risk and provide adequate appearance and function. Any risks must be weighed against potential benefits.

Implants may be contraindicated if it is determined that a patient cannot cope with the surgery, or if they are unable to cope with implant maintenance, for example, dexterity problems. All patients have their own unique set of circumstances.

The following factors need careful assessment and occasionally physician consultation before contemplating implant treatment:

General factors

- *Patient age:* Relative contraindication <20 years, >80 years
- *Pregnancy:* provide an interim treatment
- *Smoking habit:* may compromise implant survival
- *Drug dependency:* potential compliance problems
- *Psychiatric problems:* potential compliance problems
- *Alzheimer's disease and dementias:* compliance problems
- *Physical or mental disability:* ability to cooperate and maintain prostheses.

Medications of significance

- Long-term tranquilizers
- Long-term steroid therapy
- Bone antiresorptive medications, for example, bisphosphonates
- Anticoagulant or antiplatelet medications

- Heart medications
- Antihypertensive medications.

Major medical conditions

- Cardiovascular conditions:
  - Coagulation problem: anticoagulant therapy and risk of embolism
  - Hypertension
  - Angina pectoris
  - Myocardial infarction and coronary bypass surgery
  - Congestive heart failure
  - Risk of endocarditis
- Diabetes mellitus
- Compromised immune system: autoimmune disease, cancer chemotherapy, organ transplant chemotherapy, HIV, and chronic steroid medications
- Irradiated facial bones
- Antiresorptive (e.g., bisphosphonates) therapy for cancers or osteoporosis
- Psychiatric disorders and personality disorders
- Addiction to controlled drugs.

Physician consultation

A consultation with the patient's physician is recommended to clarify drug regimens or the status of a condition, such as diabetes, cancer, or anticlotting treatments (INR for anticoagulation). This information will be essential for the surgical consultation. Consultation may be needed to confirm or refute the need for endocarditis prophylaxis in joint replacement patients.

Relative contraindications for implants

- Age, that is, young growing patients and elderly patients
- Current or recent intravenous bisphosphonate therapy

- History of jaw irradiation
- Unrealistic expectations.

Absolute contraindications for implants

- Serious acute illness
- Acute oral infection
- Active chemotherapy or jaw irradiation
- Uncontrolled systemic disease, for example, diabetes mellitus
- Serious anesthetic or bleeding risk
- Pregnancy
- Inability of patient to comprehend or maintain implant therapy.

Patient age guideline

With younger patients, and when sequential orthodontic lateral skull radiographs are unavailable, it is wise to wait until the patient is aged 20 years prior to implant placement (Cronin and Oesterle 1998). At age 20 years, the jawbones are usually fully grown. Jaw growth is complete earlier for women than men (Fig. 5.2). A decision can be made after consultation with an orthodontist and surgeon. Elderly patients, for example, 80 years and older, may have lowered ability to cope with surgery and maintenance issues.

5.4 Dental history and clinical examination

One can gradually make the assessment about a patient's level of understanding, attitude, motivation, potential compliance, and ability to pay for implant treatment during history taking and examination.

Dental history

A thorough knowledge of the patient's dental experiences and treatment history will give

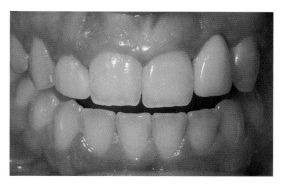

5.2. Left lateral incisor implant crown was placed in a growing patient creating a later problem in that it "submerges." The crown could be changed, but not the changing tissue line, as the implant cannot be moved orthodontically (courtesy of Dr. C. Goodacre).

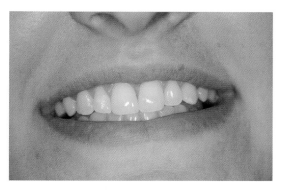

5.3. High smile line and thin scalloped gingival biotype.

valuable insight and may help predict future outcomes. How does the patient see their current dental problem and how did it arise? How is the problem influenced or related to personal/social or health problems? Is it a long-term or short-term problem? During the discussion, the dentist considers interim solutions for the patient's presenting problems for example, interim dentures, or soft linings for old dentures. Aspects to consider include the following:

- Attendance record
- Positive and negative dental experiences
- Dental knowledge, including implants
- Orthodontic, restorative, endodontic, surgical, and periodontal treatment history.

Dental examination

A thorough *examination* of oral and circum-oral soft and hard tissues is important in order to establish a baseline of the state of oral health prior to treatment and for future reference. This is usually complemented with a recent *full mouth series* and *panoramic radiograph*, and if possible clinical *photographs and study models*.

The prognosis of a single tooth cannot take place in isolation, but should be a part of a comprehensive case assessment. A tooth may have been lost, or may be about to be lost for a multitude of reasons, including trauma, caries, and periodontal disease. The clinician's first objective after assessing the presenting complaint is to evaluate plaque control, caries risk, and periodontal status. Extraoral examination of head and neck includes the following:

- Cancer screening
- Skeletal and soft tissue facial profile
- Smile line, lip line at rest and during speech (Fig. 5.3)
- Facial symmetry
- TMJs and range of motion: asymmetric movement indicative of internal joint derangement, limited opening, and TMDysfunction
- Muscles of mastication: hypertrophy indicating parafunction and dyskenesia.

Intraoral exam of an edentulous patient includes the following:

- Angular cheilosis
- Health and color of attached and reflected mucosa
- Volume of edentulous ridges

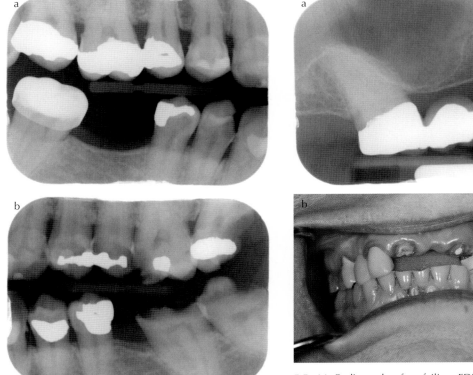

5.4. (a,b) Bitewing images of a young adult with a high caries activity.

5.5. (a) Radiograph of a failing FDP, showing antral expansion and limited bone volume. (b) FDP loss due to abutment caries and fracture. High caries rate and bruxing habit must be considered in treatment planning.

- Skeletal classification
- Amount of freeway space, relative overclosure and interarch space
- Quality of existing dentures.

The intraoral examination of a partially dentate patient (Fig. 5.4a,b, Fig. 5.5, and Fig. 5.6a,b) includes the following:

- *Ability in plaque control*: Home care, presence of plaque, and calculus—plaque control can be rated as good, average, or poor (plaque index)
- *Hard and soft tissue pathology*

- *Salivation*: xerostomia/dry mouth may be related to age, drugs, or disease. This is a major caries risk
- *Caries*: history, caries rate and activity, and caries risk
- *Condition of dentition*: dental charting of (dmf) teeth, congenital absence, impaction, existing plastic restorations, and prostheses
- *Periodontal charting and diagnosis*: plaque, calculus, bleeding on probing, pocket depths, attachment loss, mucogingival problems, localized and generalized mild, moderate, or severe periodontitis, and complicating factors (Fig. 5.6a,b)

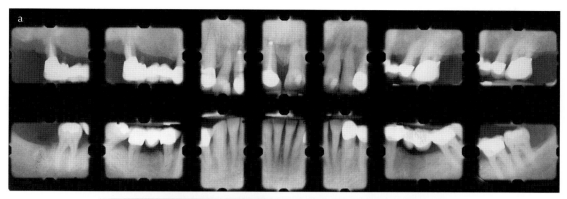

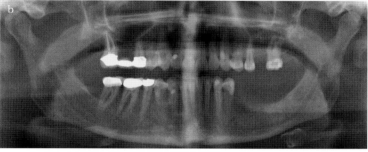

5.6. (a) Radiographic series showing advanced periodontal bone loss in a heavily restored dentition. (b) Panoramic radiograph showing severe left-side mandibular ridge atrophy in young patient.

- *Endodontic problems*: symptomatic teeth and peri-radicular pathology
- *Restorative problems*: failures, potential failures, and extractions needed
- *Edentulous spaces or potential implant site*: space dimensions, status of ridge resorption, supereruption, adjacent tooth encroachment, vital structure encroachment (Fig. 5.7 and Fig. 5.8)
- *Evidence of parafunction* (bruxism and clenching): wear, abfraction, and tooth or restoration fractures.
- *Existing occlusion* (how many teeth are in function?): arch relations and occlusal guidance, and the proportion of function the implant might support
- *TM dysfunction and myofascial pain*

- *Limited jaw opening or movement and mandibular dyskenesia* (Fig. 5.7, Fig. 5.8, Fig. 5.9, and Fig. 5.10)

5.5   Special diagnostic tests

Photographs

Photographs provide documentation of the dental status prior to treatment, including smile line and aesthetics, and can be used in discussions with the patient, consulting dentists, and the laboratory. With patient consent, one can create a practice case portfolio for general patient information. Photographs are a useful

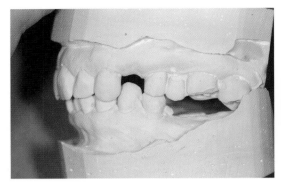

5.7. Study models showing tooth loss and supereruption.

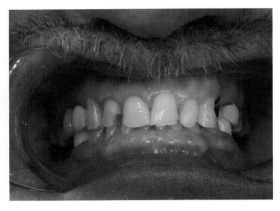

5.10. Bruxism case with posterior tooth loss, extreme vertical overlap, advanced incisor wear, and tooth loss.

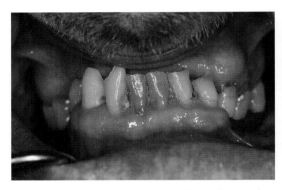

5.8. Tooth loss with extreme vertical overlap or "bite collapse."

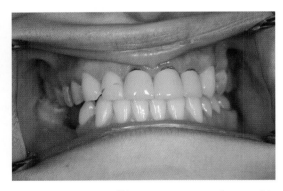

5.11. Preexisting condition: pretreatment photographic record for diagnostic, educational, and legal reasons.

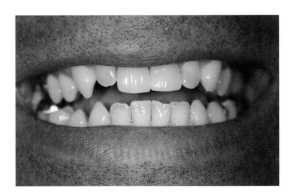

5.9. Anterior open-bite with occlusal contact only on second molars.

legal record of conditions before and after treatment (Fig. 5.11).

Study impressions and models/casts

Study models or casts are a very useful planning aid for orthodontics, restorative dentistry, and implant dentistry. They can be examined when the patient is not present, and can be used in discussions with colleagues. They may be used when giving explanations to patients, and provide a permanent record. Models can be

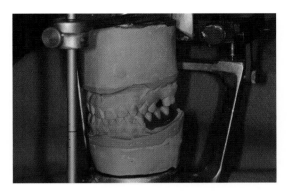

5.12. Study models mounted in a semi-adjustable articulator, and diagnostic mock-up for distal extension mandibular molar space.

presented trimmed in the orthodontic style when sufficient teeth are present, or mounted on a simple semi-adjustable articulator (Fig. 5.12). Increasingly, it will become possible to create computer-generated facial and dental interactive 3D models. Study models can be used for the following:

- Examine the horizontal and vertical maxillomandibular dental relationships
- Assess the occlusal condition (CR/MI), premature contacts, number of occluding posterior teeth, drifting, and supereruption
- Measure the vertical and mesio-distal implant space
- Estimate residual ridge volume
- Make a diagnostic mock-up of the proposed prosthetic restoration
- Fabricate radiographic and surgical guides.

Radiographs

The goal of the surgeon is to place the implant in the edentulous space and avoid damaging the adjacent vital anatomic structures. The standard diagnostic radiographs are a panoramic film and supplementary peri-apical films. As radiographs are 2D, bone volume, bony concavities, and vital anatomical structures are best visualized by means of a cone beam computed tomogram (CBCT).

Depending upon the status of the patient's current dentition, a full mouth series or a panoramic film supplemented by peri-apical films may be recorded in order to do the following:

- Show normal anatomic structures: teeth and restorations, tooth roots, and other anatomic structures—incisive canal, mandibular canal, mental foramen, maxillary sinus, and so on
- Help diagnose caries, periodontal bone loss, peri-radicular, and other bony pathologies and TMJ pathology.

The reader is referred to the current radiology guidelines of the American Academy of Oral and Maxillofacial Radiology (AAOMR) (Tyndall et al. 2012).

Peri-apical radiograph

This routine image is most often used for a single tooth implant in a region of abundant bone width. The available bone volume may be difficult to determine because the image is slightly magnified, may be distorted, and does not depict the third dimension of bone width. This film shows tooth and root alignment, periodontal bone levels, restorations, and peri-radicular radiolucency.

Panoramic radiograph

This is an excellent screening tomogram and patient education tool for the dentition and jawbones. It is a low radiation dose and presurgical diagnostic technology that is available in many general practices. However, the image routinely shows a vertical magnification (approximately 10%) and horizontal magnification (approximately 25%), as well as some

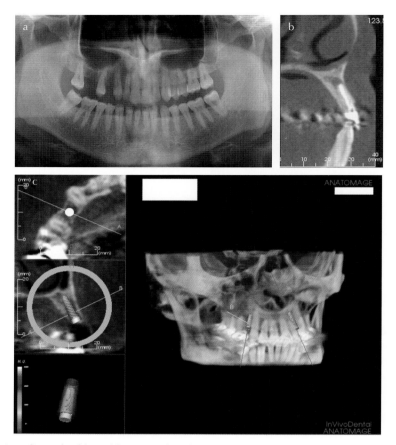

5.13. (a) Panoramic radiograph of favorable potential implant case (spaces #3 and #5). (b) CBCT section showing peri-apical radiolucency on endodontically treated maxillary central incisor (courtesy Dr. O. Ahmad). (c) Software rendering of implant treatment planning using CBCT data (Anatomage™ Interactive planning software) (courtesy of Dr. M Byarlay).

image distortion, especially anteriorly. Metal objects of known dimension may be located in the oral cavity using acrylic templates or dentures in order to more accurately assess bone height with this image (Fig. 5.13a).

Computed tomograph (CT or cone beam CT)

This is a 3D volumetric image of bone, which is graphically presented using specialized computer software (CT or CBCT scan).

Cross-sectional and reformatted panoramic images can be viewed. It is possible to create 3D volumetric images for implant sizing and virtual positioning in the jawbone (Fig. 5.13b,c).

These images are invaluable for identifying normal anatomic structures, anatomic variants, and bone volume during surgical implant planning. The CBCT has advantages over a conventional medical CT in that it has lower cost, lower dosage, and shows less artifact from metal restorations. The images are also convenient for implant team communication and for patient education on the unique attributes of their case. CT images are considered by many to be state of the art for implant case planning.

For optimum use, the CBCT scan should be used in combination with a radiographic guide or stent that utilizes radio-opaque references showing the proposed implant and restoration (tooth) position.

Relative radiation dosage

Ludlow et al. (2006) noted that the effective dose detriment of a CBCT (45–558 μSv) is a factor of 4–42 times greater than a conventional panoramic image.

Consultations and referrals

Refer for orthodontic, periodontal, endodontic, and surgical opinions and treatment when indicated.

5.6 Examination of edentulous space or potential implant site

Aesthetic zone

When the gingival line would be visible as the patient smiles, the case becomes advanced in terms of difficulty, rather than straightforward (Dawson and Chen 2009). Thin scalloped gingiva presents a greater aesthetic challenge than a thick gingival biotype (Fig. 5.14a,b).

Residual ridge (aided by using study models and radiographs)

Ridge resorption occurs rapidly after tooth extraction. Bucco-lingual socket contraction of up to 60% occurs within 6 months (Tan et al. 2012) and reduces bone volume dramatically for implant placement. The longer the delay following extraction, the greater is the

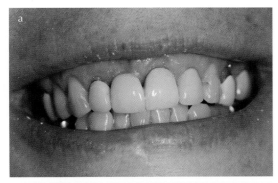

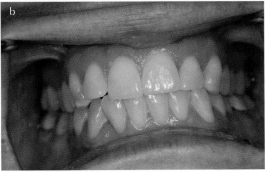

5.14. (a) Favorable thick gingival bioptype. (b) Unfavorable thin, scalloped gingival biotype.

likelihood of a need for bone grafting. The bone volume determines the diameter and length of implant that can be placed.

The initial assessment using palpation and routine radiographs (panoramic supplemented with peri-apical radiographs) yields some useful information. Definitive evaluation may be delayed until the surgical consultation, and may involve the following:

- "Ridge mapping" with a calibrated probe and local anesthesia to determine alveolar bone volume (Luk et al. 2011; NobelGuide™ 2005)
- CBCT scan when available and justified (optional radiographic guide) (Fig. 5.15 and Fig. 5.16)
- Exploratory surgery when necessary.

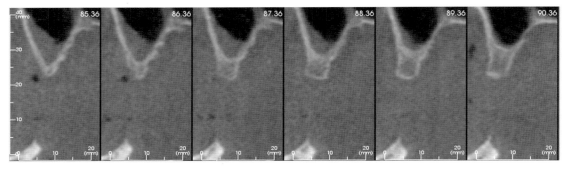

5.15. CBCT serial axial sections of an atrophic maxillary ridge showing hypertrophy of the antral lining (courtesy of Dr. O. Ahmad).

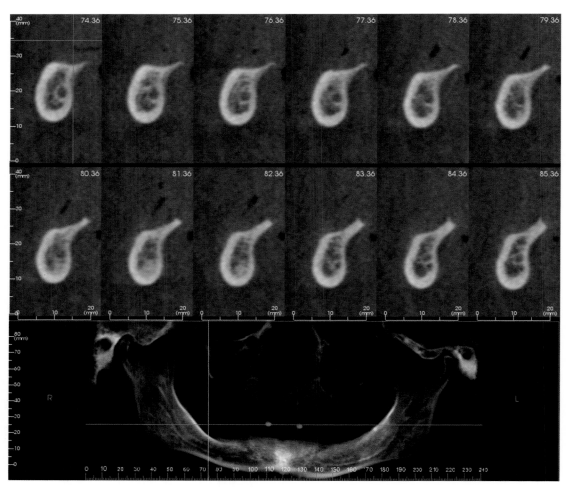

5.16. CBCT images of first molar area of atrophic mandible, showing the external oblique ridge, a prominent mylohyoid ridge with lingual concavity, and lingually positioned mandibular canal (courtesy of Dr. O.Ahmad).

Mesio-distal crown and root spacing

Clinical crowns or roots of adjacent teeth may encroach on surgical access to the potential implant site (Fig. 5.17). Even when the crowns are ideally spaced, the roots may encroach. The number and diameter of implants selected will depend on the dimension of the mesio-distal crown and root space. One may have to consider the need for orthodontics to correct crown or root alignment, or the size of spaces. When a space is large, more than one implant may be indicated. For planning purposes, the following bone dimensions must be borne in mind:

- 1.0–2.0 mm bone should surround the implant bucco-lingually and mesio-distally
- 2.0–3.0 mm bone should remain between adjacent implant platforms (Fig. 5.18a,b).

Vertical space for implant prosthesis

Space for a restoration may be limited when there is minimal ridge resorption with or without supereruption of the opposing teeth (Fig. 5.19). One must also check for bucco-lingual alignment of opposing teeth and the potential implant restoration; this is best evaluated using study models. A height of between 5.0 and 8.0 mm for crowns and bridges, and between 10.0 and 12.0 mm for overdentures is desirable from a technical restorative

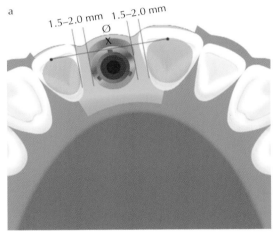

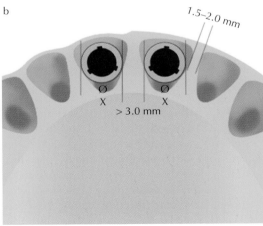

5.17. Adjacent crown encroachment on potential implant canine space.

5.18. (a, b) Mesio-distal space guidelines for single implants (courtesy of CAMLOG).

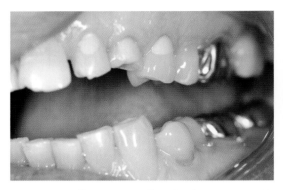

5.19. Retained but worn maxillary deciduous canine with supereruption of opposing canine, and thus limited vertical space for an implant restoration.

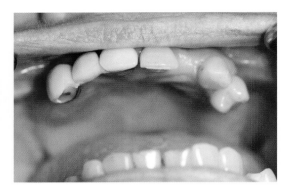

5.20. A dentition with missing posterior teeth. The missing lateral incisor must be treated as part of a comprehensive treatment plan.

perspective. This may be difficult to achieve anteriorly in a complete denture patient with little resorption. If there is too much vertical space due to ridge atrophy, there will be a poor crown/implant ratio, risking adverse moment forces (see Chapter 3). The restorative vertical space is measured from the crest of the edentulous ridge or the platform of the implant to the opposing tooth or teeth.

Opposing arch and force factors

The status of the dental arch opposing the proposed implant restoration plays a role in treatment planning (Gross 2008). The implant support must be planned in relation to the predicted forces.

- *Vertical and horizontal overlap:* severe incisor overbite in class II division 1 and division 2 presents a difficult technical challenge for anterior tooth replacement due to space limitations and off-axis forces. Class II division 2 occlusion is commonly associated with incisal wear and bruxing habits. A severe class III skeletal base has mechanical implications for an atrophic maxilla in full-arch implant restorations.

- *Implant opposing natural teeth:* natural teeth provide proprioceptive input, which is desirable, but forces will be greater than with an opposing removable prosthesis.
- *Implant opposing a removable prosthesis:* this is advantageous for force mitigation.
- *Implant opposing implant prosthesis:* the lack of proprioception and nociception may create the potential for excessive damaging forces (Tokmakidis et al. 2009).
- *Parafunction:* this is a major risk factor for conventional and implant restorations.
- *Number of teeth in occlusion:* the forces on a single implant crown should be less in an intact dentition when compared with a dentition that is limited to anterior tooth function, with or without RPDs. A shortened dental arch (no molars) will increase functional forces on the remaining teeth or implant crowns/FDPs (Fig. 5.20).

Identification of contiguous anatomic structures

The goal of implant surgery is to place the implant in good alignment in the edentulous space, while avoiding damage to the adjacent anatomic structures (tooth roots, neurovascular bundles, sinus, nasal, and sublingual space). Anatomic structures such as the mandibular lingual bony concavities are best visualized with a CBCT scan in advance of surgery, or with good surgical access during surgery. Surgical experience is paramount.

5.7   Surgical consultation

The implant treatment option will remain tentative until the surgical consultation is completed. All appropriate information is transmitted to the surgeon in advance of the consultation. This includes relevant medical and dental history, radiographs, study models, along with a tentative treatment plan. The surgeon will examine the patient in the light of the plan while assessing the feasibility of implantation and the number of implants that might be appropriate. Further radiographs and medical consultation may be required for a definitive surgical proposal. The surgeon will report findings to the patient and referring dentist. Various options will be offered to the patient depending on their unique presentation:

- One- or two-stage implant surgery
- Ridge or socket augmentation: guided bone regeneration (GBR), grafting
- Immediate implant placement after extraction
- Sedation and anesthesia options.

The confluence of ideas from the restorative dentist, surgeon, and patient will ultimately lead to a definitive treatment plan.

5.8   Synthesis of data and treatment planning

Active disease states such as mucosal or bone pathologies, caries, periodontitis, pulpitis, and others, override any implant treatment decisions. Pain problems and disease states must be diagnosed and addressed during initial phase therapy before embarking on definitive restorative work. For the patient with unsatisfactory complete dentures, initial therapy may involve tissue conditioning. Advice on smoking cessation may be appropriate for patients with periodontitis. The patient is educated on the state of health of their mouth and dentition, and any remedial treatment required. The tentative restorative plan is an ongoing educational topic during initial phase therapy.

In order to provide the patient with a comfortable and presentable dental situation, interim restorations and prostheses may need to be provided. A tentative restorative plan can be outlined for the patient contingent upon their response to disease control. The definitive treatment will depend greatly on the response to disease control.

Reevaluation

Data collection and analysis for restorative treatment continues while initial phase therapy and disease control progresses. Following initial therapy, the patient is reevaluated for progress and compliance with oral hygiene measures. At this stage, the patient may return to initial therapy or proceed to treatment planning for definitive restoration, including implants. The placement of implants piecemeal, in a failing dentition (caries, periodontal disease, or chronic wear), is not recommended unless it is part of a comprehensive long-term strategy for the dentition.

Articulated casts, a diagnostic mock-up, and interim restorations may be required for diagnostic purposes, mechanical or aesthetic, prior to determining a definitive treatment plan.

Treatment selection

Having made a diagnosis, it is necessary to discuss and present various treatment options, while simultaneously educating and informing the patient about the risks, advantages, and limitations of implant treatments and other alternatives. Procedures must be explained methodically and in words the patient can understand. The treatment plan options should be clearly explained and presented in written form, with projected treatment and maintenance costs, so as to avoid confusion later. The patient may choose implant treatment as their favored option. The key to success is formulating the simplest plan that solves the problem for the patient, does the least harm to the patient, and has the fewest short and long term risks. The patient may choose implant treatment as their favored option.

The clinician then explains the relevant surgical and prosthetic treatment procedures in detail, the costs, timeline for treatment, as well as the need for routine maintenance visits over the lifetime of the implants. Provisional restorations pre- and postsurgery will feature prominently in this discussion. The patient may find that surgical treatment can be quite complex when bone is deficient; the patient may have some difficult decisions to make especially if grafting is proposed and the treatment process significantly lengthened. The clinician must support the patient in this process and provide explanations and alternatives. An implant crown may seem like the logical solution for a particular scenario, when enough bone is available and the process is financially viable.

Conversely, a case may be complex and lengthy, involving extractions of teeth with a poor prognosis, extensive preventive therapy, periodontal referral, extensive restorative treatment and interim prostheses, prior to final deliberation on a possible implant treatment for missing teeth. Ultimately, it is important that the patient make up their own mind. If the clinician feels uncomfortable with the patient's chosen treatment at this point, it is a good time to suggest referral to a specialist colleague for a second opinion (Fig. 5.21).

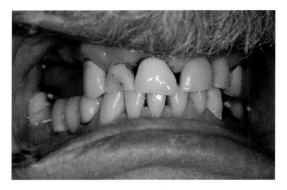

5.21. Long-term smoker, failing restorations, and advanced periodontal disease. (This is a clinical photo of Fig. 5.6a.)

Patient responsibilities

- A time commitment
- Availability for appointments
- Cooperation during treatment (follow instructions during healing and loading)
- Routine maintenance visits for evaluation and hygiene
- Commitment to good home care
- A financial commitment.

5.9   Evidence-based implant dentistry

There are many excellent sources for evidence-based dentistry (EBD) reviews and information (ADA EBD website, http://www.cebd.org, and *The Journal of Evidence-Based Dental Practice*, http://www.jebdp.com), and the general topic can be reviewed in several texts (Clarkson et al. 2003; Thomas 2009). In accordance with the principles of EBD, treatment decisions are based on three factors:

- The patient's needs and preferences
- The clinician's knowledge, training, and clinical ability
- The "best" available scientific evidence.

The overlap of these factors will help lead to an acceptable rational treatment plan for both the patient and clinician. Various sources are available for the clinician to consult for research evidence and guidance. A focused clinical question can be formulated, and databases such as PubMed searched for systematic reviews with meta-analyses on the topic, or lower forms of evidence in the evidence hierarchy. The availability of high quality evidence gives a higher level of confidence in a particular treatment. The "best" evidence does not always mean a high level of evidence, but the best available for the particular clinical question. Questions may arise, for example, as to whether implant therapy may be affected by certain systemic conditions, or whether one technique has an advantage over another, or whether grafting would increase the risk of implant failure. The patient will be interested in the prognosis for various suggested treatment options and, where evidence is lacking, will have to rely on the dentist's clinical judgment and experience, or seek a second opinion.

Clinical evidence on many topics is often inconclusive, such as for example, when it is best to extract and not restore a tooth with a questionable prognosis (Fugazzotto 2009), or when it is advisable to consider immediate placement of implants (Esposito et al. 2010, Hämmerle et al. 2011), or early loading of implants (Chiapasco and Gatti 2003; Quinlan et al. 2005; Eliasson et al. 2009). Similarly, it is difficult to give definitive answers relating to many prognostic questions relating to the success of implants and implant restorations in the numerous clinical scenarios encountered in daily practice. Research conclusions cannot always be easily extrapolated to every patient and the innumerable clinical scenarios. However, it would be wise for the clinician to keep abreast of developments in the implant field and be able to recommend the best current treatment based on the best available evidence. Dental implantology has a good research foundation, and the volume of research continues to grow.

5.10   Case selection and risk assessment

The cases selected for implant treatment must fall within the skill level of the clinician. Alternative restorative plans not involving implants must be presented to the patient, who must also be given the option to seek specialist opinions before deciding on a definitive treatment. The McGarry et al. (1999) *prosthodontic index* may prove useful in making treatment decisions for edentulous patients. Four categories are defined, ranging from Class I to Class IV, with Class I defining an uncomplicated clinical scenario, and a Class IV defining the most complex and highest risk situation.

The ITI group has produced *SAC* (straightforward, advanced, complex) *guidelines* for identifying risk factors, both restorative and surgical that determine the complexity of cases. The SAC classification (Dawson and Chen 2009) is an assessment of the potential difficulty and risk, and helps to guide case selection and treatment planning. The authors give excellent examples and illustrations of clinical cases from these SAC categories. It is difficult to predict the soft tissue outcome following implant surgery, and also the long-term stability of the peri-implant tissues. The following guidelines are helpful in case selection for treatment or referral.

Straightforward

- A nonaesthetic site with minimal aesthetic risk
- An uncomplicated restorative process
- A predictable restorative outcome
- A low risk of complications.

Advanced

- More aesthetically demanding
- Restoration involves more steps but the outcome is still predictable

- Restorative outcome can be readily visualized
- Moderate risk of complications.

Complex Cases

- High aesthetic risk, for example, several adjacent anterior teeth missing
- Restoration involves many steps and the plan may need to change depending on outcome of prior steps.
- Restorative outcome cannot be readily visualized
- High risk of complications affecting long-term outcomes (Fig. 5.21)
- Patient must understand and accept the risk of compromised outcomes.

5.11 Treatment modifiers, complicating or risk factors

In the course of data collection, diagnosis, and treatment planning, certain case factors will come to light that may play an important part in deciding the best treatment approach. The key to diagnosis and treatment is awareness of these factors. These factors will also play a key role in determining whether the patient should be referred for specialist care. No treatment is risk-free, but more complex treatments have greater potential for complications. The clinician must be aware of the key risk factors during synthesis of data. When identified, steps can be taken to minimize their effect on outcomes. Patients are educated about these risks and potential negative outcomes, which will help temper expectations in advance. A summary of risk factors includes the following:

Operator risk factors

- Inadequate knowledge, skill, and experience
- Poor case assessment, planning, and execution

- Poor implant placement: position or angle, leading to adverse forces
- Poor force management: prosthesis design, occlusion

Patient risk factors

- Patient expectations too high
- Poor compliance, for example, availability for treatment due to health, work, or family, or inability to cooperate
- Oral hygiene difficulties or dexterity issues
- Compromised general health affecting healing: diabetes and smoking
- Compromised bone healing, for example, irradiated bone, chemotherapy, antiresorption therapy
- Compromised oral health, for example, poor plaque control, high caries rate, history of or active periodontitis
- Active jaw growth in a young patient
- Poor (<10 year) prognosis of the dentition.

Biological risk factors

- Insufficient bone volume and soft tissue volume with a need for ridge augmentation
- Vital anatomic structures too close to the planned osteotomy site
- Inadequate band of attached mucosa
- Thin gingival biotype
- Parafunction.

Aesthetic risk factors

- Mucosal margin in the implant area visible upon smiling

Mechanical risk factors

- Cantilevers with moment forces
- Interarch distance is too small or too great
- Limited occlusal function of remaining dentition: number of premolars and molars in function

- Opposing dentition type: either natural teeth, implant restoration, or removable denture
- Extreme arch mismatch: either extreme horizontal or vertical overlap.

The prognosis of teeth adjacent to the implant site, and the prognosis of the dentition are central to the process of treatment planning for implant dentistry. Many of the listed risk factors preclude treatment by an implant novice. Cases with inadequate bone volume or parafunction should be referred for specialist care. Poor prognosis of some teeth may hasten their extraction and necessitate their inclusion in a prosthetic treatment plan. The patient should be in no doubt as to the prognosis of existing teeth prior to consideration of implants for missing teeth. Patients with chronic moderate to advanced periodontal disease should be referred for periodontal treatment prior to implant treatment due to the increased risk of peri-implant bone loss (Karoussis et al. 2003; Roos-Jansåker et al. 2006; Pjetursson et al. 2012; Renvert et al. 2013). Ultimately, increasing levels of complexity of surgery or prosthetics may influence implant treatment outcomes as follows (Dawson and Chen 2009):

- No effect on outcome
- A suboptimal outcome that does not reduce longevity of the implant prosthesis
- A compromised outcome with reduced long-term success or stability of the implant prosthesis
- Failure of the implant and/or prosthesis.

5.12 Patient education, expectations, and consent

The restoring dentist ensures good communication within the team and between the team and the patient, and ultimately determines how the case will progress.

The patient must be educated on the importance of plaque control, the regular maintenance visits required for implant prostheses, and the risk of peri-implant bone loss. Implant hygiene must be particularly emphasized for these patients who may have had a hygiene deficit in the past or have periodontal issues. It is easier to prevent peri-implantitis than to recover the situation when bone loss has occurred and implant threads or rough implant surfaces have been exposed. It should be emphasized to patients that restorative longevity will depend on a good preventive and maintenance strategy. There is a tendency for patients to wrongly assume that when restorative work is complete, all the work is done.

When the definitive surgical and restorative plan has been determined with the patient, written consent is obtained.

Informed consent

Following a surgical consultation and the formulation of a definitive treatment plan, and when the patient is satisfied to proceed with implant therapy, it is time for the patient to sign a *consent form* (Froum 2010). The consent form must be tailored to the treatments offered. The consent form confirms overall patient education, an adequate explanation of treatment alternatives, an outline of surgical and restorative processes, and information on possible complications with surgery, anesthesia, implant failure, and restoration failure. An example of informed consent can be seen in Appendix 1. It is not the role of the clinician to convince the patient to have a particular treatment, but to advise.

Finally, one must discuss a plan of action and proposed schedule of treatment. When the patient accepts the implant treatment plan, a definitive time line can be formalized.

Legal issues

Froum (2010) has drawn attention to good practice in implant dentistry and the avoidance of litigation problems. Many complications can be avoided when dentists are better trained and maintain high standards of clinical care. Froum reiterates the fundamental ethical principle "do no harm," and the requirement for continuous professional development in the field. Realistic expectations must be emphasized for patients regardless of preconceptions. Informed consent is a *sine qua non*.

5.13   Summary of assessment and treatment planning

- Assess the presenting problem
- Thorough data collection, and case assessment
- Understand the patient's perceived needs and expectations, and serve the patient's best interests. The patient really wants teeth, not implants
- Tentative outline of treatment plan and alternatives
- Patient education
- Consider implant therapy in the context of comprehensive care: complex treatment is not inherently better, simple treatment may be more appropriate
- Consider specialist referral depending on case complexity and risk factors
- Surgical consultation
- Discuss options, explain potential problems, and manage expectations
- Definitive plan
- Informed consent
- Manage treatment
- Stress the need for maintenance.

References

Chiapasco M, Gatti C. (2003) Implant-retained mandibular overdentures with immediate loading: a 3- to 8-year prospective study on 328implants. *Clin Implant Dent Relat Res.* 5(1):29–38.

Clarkson J, Harrison JE, Ismail AI, Needleman I, Worthington H. (eds.) (2003) *Evidence Based Dentistry for Effective Practice*. Martin Dunitz, London/New York.

Cronin RJ Jr, Oesterle LJ. (1998) Implant use in growing patients. Treatment planning concerns. *Dent Clin North Am.* 42(1):1–34.

Dawson A, Chen S. (eds.) (2009) *The SAC Classification in Implant Dentistry*. Quintessence, Berlin.

Eliasson A, Blomqvist F, Wennerberg A, Johansson A. (2009) A retrospective analysis of early and delayed loading of full-arch mandibular prostheses using three different implant systems: clinical results with up to 5 years of loading. *Clin Implant Dent Relat Res.* 11(2):134–48.

Esposito M, Grusovin MG, Polyzos IP, Felice P, Worthington HV. (2010) Interventions for replacing missing teeth: dental implants in fresh extraction sockets (immediate, immediate-delayed and delayed implants). *Cochrane Database Syst Rev.* (9):CD005968.

Froum S. (ed.) (2010) *Dental Implant Complications; Etiology, Prevention and Treatment*. Wiley-Blackwell, Ames.

Fugazzotto PA. (2009) Evidence-based decision making: replacement of the single missing tooth. *Dent Clin North Am.* 53(1):97–129.

Gross MD. (2008) Occlusion in implant dentistry. A review of the literature of prosthetic determinants and current concepts. *Aust Dent J.* 53(Suppl 1): S60–8.

Hämmerle CH, Araújo MG, Simion M; Osteology Consensus Group. (2011) 2012) Evidence-based knowledge on the biology and treatment of extraction sockets. *Clin Oral Implants Res.* 23(Suppl 5): 80–2.

Karoussis IK, Salvi GE, Heitz-Mayfield LJ, Brägger U, Hämmerle CH, Lang NP. (2003) Long-term implant prognosis in patients with and without a history of chronic periodontitis: a 10-year prospective cohort study of the ITI Dental Implant System. *Clin Oral Implants Res.* 14(3):329–39.

Ludlow JB, Davies-Ludlow LE, Brooks SL, Howerton WB. (2006) Dosimetry of 3 CBCT devices for oral and maxillofacial radiology: CB Mercuray, NewTom 3G and i-CAT. *Dentomaxillofac Radiol.* 35(4):219–26.

Luk LC, Pow EH, Li TK, Chow TW. (2011) Comparison of ridge mapping and cone beam computed tomography for planning dental implant therapy. *Int J Oral Maxillofac Implants.* 26(1):70–4.

McGarry TJ, Nimmo A, Skiba JF, Ahlstrom RH, Smith CR, Koumjian JH. (1999) Classification system for complete edentulism. The American College of Prosthodontics. *J Prosthodont.* 8(1):27–39.

NobelGuide™: *Genieoss* (2005). http://genieoss .com/acrobat/nobelCTManual.pdf

Pjetursson BE, Helbling C, Weber HP, Matuliene G, Salvi GE, Brägger U, Schmidlin K, Zwahlen M, Lang NP. (2012) Peri-implantitis susceptibility as it relates to periodontal therapy and supportive care. *Clin Oral Implants Res.* 23(7):888–94.

Quinlan P, Nummikoski P, Schenk R, Cagna D, Mellonig J, Higginbottom F, Lang K, Buser D, Cochran D. (2005) Immediate and early loading of SLA ITI single-tooth implants: an in vivo study. *Int J Oral Maxillofac Implants.* 20(3):360–70.

Renvert S, Aghazadeh A, Hallström H, Persson GR. (2013) Factors related to peri-implantitis—a retrospective study. *Clin Oral Implants Res.* doi: 10.1111/ clr.12208. [Epub ahead of print].

Roos-Jansåker AM, Renvert H, Lindahl C, Renvert S. (2006) Nine- to fourteen-year follow-up of implant treatment. Part III: factors associated with peri-implant lesions. *J Clin Periodontol.* 33(4):296–301.

Tan WL, Wong TL, Wong MC, Lang NP. (2012) A systematic review of post-extractional alveolar hard and soft tissue dimensional changes in humans. *Clin Oral Implants Res.* 23(Suppl 5): 1–21.

Thomas MV. (ed.) (2009) *Evidence-Based Dentistry. Dental Clinics of North America,* January 2009, Vol. 53, Number 1. Saunders, St. Louis.

Tokmakidis K, Wessing B, Papoulia K, Spiekermann H. (2009) Load distribution and loading concepts on teeth and implants. *J Dent Implantol.* 25(1): 44–52.

Tyndall DA, Price JB, Tetradis S, Ganz SD, Hildebolt C, Scarfe WC; American Academy of Oral and Maxillofacial Radiology. (2012) Position statement of the American Academy of Oral and Maxillofacial Radiology on selection criteria for the use of radiology in dental implantology with emphasis on cone beam computed tomography. *Oral Surg Oral Med Oral Pathol Oral Radiol.* 113(6):817–26.

6

Essentials for Implant Treatment

6.1 Brånemark osseointegration protocol	**6.5** Implant treatment outcomes
6.2 Other surgical protocols	**6.6** Criteria for patient outcomes
6.3 Different treatment presentations and arch configurations	**6.7** Implant maintenance
6.4 Prosthetic options: screw fixation, cementation, and retentive anchors	**6.8** Peri-implant health assessment and treatment

6.1 Brånemark osseointegration protocol

Originally, the Brånemark team outlined the principles and procedures for achieving predictable implant osseointegration and rehabilitation in edentulous patients (Zarb 1983; Brånemark et al. 1985; Albrektsson and Lekholm 1989; Lekholm et al. 1999). The guiding principles still hold well today, some 30 years later. Although some technical aspects have been refined, Brånemark's work is still the reference protocol for placing dental implants. Brånemark described the technique in detail, from patient and surgical field preparation to the final prosthesis delivery. Three major principles underpin successful outcomes for osseointegration: atraumatic surgery to create the osteotomy, implant immobilization during healing, and well-managed delayed functional loading. Brånemark's approach is referred to as a *two-stage* or *submerged* implant surgery.

First-stage surgery

- Preoperative antibiotics
- Aseptic surgical field
- Full-thickness muco-periosteal flap access
- Standardized atraumatic osteotomy preparation: drill speed 45 < 2000 rpm, staged drilling, pumping drill action, copious saline irrigation, direction indicators, and depth indicators. Dense cortical bone needs careful, slow drilling and sharp burs to avoid overheating, followed by thread formation. Excessive heat generation leads to bone damage with sequestra, infection, connective tissue scarring, lack of integration, and early failure. Soft-bone osteotomy may be of reduced diameter, allowing for thread engagement in unprepared bone. Similarly, osteotome techniques have been adopted to compress bone rather than removing it from the osteotomy site (Fig. 6.1a–c).
- Correctly manufactured implants

Fundamentals of Implant Dentistry, First Edition. Gerard Byrne.
© 2014 John Wiley & Sons, Inc. Published 2014 by John Wiley & Sons, Inc.
Companion website: www.wiley.com/go/byrne/implants

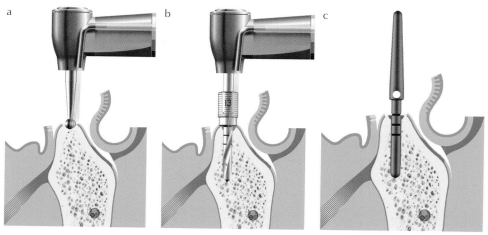

6.1. Diagrams of submerged surgery protocol: first-stage surgery. (a, b) Pilot drills (courtesy of CAMLOG). (c) Guide post or direction indicator (courtesy of CAMLOG).

- Noncontamination of implant surfaces
- Tapping of osteotomy site in dense bone to ensure precise fit of a screw implant
- Implant insertion at 15–20 rpm
- Cover screw approximately flush with bone crest
- Flap sutured with suture line away from the implant position
- Healing for 2 weeks without any loading, direct or indirect
- Postoperative antibiotic for 10 days, saline mouthrinses, and analgesics
- Healing time of between 3 and 6 months, as set by the Brånemark group, based on their long-term clinical trails (Fig. 6.1a–c and Fig. 6.2a–d).

NB: Early loading or micro-motion increases the risk of nonintegration or fibrous tissue scarring. The surgical placement technique is very important, and implant success depends greatly on the skill of the individual surgeon.

Atrophic maxillae

The Brånemark team also presented technique modifications for the unique challenges of working on the porous bone of the maxillae. The mandible is a long bone with a dense cortex and a porous inner core of trabecular bone. The maxillae are quite different and consist almost entirely of fine trabecular bone with a very thin or no cortical layer (Sennerby and Roos 1998). Lekholm and Zarb (1985) classified bone density and ridge resorption to help standardize the surgical approach. Reported success rates are lower for atrophic maxillae than for the mandible (Sorní et al. 2005).

Second-stage surgery

- Expose the implant platform and remove overlying soft tissue or bone.
- Attach a transmucosal healing abutment to the implant body, bringing the implant into contact with the oral environment for the first time (Fig. 6.3a,b).

Prosthetic rehabilitation

- Between 3 and 6 months healing prior to loading (*delayed loading*)

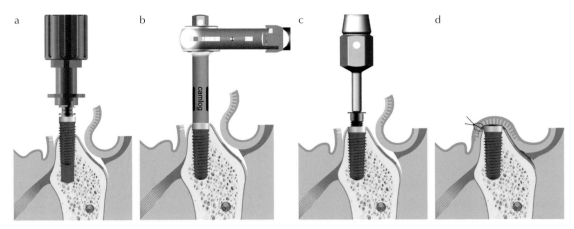

6.2. Diagrams of submerged surgery protocol continued. (a) Finger driving the implant (courtesy of CAMLOG). (b) Torque driving the implant to final position (courtesy of CAMLOG). (c) Cover screw (courtesy of CAMLOG). (d) Flap sutured (courtesy of CAMLOG).

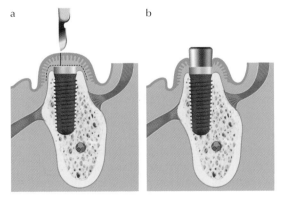

6.3. Second-stage surgery. (a) Exposing the implant (courtesy of CAMLOG). (b) Removal of cover screw and placement of a healing abutment (courtesy of CAMLOG).

- Restorative procedures with well-balanced functional forces that promote maintenance of long-term osseointegration
- Significant remodeling continues for approximately 1 year after loading,
- Functional bone remodeling continues over the lifetime of the implant.

The implant platform is positioned flush with the bone crest at first-stage surgery. Brånemark and his team observed that bone loss occurred at the bone crest around the implant, following second-stage surgery and abutment connection. Bone recedes from the implant–abutment junction (IAJ) by up to 2.0 mm in the first year. After the first year in function, an annual bone loss rate of 0.2 mm/year was predicted (Brånemark et al. 1985; Albrektsson et al. 1986). Early bone loss is considered to be related to the placement of the implant platform flush with the bony crest, reentry surgical trauma, and the presence of a bacteria-harboring implant-abutment junction (IAJ).

Remodeling of bone proceeds during functional loading, and the process is predicated upon the magnitude and direction of the functional loads. After 18 months, a steady state of bone remodeling is achieved. When loading is within physiologic limits, the bond between implant and bone (osseointegration) becomes stronger over time. Peri-implant disease, excessive loading, or functional overload may cause the breakdown of osseointegration with bone loss and eventually, implant loss.

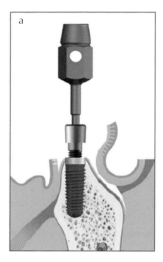
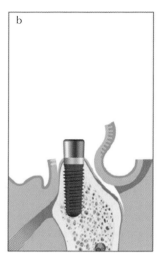
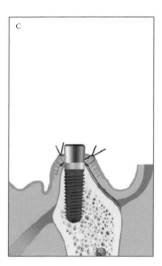

6.4. Diagram of nonsubmerged, one-stage surgery technique with transmucosal healing. (a) Inserting the CAMLOG® healing abutment. (b) CAMLOG Screw-Line implant with healing abutment. (c) Wound closure. (courtesy of CAMLOG).

6.2 Other surgical protocols

One-stage surgery with transmucosal healing

During the 1980s, Schroeder and colleagues presented in the German literature a one-stage surgery protocol for Straumann/ITI/Bonefit® implants. These implants had an integral polished transmucosal collar or abutment, which remained open to the oral environment after surgery (Fig. 6.4). Later publications (Schroeder et al. 1991, 1996) in English brought the system to a larger readership. Schroeder's one-stage surgical technique is well documented and is currently well established (Jokstad 2009). One-stage surgery is efficient and effective and may be appropriate for elderly or medically compromised patients. The reported success rate for this technique is comparable with that of two-stage surgery (Dawson and Chen 2009).

Other surgical protocols and shortened loading protocols

Some implant protocols allow for immediate placement of implants into extraction sockets. Immediate implant placement is gaining in popularity due to the promise of reduced treatment times and bone preservation. The earliest example was the Tübingen implant, which was placed immediately into extraction sockets (D'Hoedt and Schulte 1989). Other technique variants include early placement after early socket healing, and implantation combined with grafting, guided bone regeneration (GBR), or sinus lift. These new techniques present unique challenges and require careful long-term clinical evaluation before they can be recommended with confidence. Additionally, shortened loading protocols have been introduced to accelerate implant treatment (see Chapter 12) (Fig. 6.5).

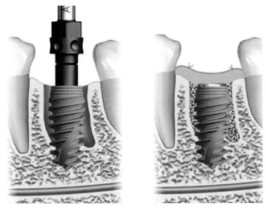

6.5. Diagram of immediate implant placement in an extraction socket with in-fill using a graft material and flap closure (courtesy of Nobel Biocare).

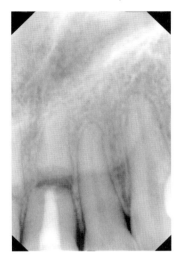

6.6. Fractured central incisor, which will be extracted.

6.3   Different treatment presentations and arch configurations

In most cases, standard (4.0 mm) or small-diameter (3.0–3.5 mm) implants are more readily accommodated within the edentulous ridge, than wide-diameter implants. Thus, for implant restorative planning purposes, one can think in terms of central incisor or premolar size implant arch segments on standard implants, as a reference, unless wide-body implants can be used in molar segments. Such an implant needs a minimum of between 6.0 and 8.0 mm of bone mesio-distally. The reader is referred to Chapters 8–10 for specifics of treatments.

The single-implant crown

The tooth position, the condition of the residual ridge, adjacent teeth and arch, and the opposing teeth determine the feasibility of implant treatment. A single missing maxillary incisor represents a significant aesthetic challenge in patients with a high smile line and thin gingival biotype. However, the advantages of a well-executed implant crown should outweigh the preparation of adjacent healthy teeth to support a conventional fixed bridge. Replacement of a single tooth is easier when the original tooth or root is still present and bone levels are good. Depending on the cause of tooth loss or impending extraction, socket damage and ridge resorption may compromise implant placement (Fig. 6.6). Consideration of immediate implant placement should be cautiously weighed, as long-term success data are limited. When a tooth is congenitally absent, alveolar bone is often poorly developed, and there may be proximity issues with adjacent roots and crowns. Orthodontics or ridge augmentation may have to be considered. Implant treatment may need to be postponed until jaw growth is complete. Additionally, space maintenance and prevention of supereruption of opposing teeth may be necessary before and during implant treatment.

The loss of a lower premolar, first molar, or the most distal tooth in an arch may not be perceived as a problem by elderly patients, but may be very significant for a young patient. Many arguments can be made for *not* replacing second molars with implants due to the quality of bone, the potentially large

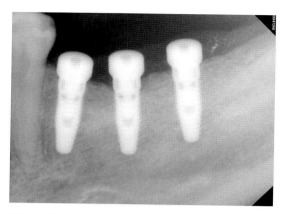

6.7. Multiple tooth loss in one quadrant and implant replacements.

occlusal force in this area, poor accessibility, and the relatively minor aesthetic consequence. However, in an otherwise excellent dentition, placement of such a second molar implant restoration restores form and function of the dentition. It is also arguable that first molars or other teeth with a poor prognosis should be maintained in teenagers, thus enabling bone retention for possible implant placement at a later date.

Multiple missing teeth

Multiple missing units may indicate a caries or periodontal problem. Alternatively, teeth may have been removed as a matter of urgency, expediency, or economy in various circumstances. Often, the tooth loss has been restored with an FDP or an RPD, which may be failing or need replacement. Traditional treatments with tooth borne bridges or removable prostheses are valid, but implant restorations are viable provided there is an adequate volume of bone. Guided bone regeneration (GBR) is becoming more feasible for deficient ridges. When multiple contiguous teeth are missing in an arch, one can classify the tooth loss

in broad terms as with removable partial dentures:

Kennedy Class I and II (distal extension RPD): Many partially edentulous cases may result from failure of previous crown and bridgework and involve edentulous distal extension "saddle" areas. In the case of preexisting FDPs and RPDs, there will be significant ridge atrophy. Natural abutments may be unusable for a conventional FDP due to endodontic, caries, or periodontal bone loss. Often, a choice remains between an RPD and an implant fixed multi-unit restoration. The concept of a shortened dental arch or premolar occlusion should be considered in many of these scenarios (Carlsson 2009). It may be more appropriate, when possible, to replace a molar segment with one or two implant crowns than with an RPD (Fig. 6.7).

Kennedy Class III: In dealing with Class III cases, the chief problems with implant treatment relate to ridge volume and supereruption of opposing teeth in pontic areas. When the residual ridge is favorable, these cases are relatively straightforward with decisions needed on the number of implants and prosthesis design. Atrophic ridges pose an implant placement problem.

Kennedy Class IV: Missing anterior teeth as a consequence of trauma or loss of an old fixed prosthesis presents many potential difficulties with occlusion and aesthetics. There will often be significant tissue loss so that the prosthesis has to compensate for missing pink "gum" tissue without extensive ridge grafting. There may also be supereruption of opposing teeth. A simple removable partial denture may be an excellent interim diagnostic choice for such a case, with referral to a more experienced colleague for subsequent implant treatment (Wittneben and Webber 2013). Such cases would benefit from a *radiographic guide* and diagnostic CBCT with a view to optimum implant placement with

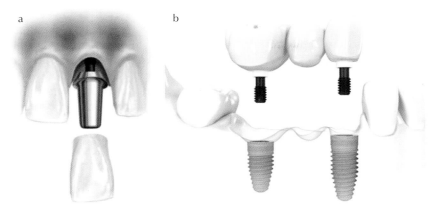

6.8. (a) Diagram of a screw-retained abutment and cement-retained crown (courtesy of Nobel Biocare). (b) Diagram of direct screw-retained (one-piece with integral abutments) three-unit fixed implant prosthesis (courtesy of Nobel Biocare).

further options of GBR and guided implant placement (see Chapter 11)

One edentulous arch opposing a natural arch or partial arch with or without significant restoration

These may be regarded as complex cases and present the implant treatment option of an implant overdenture or an implant fixed full arch prosthesis. With failed single dental arches, one should suspect a history of parafunction. Technical complications are likely due to super-eruption and unfavorable force factors.

Complete edentulism

A patient who wears existing dentures with which they are unhappy should be carefully assessed for replacement dentures. This also applies to dentate patients who have no recourse but complete dentures because of extreme wear, caries, or periodontal breakdown. A mandibular implant-supported overdenture opposing a maxillary complete denture becomes a viable treatment option for many of these patients. Alternatively, both mandibular

and maxillary implant overdentures or implant fixed prostheses may be considered.

6.4 Prosthetic options: Screw fixation, cementation, and retentive anchors

Fixed implant restorations are retained with abutment screws, prosthetic screws or cement (Fig. 6.8a,b). There is no evidence determining which is the better approach, and patient and operator preference dictates which method to use. Screw-retained prostheses allow retrievability. Cemented crowns are generally indicated for maxillary incisors and canines due to the bony anatomy and implant angulation relative to the crown. Similarly, adverse implant angulation precludes screw-retained crowns. Patients must be educated on the positives and negatives of each option during treatment planning. Some clinicians favor the use of temporary cements with a view to prosthesis retrieval, but it is likely that such restorations would still be difficult to remove should abutment screws come loose.

Removable implant prostheses are retained with round/oval bar and clip devices or individual implant clips, such as Dalbo®-Plus ball or Zest Locator® attachments. Both approaches work well. Individual attachments are simpler, less expensive to fabricate, and easier to clean than bar attachments. Bars are favored in the maxilla due to problems with implant angulation and the possible biomechanical advantage of splinting implants in softer bone.

NB: Accurate clinical records must be maintained for the implant (implant data label), the torque value of abutment fixation, and details of the type of restoration utilized.

6.5 Implant treatment outcomes

Clinical implant success has been widely validated (Adell et al. 1981; Adell 1985; Van Steenberghe et al. 1991; Buser et al. 1997). Sennerby and Roos (1998) reported that high implant failure rates were associated with poor bone quality, short implants in areas of reduced bone volume, lack of presurgical antibiotics, smoking, and limited clinician experience. Certain terms are used in defining success and failure:

- Implant success
- Implant survival
- Early failure, that is, failure to osseointegrate
- Late failure, that is, failure during function
- Prosthesis survival.

Implant success

Implants are considered successful if they fulfill a list of criteria considered essential for long-term survival. These criteria were first presented by Albrektsson et al. (1986). Modified criteria were later proposed by Roos et al. (1997). The further criterion of acceptable restorative aesthetics is currently accepted.

The updated criteria include:

- No mobility of the implant
- No radiographic peri-implant radiolucency
- ≤ 1.0 mm bone loss during the first year of function
- ≤ 0.2 mm annual bone loss thereafter
- No pain or infection at the site
- Functional survival of the implant for 5 years in 90% cases
- Functional survival of the implant for 10 years in 85% cases.

Implant survival or cumulative survival rate (CSR)

If an implant exhibits characteristics that may lead to eventual loss (e.g., the progressive bone loss of peri-implantitis or other severe osseous defect), it would not be considered successful (Jokstad 2009; Froum 2010), and as such may be regarded as a failing implant.

An implant may be considered a failure if it is unusable for its intended purpose for the following reasons:

- It has lost, or is losing, its osseointegration.
- It is malpositioned, making it unusable.
- It is impinging on vital anatomic structures (requiring removal).
- It has fractured.

Primary or early failure occurs prior to functional loading and means that the implant has failed to integrate, or integration has broken down. This is most likely the result of excessive surgical trauma, an unstable implant in the osteotomy at the time of surgery, or inadvertent loading during healing (Fig. 6.9).

Secondary or late failure occurs after osseointegration and following functional loading. It may occur as a result of peri-implantitis and/or overload (Sennerby and Roos 1998). Smoking is often a predisposing factor (Fig. 6.10).

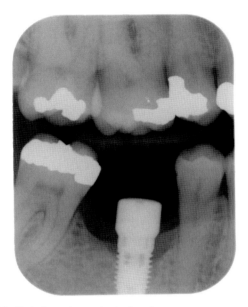

6.9. Early bone loss prior to function.

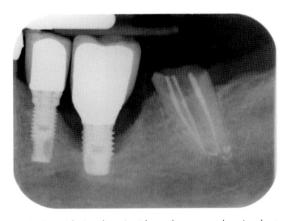

6.10. Late (during function) bone loss around an implant with a poor crown-to-implant ratio.

Prosthesis survival

Prosthesis survival implies a functioning prosthesis. A multi-unit fixed prosthesis or an implant-supported denture can remain functional despite the loss of one or more supporting implants.

6.6 Criteria for patient outcomes

Certain outcomes are important from the patient's perspective. Whether a patient receives a single crown or a complex full-arch fixed prosthesis, the expectations will be similar. Each patient will have his or her own focus. Good aesthetics is an overriding expectation in restorative dentistry. Function and comfort may be the primary concerns for a patient with complete dentures, whereas aesthetics may be more important for the partially dentate patient.

Positive outcomes from a patient perspective

- Good aesthetics leading to improved quality of life
- Good comfort and function leading to improved nutrition and quality of life
- Good cost:benefit ratio for implant treatment
- Good implant longevity
- Good prosthesis longevity
- Low incidence of implant and prosthetic complications
- Low cost of maintenance.

Dentists have relied for some time on the outcome criteria listed previously in the section "Implant Success" as a measure of implant success and failure. Given our experience thus far with endosseous implants, it may be reasonable to expect indefinite long-term success of implant osseointegration for a healthy patient with good plaque control and favorable biomechanical factors. More information, from long-term clinical research, is needed on the incidence of peri-implantitis and the roles of other systemic and local factors in progressive peri-implant bone-loss and implant failure.

The relatively high cost of implant treatments may sharpen patient focus, and often elevates expectations. As with traditional restorative dentistry, it is reasonable to expect a period of between 10 and 15 years of trouble-free function for a prosthesis. Routine wear and tear demands may determine the need to remake the prosthesis or to repair a damaged prosthesis.

6.7   Implant maintenance

From the clinician's viewpoint, expectation of longevity is dependent on maintenance of good general health, regular dental mainte-nance checks, and excellent plaque control. Many peri-implant problems relate to poor plaque control and overloading (Schou et al. 1992). These factors will have been explained to the patient at the outset. For dentate patients, the necessity for maintenance is viewed as a routine issue. However, the edentulous patient, especially the overdenture patient, is less likely to see the reasoning for regular recall and good oral hygiene, although their implant mainte-nance needs are likely to be greater due to muco-gingival problems, retentive clip prob-lems, and relining needs. Problems, such as recession with implant exposure, inflammatory soft tissue overgrowth with or without peri-implant bone loss, become more problematic to treat when neglected (Heitz-Mayfield 2008).

It is the responsibility of the dentist to emphasize maintenance procedures, advise the patient and reiterate risks, and conse-quences of neglect. It is also important to be vigilant for possible underlying systemic health conditions. The patient must be advised about limiting forces during the remodeling phase (6–12 months after implant placement), when the bone remodels in response to functional forces. Parafunctional activity and the potential for overload of implant components should be managed in a palliative manner, with protec-tive occlusal devices, and with the understand-ing that the underlying etiology cannot be eliminated.

Difficulties will arise in cases where a patient's dexterity deteriorates, as occurs with Alzheimer's disease (AD), Parkinson's disease (PD), and multiple sclerosis (MS), or when vision becomes impaired or when a patient's living circumstances change dramatically (e.g. confinement to bed, rest homes, and hospitals). In these circumstances, detailed instructions must be given to carers for implant prosthesis care.

Recall schedule

A 6- to 12-monthly follow-up regime is recom-mended to monitor the hard and soft tissue health of the implants and the functional aspects of the prosthesis. Routine professional cleaning of the implants and hygiene advice is necessary. Peri-apical radiographs may be recorded annu-ally or as indicated for the implant restoration; if the implant appears in bite-wing radiographs, these usually suffice. Cases of peri-implantitis with or without implant thread or textured surface exposure should be discussed with, or referred to, the surgeon of record. Preexisting periodontal disease is considered a risk factor (Roos-Jansåker et al. 2006, Schou et al. 2006; Mombelli et al. 2012).

Prosthetic stability

It is important that restoration seating, screw torquing, and occlusion are optimal at the outset.

Routine checks at 6-monthly intervals:

* Warn the patient about initial *1-year period of bone remodeling* and the need to moderate biting forces during this time.
* Verify positive *proximal contacts*.
* Check *occlusion* on implant restorations for changes in maximum intercusping and eccentric glide contact.
* Replace or activate *retentive clips/matrices*.
* Monitor resorption of residual ridges and *denture stability*.

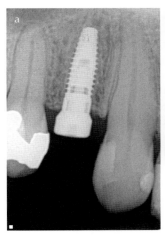
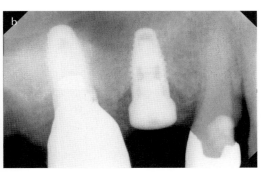

6.11. (a) Favorably angled diagnostic radiograph showing threads, connection detail, and bone level. (b) Poorly angled radiograph.

- Verify the fit of protective *occlusal devices* and patient compliance in wearing them.

6.8   Peri-implant health assessment and treatment

Peri-implant health assessment, professional cleaning of the implants, and oral hygiene advice is recommended at 6-monthly intervals, or more often in cases with ongoing periodontal problems, on a case-by-case basis (Schou et al. 1992; Lang et al. 1997, 2000; Weber and Cochran 1998).

The following should be assessed:

- *Plaque control:* use plaque indices.
- *Peri-implant soft tissue health—bleeding on probing (BOP) and pocket depths:* gentle probing (nylon probe) should not elicit bleeding. Bleeding may indicate mucositis, or peri-implantitis, that is, pocketing and bone loss.
- *Peri-implantitis:* where bone loss is suspected, probing depths should be recorded.
- *Purulent discharge.*
- *Hyperplastic tissue growth.*

- *Fistula formation:* a fistula is often related to incomplete seating of cover screws or abutments. A postoperative radiograph helps confirm complete abutment seating.
- *Gingival recession.*
- *Mobility:* perceptible mobility is likely to be due to restoration loosening. An implant that is mobile has failed and will have inflammatory signs and symptoms.
- *Radiographs:* peri-implant bone level should be checked with perpendicular radiographs (bitewing and peri-apical) in the presence of pockets greater than 5.0 mm and adverse soft tissue signs. *Radiographs do not show buccal or lingual bone levels.* (Roos et al. 1997) (Fig. 6.11a,b).

Implant surfaces and biofilms

The implant collar, IAJ, ledges seen in platform-switching, implant threads and textured surfaces, all have implications for biofilm removal (Fig. 6.12). The daily removal of bacterial plaque around implants is essential for soft tissue health. This is analogous to maintaining

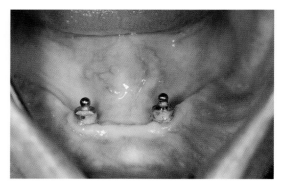

6.12. Plaque deposits on ball abutments, but relatively healthy adjacent mucosa.

periodontal health around natural teeth (Heydenrijk et al. 2002).

The presence of deposits of plaque and calculus causes an immune-mediated chronic inflammatory response (mucositis and peri-implantitis) analogous to gingivitis and periodontitis (Lang and Berglundh 2011). Peri-implantitis may lead to tissue recession and implant thread exposure, which further compounds the plaque control problem. It is difficult to remove biofilms from exposed threads, ledges, and textured surfaces.

As a profession, we must develop effective strategies for debridement and maintenance of exposed implant surfaces that result from bone loss and tissue recession (Klinge and Meyle 2012).

Peri-implant probing

It is generally accepted in periodontics that a 2.0 to 3.0 mm sulcus is easy to maintain, whereas a sulcus of 5.0 mm or greater, is more problematic due to oxygen deficit and growth of anaerobic organisms. However, sulcus depth around healthy implants can range between 2.0 and 6.0 mm. This variable sulcus depth is due to the varied thicknesses of ridge mucosa surrounding the implant and abutment collar caused by scarring following extractions (Ericsson and Lindhe 1993). The deeper sulcus does not imply a disease state, and the presence of the deeper pockets is not necessarily accompanied by inflammation or bone loss. When probing the peri-implant sulcus, access can be complicated by bulbous restorations and platform-switched designs (Fig. 6.13a–d).

Probing depths are shown to be more inconsistent around implants than natural teeth in controlled research conditions (Mombelli and Lang 1998). It is important to be aware of this difference in probing between the natural periodontium and implants. It is widely accepted that there is no direct fibrous attachment to the implant, as with a natural tooth, and that the tissue in the base of the sulcus can easily be penetrated by a probe, causing bleeding (Gerber et al. 2009; Lang and Tonetti 2010).

Keratinized (attached), nonkeratinized peri-implant cuff/mucosa

While it is accepted that implants survive without a band of keratinized peri-implant tissue, it is also accepted that such a band is highly desirable (Schrott et al. 2009; Lin et al. 2013). In cases with nonkeratinized mucosa, there may be an increase in plaque accumulation and peri-implant tissue inflammation, but not necessarily bone loss (Fig. 6.14). Keratinized attached mucosa has several advantages over nonkeratinized mobile tissue:

- It resists plaque removal trauma better.
- It resists abrasion during mastication better.
- It is less likely to collapse over the implant platform during prosthetic work.
- There is less likelihood of gingival recession.

Treatment of soft tissue problems and peri-implant infection

Implants without plaque or calculus deposits with adjacent healthy peri-implant soft tissue

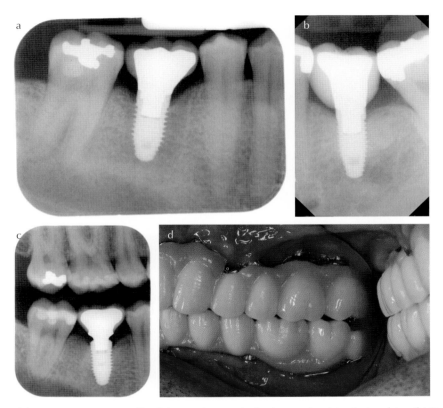

6.13. (a) Favorable crown emergence profile giving good access for hygiene and peri-implant probing. (b) Overcontoured crown restricting hygiene and peri-implant probing. (c) Platform-switched crown creating hygiene and peri-implant probing difficulty. (d) Complex fixed prostheses restricting access for hygiene and peri-implant probing (courtesy of Dr B. Kim).

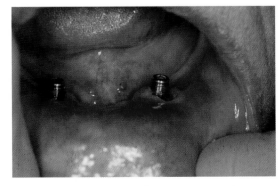

6.14. Mobile nonkeratinized mucosa surrounding overdenture abutments.

(no BOP, no suppuration, pocket depth 3.0–4.0 mm) may be considered clinically stable. Routine care, including *scaling and prophylaxis*, can be performed by the dentist or hygienist. Nylon or carbon fiber scalers are recommended in order to avoid scratching implant surfaces (Lang and Tonetti 2010).

More severe cases of mucositis, excessively mobile peri-implant tissue, hyperplasia, recession, or peri-implantitis should be referred to a periodontist for monitoring and treatment. General health issues and smoking must be taken into account and monitored.

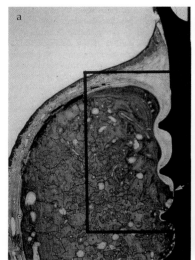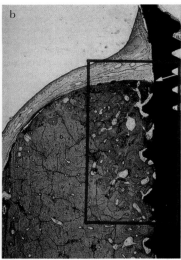

6.15. Peri-implantitis treatment in an animal model. Histologic documentation of cumulative interceptive supportive therapy (CIST): regimens A + B + C + D: mechanical, antiseptic cleaning, administration of systemic antibiotics plus regenerative surgical therapy in a dog model. (a) Bone fill within the red frame (new bone in darker stain), but very limited reosseointegration in the apical portion of an experimental peri-implantitis lesion (white arrow) on a turned titanium implant surface. (b) Bone fill within the red frame (new bone in darker stain), but almost complete (>80%) reosseointegration of an experimental peri-implantitis lesion (white arrow) on a microroughened (SLA) titanium implant surface. Lang NP, Tonetti MS, in Froum S [ed.] *Dental Implant Complications: Etiology, Prevention, and Treatment.* Wiley-Blackwell, p. 130 (adapted from Persson et al. [2001] *Clin Oral Implants Res.* 12: 595–603.)

There are many approaches to the treatment of peri-implant infection. The reader is referred to Heitz-Mayfield (2008), Froum (2010), and Schwarz and Becker (2010) for detailed discussion on treatment of mucositis, fistulae, hyperplasia, bone dehiscence and fenestration, and peri-implantitis. Treatment of peri-implantitis is a problematic evolving situation. A sequence of therapeutic measures from debridement (A) through antiseptic (B) and antibacterial therapy (C) to resective (D) or regenerative therapies, is referred to as cumulative interceptive supportive therapy (CIST). Treatment depends on the severity and extent or the peri-implant lesion.

Conservative therapy should be instituted to improve plaque control, along with scaling and antibiotics, before more complex guided bone regeneration techniques are considered. More complex GBR treatments may not ultimately be successful (Chiapasco and Zaniboni 2009;

Esposito et al. 2012). Regenerative success has been documented with a Straumann SLA® surface (Persson et al. 2001) (Fig. 6.15).

A summary of CIST treatment approach to peri-implantitis:

- Plaque control emphasis
- Mechanical debridement (A) (carbon fiber curettes) and polishing
- Antiseptic treatment (B) (chlorhexidine digluconate daily rinse 0.1%, 0.12%, 0.2%, or gel application to the site for 3–4 weeks)
- Systemic or local antibiotics (C) for pockets of ≥6.0 mm: metronidazole (350 mg/t.i.d./10 days) in conjunction with antiseptic therapy
- Regenerative or resective surgery (D) supplemented by polishing of textured surfaces and removal of threads. (*There is inadequate documentation on such therapies to date.*)
- Implant removal when the implant is mobile.

References

Adell R. (1985) Tissue integrated prostheses in clinical dentistry. *Int Dent J.* 35(4):259–65.

Adell R, Lekholm U, Rockler B, Brånemark P-I. (1981) A 15-year study of osseointegrated implants in the treatment of the edentulous jaw. *Int J Oral Surg.* 10(6):387–416.

Albrektsson T, Lekholm U. (1989) Osseointegration: current state of the art. *Dent Clin North Am.* 33(4):537–54.

Albrektsson T, Zarb G, Worthington P, Eriksson AR. (1986) The long-term efficacy of currently used dental implants: a review and proposed criteria of success. *Int J Oral Maxillofac Implants.* 1(1):11–25. Review.

Brånemark P-I, Zarb GA, Albrektsson T. (eds.) (1985) *Tissue-Integrated Prostheses: Osseointegration in Clinical Dentistry.* Quintessence, Chicago.

Buser D, Mericske-Stern R, Bernard JP, Behneke A, Behneke N, Hirt HP, Belser UC, Lang NP. (1997) Long-term evaluation of non-submerged ITI implants. Part 1: 8-year life table analysis of a prospective multi-center study with 2359 implants. *Clin Oral Implants Res.* 8(3):161–72.

Carlsson GE. (2009) Dental occlusion: modern concepts and their application in implant prosthodontics. *Odontology.* 97(1):8–17.

Chiapasco M, Zaniboni M. (2009) Clinical outcomes of GBR procedures to correct peri-implant dehiscences and fenestrations: a systematic review. *Clin Oral Implants Res.* 20(Suppl 4):113–23.

Dawson A, Chen S. (2009) *The SAC Classification in Implant Dentistry.* Quintessence, Berlin.

D'Hoedt B, Schulte W. (1989) A comparative study of results with various endosseous implant systems. *Int J Oral Maxillofac Implants.* 4(2): 95–105.

Ericsson I, Lindhe J. (1993) Probing depth at implants and teeth. An experimental study in the dog. *J Clin Periodontol.* 20(9):623–7.

Esposito M, Maghaireh H, Grusovin MG, Ziounas I, Worthington HV. (2012) Soft tissue management for dental implants: what are the most effective techniques? A Cochrane systematic review. *Eur J Oral Implantol.* 5(3):221–38.

Froum S. (ed.) (2010) *Dental Implant Complications: Etiology, Prevention, and Treatment.* Wiley-Blackwell, Ames.

Gerber JA, Tan WC, Balmer TE, Salvi GE, Lang NP. (2009) Bleeding on probing and pocket probing depth in relation to probing pressure and mucosal health around oral implants. *Clin Oral Implants Res.* 20(1):75–8.

Heitz-Mayfield LJ. (2008) Peri-implant diseases: diagnosis and risk indicators. *J Clin Periodontol.* 35(8 Suppl):292–304.

Heydenrijk K, Meijer HJ, van der Reijden WA, Raghoebar GM, Vissink A, Stegenga B. (2002) Microbiota around root-form endosseous implants: a review of the literature. *Int J Oral Maxillofac Implants.* 17(6):829–38.

Jokstad A. (2009) *Osseointegration and Dental Implants.* Wiley-Blackwell, Ames.

Klinge B, Meyle J; Working Group 2. (2012) Peri-implant tissue destruction. The Third EAO Consensus Conference 2012. *Clin Oral Implants Res.* 23(Suppl 6):108–10.

Lang NP, Berglundh T; Working Group 4 of Seventh European Workshop on Periodontology. (2011) Periimplant diseases: where are we now?: Consensus of the Seventh European Workshop on Periodontology. *J Clin Periodontol.* 38(Suppl 11): 178–81.

Lang NP, Tonetti MS. (2010) Peri-implantitis: etiology, pathogenesis, prevention, and therapy. In: SJ Froum (ed.), *Dental Implant Complications: Etiology, Prevention, and Treatment.* Wiley-Blackwell, Ames, pp. 119–33.

Lang NP, Mombelli A, Tonetti MS, Brägger U, Hämmerle CH. (1997) Clinical trials on therapies for peri-implant infections. *Ann Periodontol.* 2(1): 343–56.

Lang NP, Wilson TG, Corbet EF. (2000) Biological complications with dental implants: their prevention, diagnosis and treatment. *Clin Oral Implants Res.* 11(Suppl 1):146–55.

Lekholm U, Zarb GA. (1985) Patient selection and preparation. In: P-I Brånemark, GA Zarb, T Albrektsson (eds.), *Tissue-Integrated Prostheses: Osseointegration in Clinical Dentistry.* Quintessence, Chicago.

Lekholm U, Gunne J, Henry P, Higuchi K, Lindén U, Bergström C, van Steenberghe D. (1999) Survival of the Brånemark implant in partially edentulous jaws: a 10-year prospective multicenter study. *Int J Oral Maxillofac Implants.* 14(5):639–45.

Lin GH, Chan HL, Wang HL. (2013) The significance of keratinized mucosa on implant health: a systematic review. *J Periodontol.* 84(12):1755–1767.

Mombelli A, Lang NP. (1998) The diagnosis and treatment of peri-implantitis. *Periodontol 2000.* 17:63–76.

Mombelli A, Müller N, Cionca N. (2012) The epidemiology of peri-implantitis. *Clin Oral Implants Res.* 23(Suppl 6):67–76.

Persson LG, Berglundh T, Lindhe J, Sennerby L. (2001) Re-osseointegration after treatment of peri-implantitis at different implant surfaces. An experimental study in the dog. *Clin Oral Implants Res.* 12(6):595–603.

Roos J, Sennerby L, Lekholm U, Jemt T, Gröndahl K, Albrektsson T. (1997) A qualitative and quantitative method for evaluating implant success: a 5-year retrospective analysis of the Brånemark implant. *Int J Oral Maxillofac Implants.* 12(4):504–14.

Roos-Jansåker AM, Renvert H, Lindahl C, Renvert S. (2006) Nine- to fourteen-year follow-up of implant treatment. Part III: factors associated with peri-implant lesions. *J Clin Periodontol.* 33(4):296–301.

Schou S, Holmstrup P, Hjørting-Hansen E, Lang NP. (1992) Plaque-induced marginal tissue reactions of osseointegrated oral implants: a review of the literature. *Clin Oral Implants Res.* 3(4):149–61.

Schou S, Holmstrup P, Worthington HV, Esposito M. (2006) Outcome of implant therapy in patients with previous tooth loss due to periodontitis. *Clin Oral Implants Res.* 17(Suppl 2):104–23.

Schroeder A, Sutter F, Krekeler G. (1991) *Oral Implantology: Basics—ITI Hollow Cylinder.* Thieme, New York.

Schroeder A, Sutter F, Buser D, Krekeler G. (1996) *Oral Implantology: Basics—ITI Hollow Cylinder.* Thieme, New York.

Schrott AR, Jimenez M, Hwang JW, Fiorellini J, Weber HP. (2009) Five-year evaluation of the influence of keratinized mucosa on peri-implant soft-tissue health and stability around implants supporting full-arch mandibular fixed prostheses. *Clin Oral Implants Res.* 20(10):1170–7.

Schwarz F, Becker J. (2010) *Peri-Implant Infection: Etiology, Diagnosis and Treatment.* Quintessence, London.

Sennerby L, Roos J. (1998) Surgical determinants of clinical success of osseointegrated oral implants: a review of the literature. *Int J Prosthodont.* 11(5):408–20.

Sorní M, Guarinós J, García O, Peñarrocha M. (2005) Implant rehabilitation of the atrophic upper jaw: a review of the literature since 1999. *Med Oral Patol Oral Cir Bucal.* 10(Suppl 1):E45–56. [Article in English, Spanish].

Van Steenberghe D, Brånemark PI, Quirynen M, De Mars G, Naert I. (1991) The rehabilitation of oral defects by osseointegrated implants. *J Clin Periodontol.* 18(6):488–93.

Weber HP, Cochran DL. (1998) The soft tissue response to osseointegrated dental implants. *J Prosthet Dent.* 79(1):79–89.

Wittneben JG, Webber HP. (2013) *ITI Treatment Guide-Volume 6: Extended Edentulous Spaces in the Esthetic Zone.* (eds. D Wismeijer, S Chen, D Buser). Quintessence, Berlin.

Zarb GA. (1983) *Proceedings of the Toronto conference on osseointegration in clinical dentistry.* (Reprinted from the *J Prosthet Dent.* [1983] 49 and 50: 1–84.). Mosby, St Louis.

7 Surgical Planning and Procedures

7.1   Introduction

The literature has reported consistently high implant success rates in varied oral scenarios. The basic two-stage surgical protocol is well established. Immediate placement following extraction and early loading protocols have become increasingly popular, but place greater demands on the surgeon and restorative dentist. Implant surgery is a demanding procedure and implant outcome depends on surgical skill, experience, and careful planning. High implant failure rates have been linked to limited surgical experience (Sennerby and Roos 1998). Specialized surgical training or mentoring is strongly advised for the general dentist contemplating implant surgery.

When a patient is referred for a surgical implant opinion, a case history, radiographs, study models, and a tentative plan should be forwarded to the surgeon in preparation for the consultation. A joint consultation would be ideal but is not always possible. The surgeon may choose to have further medical consults and specific radiographs before giving a diagnosis, treatment plan, and prognosis. Should the consultation prove inconclusive, it will be necessary for the dentist, surgeon, and patient to further discuss the case. The benefits and risks of implant surgery should be discussed, while presenting alternative treatment possibilities and available evidence.

When the decision has been made to proceed with surgery, a consent form is signed and the patient is scheduled for surgery after preliminary care is completed. It is necessary to plan a surgical guide and a provisionalization method that works for the patient. Good communication between the restorative dentist and the surgeon is an important factor for a successful

Fundamentals of Implant Dentistry, First Edition. Gerard Byrne.
© 2014 John Wiley & Sons, Inc. Published 2014 by John Wiley & Sons, Inc.
Companion website: www.wiley.com/go/byrne/implants

outcome. Responsibility for maintenance and complications must be clear within the treatment group.

7.2 Patient education and expectations

Surgical risks, postsurgical complications, anesthesia, sedation, antibiotic therapy, and provisionals are all discussed in advance of surgery. General health issues are discussed in relation to proposed implant surgery, especially issues that may affect bone healing. The aesthetic and functional limitations of implant therapy are explained. Emphasis is given to the challenges of replacing soft tissue or augmenting bone for the aesthetic zone. Techniques for grafting and bone regeneration are presented as needed. Expectations are tempered by the explanation of risk factors.

The sequence of presurgical assessment and treatment may be outlined as follows:

- Medical and dental history
- Clinical examination
- Special tests and medical consultations
- Diagnosis
- Consideration of treatment options
- Surgical treatment plan
- Informed consent
- Implant surgery
- Surgery review
- Second-stage surgery as needed.

7.3 Medical assessment and management

A thorough medical history and assessment is essential. After a thorough assessment, the surgeon should be satisfied that the patient is physically and psychologically ready for the implant procedures. The surgeon can then focus on the technical details of the implantation.

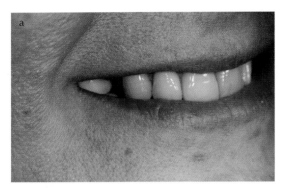

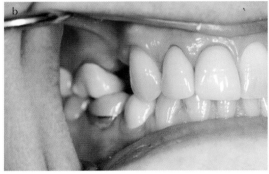

7.1. (a) Favorable aesthetic scenario for implant tooth placement in a case with relatively low smile line. (b) There is some ridge volume loss but reasonable ridge height.

The surgeon reviews the medical history and the radiographs, takes additional radiographs or a CT image, and devises a surgical strategy in concert with the referring dentist. Discussion with the patient follows, explaining such factors as: potential surgical complications, sedation, grafting, socket augmentation, immediate placement, delayed placement, one- or two-stage surgery, loading time, and other possibilities and eventualities. Interim restorations will feature prominently in this discussion, as well as postsurgical management (Fig. 7.1a,b).

Medical management

The referring dentist makes a thorough assessment of the prevailing health condition of the patient prior to referral, and relates pertinent health issues and tentative restorative possibilities to the surgeon. The surgeon focuses on the risks presented by general medical conditions, and local conditions that might lead to increased postoperative morbidity. The surgeon decides whether the risks pose a threat to patient health and to implant survival. Any condition that adversely affects the ability to heal following surgery increases the risk of implant failure. Consultation with the patient's physician is necessary to ascertain the status of specific medical conditions. The potential risks are weighed against benefits for the individual patient. Quality of life improvement from implants may be important for the patient who has had complete tooth loss and jaw irradiation for cancer despite any moderate risks. The following conditions need careful assessment and physician consultation in terms of surgical management:

- Cardiovascular conditions:
  - Coagulation problem with anticoagulant therapy
  - Hypertension
  - Angina pectoris
  - Myocardial infarction
  - Congestive heart failure
  - Risk of endocarditis.
- Diabetes mellitus
- Compromised immune system caused by immunodeficiency, autoimmune disease, cancer treatment, and organ transplants
- Irradiated facial bones
- Bone antiresorptive (bisphosphonate) therapy
- Psychiatric disorders, personality disorders
- Addiction to controlled drugs.

The risk of excessive bleeding during or after surgery is a management issue for patients with coagulation problems or who are taking *oral anticoagulants*. The patient's physician must be consulted and a recent international normalized ratio (INR) test and INR history

obtained. Implant surgery or withdrawal of Coumadin® therapy should only take place in concert with the patient's physician. The INR value for normal prothrombin time is "1." A therapeutic INR value for minor oral surgery is between 2 and 3 (Scully and Wolff 2002). Madrid and Sanz (2009a), in a systematic review, showed that patients with an INR of between 2 and 4 who continued with Coumadin therapy, did not have a significantly higher risk of postoperative bleeding than patients who discontinued the medication. Furthermore, postoperative bleeding events were effectively controlled with local hemostatic measures. More implants, more complex surgery, and grafting may indicate anticoagulant intervention. The INR should be checked on the day of the procedure and surgical trauma kept to a minimum.

Other cardiovascular conditions, such as hypertension, atherosclerosis, and angina, are relatively common in western adult populations and must be managed appropriately for elective minor oral surgery. Additionally, many patients will have had antiresorptive therapy, joint replacements, or be immuno-compromised. Patients with psychiatric issues or history of substance abuse must be carefully screened for their ability to understand and cooperate in the implant therapy process. Similarly, elderly and infirm patients may not be suitable for the rigors of implant treatment. Level of understanding and the ability to cooperate may also be an issue for elderly and institutionalized patients with or without dementia.

7.4 Implications of medical conditions and medications

There are many general medical issues that impinge on elective minor oral surgery, and they can be found in oral surgery textbooks. Additionally this area of surgical interest is thoroughly covered in other implant textbooks (Misch 2007; Block 2011) Prophylactic antibiotics are indicated to reduce the risk of postoperative infection (Esposito et al. 2010a). Certain systemic conditions and medications are relative contraindications to implant surgery due to compromised healing and possible risk to osseointegration (Mombelli and Cionca 2006; Froum 2010). These conditions include:

- Diabetes mellitus
- Immunodeficiency: immunosuppression or chemotherapy
- Bisphosphonate treatment for osteoporosis
- Irradiation of the jawbones
- Smoking.

Diabetes mellitus

Diabetes mellitus is medically managed through a combination of diet, exercise, and medication. Medication may involve multiple daily injections of insulin (slow/medium/fast-acting) or an insulin pump. Poor glycemic control is a risk for postsurgical infection and hence may have a negative impact on implant survival in the short or long term. If there is a concern about glycemic control, a physician consultation is required. Glycemic control is assessed by the patient's physician using glycosylated hemoglobin values (HBAic). Infection risk should be relatively normal when glycemic control is good; however, prophylactic use of antibiotics is recommended. The surgeon will also be aware of the increased risk of hypoglycemic episodes with the possibility of seizure or coma and will plan the surgery accounting for food intake and insulin dosage (peak activity) timing. Poor glycemic control reduces implant survival rate, whereas there is no difference with good glycemic control (Mellado-Valero et al. 2007; Javed and Romanos 2009).

Immunodeficiency

Basic wound healing processes and the ability to fight infection are a function of the patient's immune system that may be compromised in many ways. An example of such immune compromise is with human immunodeficiency virus (HIV) infection, although the use of highly active antiretroviral therapy (HAART) has limited the impact of this condition on wound healing (Shetty and Achong 2005). Autoimmune conditions, such as systemic lupus erythematosus (SLE), rheumatoid arthritis, Sjögren's syndrome, and their associated therapeutic steroids, may also increase surgical and healing risks. Immunosuppressant therapy is commonly used for cancer treatment and organ and bone marrow transplants. Active chemotherapy for cancer is an absolute contraindication for implant surgery.

Antiresorptive therapy for bone dysplasias, cancer, and osteoporosis

Bisphosphonates offer major benefits to certain cancer patients with bone involvement and osteolysis (multiple myeloma of bone and metastatic carcinomas), Paget's disease of bone, and osteoporosis. Bisphosphonates suppress osteoclast function, resulting in increased bone density and mineralization. Bisphosphonates also lead to an increased risk of jaw osteonecrosis; the risk is higher for intravenous than oral administration. Other associated risk factors are chemotherapy and steroid therapy. According to Dibart and Dibart (2011) oncology treatment accounts for 94% of osteonecrosis cases, implicating *intravenous bisphosphonates*. Implant surgery should be avoided for patients being treated with intravenous bisphosphonates, whereas it may be feasible to operate on patients taking oral bisphosphonates after withdrawal of the drug for 3 months and with physician consultation; the withdrawal time is indeterminate. The American Academy of Oral and

Maxillofacial Surgeons (AAOMS 2007) have issued guidance strategies for dealing with patients on bisphosphonates and for treatment of bisphosphonate-related necrosis of the jaws. Madrid and Sanz (2009b) consider that the placement of an implant may be a safe procedure in patients taking oral bisphosphonates for less than 5 years.

Osteoporosis is a secondary consequence of menopause. Patients with osteoporosis have low bone mass and increased incidence of bone fracture. These patients may be on oral bisphosphonates, have limited bone volume, may need grafting, and require careful management of loading conditions. An implant design that is favored for soft bone should be chosen. Smoking is also considered a significant risk factor for these patients.

Irradiation of jawbones

Radiation treatments for cancer of the head and neck carry significant risks for osseointegration of implants. High dose radiation damages the vascular supply of bone and compromises bone healing. Vascularity may be further damaged by the surgery. Changes in irradiated bone increase the risk of postradiation osteonecrosis from implant placement. A systematic review by Colella et al. (2007) showed that:

- No implant failures occurred when radiation dosage was <45 Gy (Gray unit).
- Placement of implants pre- or postradiation did not affect failure rates.
- In irradiated jaws, mandible outcomes were better than the maxilla outcomes.
- The overall implant failure rate in irradiated patients ranged between 1.4% and 12.6%.

Javed et al. (2010) reviewed oral cancer patients and concluded that dental implants can osseointegrate and remain functionally stable in patients having undergone oral cancer treatment.

Smoking

The by-products of smoking: nicotine, carbon monoxide, and hydrogen cyanide have a negative effect on the immune-inflammatory response. The relative risk is greater for the maxillae, grafted sites, and machined screw-type implants. Studies show a twofold higher failure rate in maxilla and a 3.6-fold higher failure rate in bone augmentation cases (Baig and Rajan 2007; Cavalcanti et al. 2011). Additionally, there may be an increased risk of peri-implantitis bone loss during function (Heitz-Mayfield 2008; Lindhe and Meyle 2008). Patients with tobacco habits must be informed of the increased risk, and encouraged toward cessation before implant treatment begins.

Contraindications to implant surgery

- Unrealistic patient expectations
- Poor oral health
- Pregnancy
- Age, that is, patients <20 years and still growing, patients >80 years
- Acute illness
- Chemotherapy
- IV bisphosphonates
- Uncontrolled metabolic disease
- Poor understanding of treatment or compliance issues due to ill health or age.

7.5   Surgical site assessment (see Chapter 5)

Overview of dental status

Supported by:

- Photographs
- Dental examination

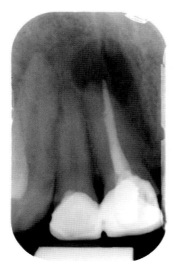

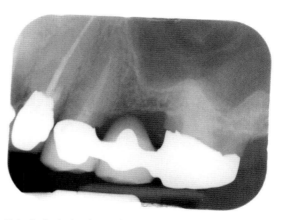

7.4. Periapical radiograph showing limited bone height in pontic area and invagination of the sinus space between and around the molar roots.

7.2. Central incisor with failed endodontic therapy and large peri-apical radiolucency; canine has an apical radiolucency.

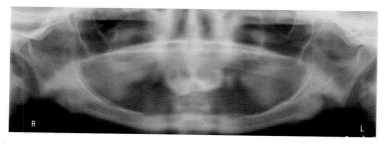

7.3. Panoramic radiograph showing advanced mandibular atrophy.

- Full mouth series and/or panoramic radiograph (Fig. 7.2, Fig. 7.3, and Fig 7.4)
- Study models.

  Assessment of:

- Smile line (see Chapter 5)
- Gingival tissue biotype (see Chapter 5)
- Active infection, pathology
- Adequate opening for surgery
- Occlusion, interarch space, super-eruption, parafunction
- Restorative, endodontic and periodontal condition
- TM dysfunction.

Applied anatomy

Inadequate bone volume focuses the surgeon on the increased risk to vital anatomical structures. Panoramic and peri-apical radiographs give a valuable diagnostic overview of the jaws. A computed tomogram (CT or CBCT) is ideal prior to surgery to assess bone volume. Anatomic features that need to be respected when planning surgery include:

- Root convergence
- Mandibular canal and neurovascular bundle
- Naso-palatine canal and neurovascular bundle

- Greater palatine foramina and neurovascular bundles
- Submental, sublingual, and submandibular fossae with neurovascular bundles
- Mental foramina and neurovascular bundles
- Facial and sublingual blood vessels
- Maxillary sinus, contiguous nerves and blood vessels
- Floor of nose.

Radiographs

A panoramic radiograph is the standard diagnostic film; it gives a good overview. Usually, peri-apical and bitewing films will also be taken prior to referral to the surgeon. Other radiography may be desirable and should be chosen by the surgeon for the assessment of the cross-sectional bone configuration and bone quality (Tyndall et al. 2012). When a CBCT is planned, then a *radiographic guide* should be fabricated. This uses radio-opaque teeth or inserts/occlusal holes to indicate proposed final prosthetic implant and tooth position relative to available bone. It serves to illustrate whether the proposed implant position and reconstruction are feasible without ridge grafting or guided bone regeneration.

- A *panoramic film* should be recorded to check for bone abnormality and to assess bone height for implant placement, keeping in mind image distortion and magnification of approximately 25%. Metal markers can be attached to an existing denture to determine the magnification ratio. Panoramic examination can be considered a safe, low radiation-dose preoperative evaluation procedure for routine posterior mandibular implant placement. A safety margin of ≥ 2.0 mm above the mandibular canal should be maintained (Vazquez et al. 2008).
- A *lateral skull film* may prove useful to the surgeon for assessment of mandibular cross-sectional dimensions, particularly if tomography is unavailable.

- *Cone beam computed tomography (CBCT)* is now becoming widely available. The AAOMR recommends CBCT imaging as the current method of choice for cross-sectional imaging as it provides the greatest diagnostic yield at an acceptable radiation dosage risk. It permits accurate 3D volumetric rendering of bone anatomy at the proposed implant sites, such as the extent of a "knife edge" bony ridge, mandibular concavities, and the location of contiguous anatomic structures (Fanning 2011; Cavézian and Pasquet 2012). Although CT technology has not been shown to definitively improve implant outcomes or decrease morbidity, it is gradually becoming an indispensable aid for implant surgery (Fig. 7.5, Fig. 7.6, Fig. 7.7, and Fig. 7.8).

Bone volume (height, width, and shape)

The implant site may still contain teeth or it may be a residual ridge. When extraction is planned, an assessment must be made of existing bone loss, peri-radicular infection, and the potential for alveolar damage during extraction. A decision must be made as to whether to allow natural socket healing prior to implantation, or to conduct immediate implantation at the time of extraction.

Resorption of the alveolar bone is variable and is related to many factors including: extraction trauma, periodontal bone loss, duration of tooth absence, and the wearing of removable prostheses. Bone resorption of the alveolus is dramatic during the first year following tooth loss. Tan et al. (2012) reported rapid ridge shrinkage within 6 months of extraction of between 29% and 63% horizontally, and between 11% and 22% vertically. Bone resorption is exacerbated by denture wear (Tallgren et al. 1980). Some patients have minimal bone resorption due to recent atraumatic tooth loss or tooth loss in older patients with no periodontal disease. Advanced periodontal disease may

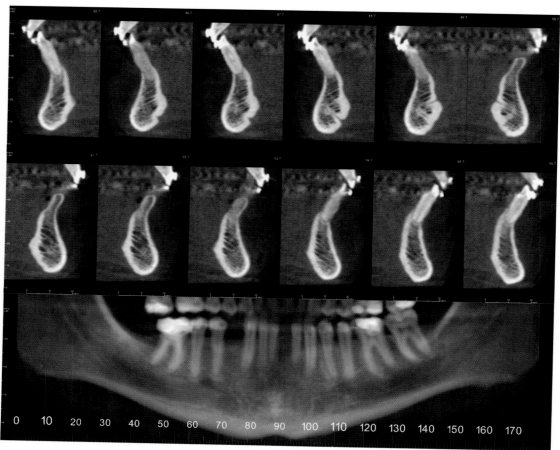

7.5. CBCT images showing a reformatted panoramic image and sections from anterior mandible #85 to 96; note cortical plate thickness around tooth roots and lingual foraminae (courtesy of Dr. S. Gonzalez).

leave little alveolar bone height after extraction and healing. Some cases with little bone loss may require ridge reduction, crest flattening or "tabling," prior to implant surgery. This is most likely in the case of extraction and simultaneous placement of mandibular overdenture implants.

The bone configuration determines the diameter and length of implant that can be placed. Traditionally, bone volume was assessed using clinical palpation, and *bone mapping* with periodontal probing of the bone

through the mucosa under local anesthesia. Bone height can be assessed with peri-apical and panoramic radiographs using metal reference markers for magnification ratios. Bone volume is most easily determined with the use of CBCT images. In some cases, there may be adequate bone for placing an implant, but the bone may not be in the ideal aesthetic or mechanical zone. It must be determined as to whether bone grafting is needed or whether to compromise on implant length, diameter, or position.

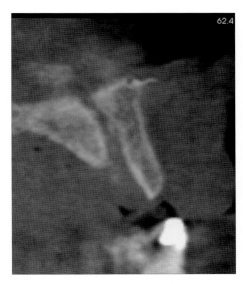

7.6. CBCT cross-sectional image of the pre-maxilla showing the naso-palatine canal (courtesy of Dr. S. Gonzalez).

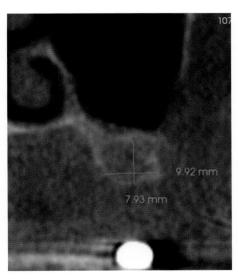

7.7. CBCT cross-sectional image of the posterior maxilla (first molar) showing ridge dimensions (courtesy of Dr. S. Gonzalez).

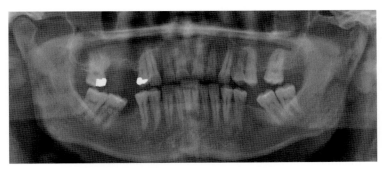

7.8. Severe bone deficiency in the maxillary right edentulous space caused by molar extraction with subsequent oro-antral fistula repair.

Bone density or quality

Bone density or quality is more difficult to assess definitively preoperatively, although this aspect is likely to change with better diagnostic imaging technology. Currently, bone quality is best assessed by the surgeon's tactile sensitivity intraoperatively, while preparing the osteotomy. Bone density varies depending on the oral location, and this has implications for surgical protocol, type of implant, healing, and loading times. High implant failure rates have been associated with poor bone quality and short implants in atrophic maxillae. Lekholm and Zarb's (1985) description and diagrams classify the types of jaw bone encountered, based on the thickness of the cortical plates, the structure of the cancellous bone core, and the degrees of edentulous ridge resorption. For communication within the profession, their classification of bone density and quality has become accepted (Fig. 7.9):

- *I*: Homogeneous compact bone (e.g., anterior mandible)
- *II*: A thick layer of compact bone surrounds a core of dense trabecular bone (e.g., anterior and posterior mandible)
- *III*: A thin layer of cortical bone surrounds dense trabecular bone (e.g., posterior mandible, anterior maxilla)
- *IV*: A thin layer of cortical bone surrounds a core of low density trabecular bone (e.g., posterior maxilla)

Misch (2007) has developed an alternative bone density classification D1 to D4 based on his extensive experience in implant surgery over three decades. His classification is as follows:

- *D1 bone (like oak or maple)*: dense cortical bone as in the anterior mandible
- *D2 bone (like pine wood)*: dense-to-thick porous cortical bone and coarse trabecular bone, usually in the anterior mandible
- *D3 bone (like compressed balsa wood)*: porous cortical and fine trabecular bone in the posterior mandible and anterior maxilla
- *D4 bone (like soft balsa wood or dense styrofoam)*: posterior maxilla.

Misch estimates a much greater bone-to-implant (BIC) contact for D1 bone, at the time of surgery, decreasing dramatically to D4 bone. This has implications for bone preparation and implant shape selection. Slow, staged drilling and a bone tap will be required in dense D1 and D2 bone in order to achieve an optimum result. An osteotome or a slightly smaller diameter drill may be used for final sizing of the osteotomy in D4 bone. Misch's surgical insights are a useful reference for the practicing implant surgeon. Misch enumerates

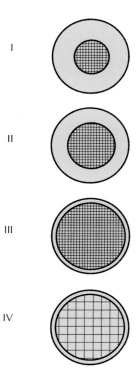

7.9. Diagram of bone quality as defined by Lekholm and Zarb (1985) for implants. I: Homogeneous compact bone. II: A thick layer of compact bone surrounds a core of dense trabecular bone. III: A thin layer of cortical bone surrounds dense trabecular bone. IV: A thin layer of cortical bone surrounds a core of low density trabecular bone (courtesy of H. Byrne).

guidelines for osteotomy preparation and implant size for each type of bone density. The initial stability of the implant is a function of precise surgery while taking into account bone quality.

Spatial factors

Space between adjacent crown and roots

The minimum mesio-distal space for implant placement between adjacent crowns and roots is the greatest diameter of the implant plus 1.0 to 1.5mm mesially and distally (Fig. 7.10a,b).

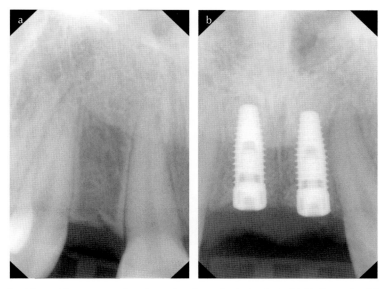

7.10. (a) Radiograph of favorable crown and root spacing for a single implant. (b) Radiograph of favorable crown and root spacing for two implants.

Hence, the minimum mesio-distal space required for a 4.0 mm implant is 6.0 mm. It is important for the surgeon to bear in mind the proximity and angle of roots in relation to the above safety margin when planning surgery. A bone thickness of between 2.0 and 3.0 mm is recommended between two adjacent implants. It is necessary to plan narrow, regular, or wide diameter implants, or a combination, depending on the space, the restorative needs, and the number of teeth that are missing. The restorative dentist apprises the surgeon of such issues on radiographs, on study models and interim restorations.

Vertical space for crown/denture (from occlusal contact to implant platform)

The *vertical space* or height available for the implant prosthesis inclusive of implant abutments and retentive components must be assessed. A space of at least 5.0 to 7.0 mm between the proposed implant platform and the opposing teeth is desirable for crown and bridgework. A minimum of 10.0 mm from the implant platform, or bony ridge crest, to the occlusal plane is needed to fabricate an implant overdenture. Cases that have limited interarch space, as with recent extractions or little or no bone loss require careful evaluation for possible ridge reduction before proceeding.

Bucco-lingual bone volume

A minimum bucco-lingual ridge width of 6.0 mm is required for a 4.0 mm implant, allowing at least 1.0 mm of bone to remain buccally and lingually after implant insertion. Sometimes, the ridge may need to be flattened to accommodate the implant collar diameter. If the remaining facial or lingual bone is less than 1.0 mm, there is an increased risk of bone dehiscence or fenestration during surgery. Ridge grafting should be considered with narrow ridges.

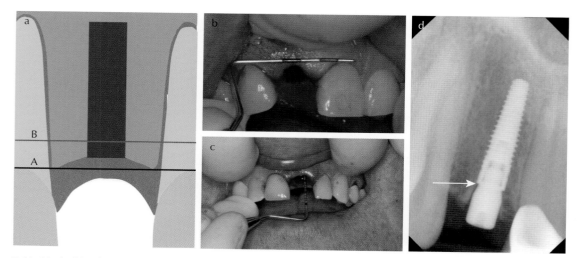

7.11. Vertical implant position: (a) Diagram showing "safety" zone for vertical position of an implant platform (distance A to B = 3.0 mm). The implant platform is depicted at bone crest level (courtesy of H. Byrne). (b) Line A from 7.11b transferred to a clinical scenario with a periodontal probe (courtesy Dr. S. Whitney). The implant platform should be positioned at the bone crest, or 2.0–3.0 mm apical to the probe position (courtesy Dr. S. Whitney). (c) Immediate implant placement: a periodontal probe indicates the implant platform is 2.0–3.0 mm apical to the adjacent cervical lines and labial gingival margin. (d) An implant platform placed too far apically (arrow) leads to crestal bone loss of 1.0–2.0 mm apical to the implant platform (courtesy Dr. S. Whitney).

3D implant positioning

Generally, implants will follow the alignment of adjacent teeth whether anterior or posterior (Fig. 7.11a–d). Occasionally, bucco-lingual positioning is compromised by bone resorption. From a biomechanical perspective, implants should be placed in line with occlusal forces when possible, symmetrically relative to the midline, parallel to each other, and at the same occlusal height. It is generally desirable to position the implant platform flush with the bony ridge crest. Placement of implants in poor positions or at bad angles can be avoided with careful planning.

Implant position: Aesthetic and safety guidelines

As a guideline, where a single healthy tooth has been lost, the implant platform must be positioned between 1.0 and 2.0 mm lingual to a line drawn between cervical lines of adjacent teeth, and at the bony crest or between 2.0 and 3.0 mm apical to the adjacent (labial) cervical line. This positioning facilitates good emergence profile and thus optimal gingival contour, while conserving bone around adjacent teeth. Poor positioning and angulation creates potential aesthetic, biological and mechanical complications. The following guidelines should be adhered to:

- Ensure that the implant platform is flush with the alveolar bone crest (which may need flattening). Polished necks are designed to extend above the crest.
- Between 1.0 and 2.0 mm of bone should surround the implant bucco-lingually and mesio-distally.
- Between 2.0 and 3.0 mm of bone should remain between adjacent implant platforms.
- The implant must be positioned at least 2.0 mm away from nerve canals.

- Between 1.0 and 2.0 mm bone should remain between the implant and the maxillary antrum, the floor of the nose, and the mandiblular inferior border or cortical plates.
- Allow 5.0 mm between an anterior implant and the mental foramen to allow for the posterior loop of the mental nerve.

Gingival biotype and the band of attached gingiva

An implant or implant abutment, should ideally be surrounded by a band of attached gingiva. With a thin gingival biotype, it is difficult to retain the interdental scalloping seen between natural teeth, and labial recession is more likely. Wearing an RPD in such cases during healing is not recommended. An immediate provisional restoration in infraocclusion may be fabricated to help maintain soft tissue contour and position. Although the presence or absence of attached gingiva may not directly affect implant prognosis, attached gingiva facilitates implant hygiene and marginal tissue stability. By facilitating implant maintenance, the long-term prognosis of the implant is enhanced. During surgical flap reflection, the attached band may be split evenly labio-lingually to give the optimum result. This can be quite challenging in cases of severe ridge resorption. Alternatively, papillae may be left undisturbed, or a flapless procedure may be used (Chen and Buser 2008). Esposito et al. (2012) have reviewed various approaches for flap management and corrective soft tissue surgery.

7.6 Implant surgery

Patient preparation and informed consent

Prior to surgery, the restorative dentist and surgeon should have a final discussion with the patient. It is important that the patient fully understands the procedures, including the use of analgesia, anesthesia, sedatives, anxiolytics, and antibiotics. When the patient is satisfied to proceed with implant surgery and the restorative treatment, an *informed consent* form should be signed.

The surgeon carefully plans for certain conditions and medications, such as anticoagulants, bisphosphonate therapy, cancer treatment, chronic steroid therapy, and cardiovascular disease. When risk is very high, as with coagulation problems, it may be wise to treat the patient in a hospital setting. Generally, a dedicated surgical operatory without operative dental equipment, is recommended. An aseptic environment and dedicated assisting are paramount. Antibiotic prophylaxis is required for patients who are at risk of endocarditis, for patients who are at higher risk of infection postoperatively, and when more complex surgery is undertaken. There is some evidence to show that 2 g amoxicillin given 1 hour preoperatively significantly reduces failures of dental implants placed in routine cases. (Esposito et al. 2010a). Wagenberg and Froum (2006) showed that failure to use postoperative amoxicillin with immediate implant placement led to higher implant failure rates.

Surgical operating field

- Chlorhexidine mouthrinses 0.12% for 30 seconds
- Standard aseptic surgical technique: sterile drapes and lavage of surgical field with betadine or chlorhexidine
- Sterile instruments
- Dedicated implant surgical handpiece
- Good illumination
- X-ray unit for intraoperative radiographs.

The surgical guide

Following the surgical consultation and formulation of a definitive plan with the surgeon, the

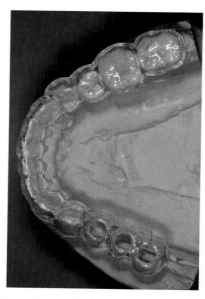

7.12. A surgical guide for guiding the surgeon with implant pilot drills.

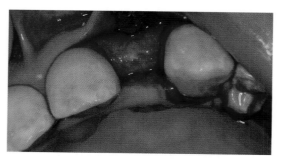

7.13. A conservative mucoperiosteal flap (courtesy of Dr. S. Whitney).

restorative dentist provides the surgeon with a surgical guide (Fig. 7.12). The surgical guide is generally fabricated on a cast with a diagnostic wax-up of the planned restoration. Alternatively, it may be a modified interim partial or complete denture. The surgical guide allows the surgeon to visualize the final restoration and the preferred restorative implant site with reference to the proposed tooth position. Generally, it acts as a guide to implant positioning facio-lingually and mesio-distally, which has important aesthetic and mechanical implications. It should not interfere with flap reflection and should allow the surgeon flexibility with drill and guide pin positioning. More advanced techniques use computer generated precision guides that determine the exact position and depth of implants (see Chapter 11).

Flap management

Muco-periosteal flap elevation gives optimal surgical access (Fig. 7.13) (Esposito et al. 2012).

Punch or flapless access may be suitable for immediate placement or guided placement techniques.

- Usually, a crestal incision is made that splits the attached gingiva bucco-lingually. A full-thickness muco-periosteal flap is elevated. Some flap incisions maintain papillae for aesthetics with single implants. Flap releasing incisions are used as needed.
- Large lingual flaps should be sutured back.
- Avoid mental neuro-vascular bundles during incisions and protect them during flap elevation.
- Maintain attached mucosa if possible for the future restoration.
- Preserve marginal bone and soft tissue height by avoiding adjacent teeth.
- Create an optimum emergence profile and papilla height with immediate provisional crowns (if used).

Implant osteotomy site, placing the implant

Most implant companies provide detailed guidance on osteotomy preparation and implant insertion (Fig. 7.14a,b). There should be detailed guidance on drill length, diameter, and implant size. The surgical technique varies

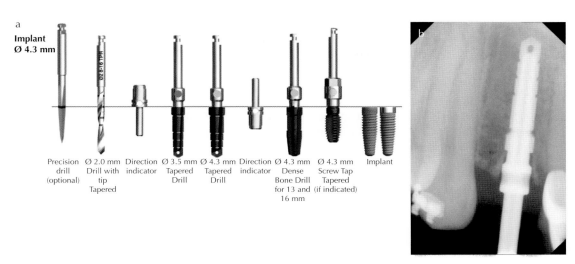

a

Implant Ø 4.3 mm

| Precision drill (optional) | Ø 2.0 mm Drill with tip Tapered | Direction indicator | Ø 3.5 mm Tapered Drill | Ø 4.3 mm Tapered Drill | Direction indicator | Ø 4.3 mm Dense Bone Drill for 13 and 16 mm | Ø 4.3 mm Screw Tap Tapered (if indicated) | Implant |

7.14. (a) A surgical drill sequence (courtesy of Nobel Biocare). (b) Intraoperative radiograph of a drill; note length of drill tip triangle (courtesy of Dr. S. Whitney).

according to bone quality. Rigorous technique is required to ensure a precise fit and good initial stability of the implant. The following guidelines should be adhered to:

- Use sharp drills, correct drill sequence, incremental drilling, limited pressure, pumping action, especially in dense bone.
- Use the drill speed stated in the implant company guidelines, <2500 rpm, depending on bone density.
- Use copious saline irrigation.
- Use direction indicators.
- Take intra-operative X-rays to check direction and proximity to vital structures.
- Use a surgical guide for correct implant positioning.
- Be aware of the added length of the "V" shaped apex of drills especially when drilling next to vital structures.
- Use side-cutting drills to change direction.
- The final drill size is critical.
- Take a postoperative X-ray to check for impingement on vital structures. A postoperative radiograph should confirm non-encroachment on the mandibular nerve canal. If there is canal encroachment, the implant must be backed away from the canal or removed.
- Perform primary flap closure with nonabsorbable or absorbable sutures, for example, Vicryl Plus™ (polyglactin 910®) (Ethicon®).
- Leave existing denture out for 10 days or provisionalize using adjacent teeth.

Screw tapping, osteotomes, final drill size, and insertion

The final drill that is used is often slightly smaller in diameter than the implant in order to ensure a good stable fit of the implant screw in the bone. Surgeons occasionally favor the use of osteotomes for the final preparation of soft bone (Type IV bone) osteotomies. Tapered implant shape and deep thread designs help to achieve better initial stability than parallel screw implants in soft bone. Dense bone needs to be screw-tapped to receive threaded implants. A threaded implant is inserted by using a drill handpiece at very low RPM (<50), with the final tightening done by hand ratchet or torque driver. The insertion torque value gives an indication of the initial implant stability. High insertion torque (>45 Ncm) is desirable in cases where the implant is to be loaded immediately. Implant companies may recommend an upper limit for implant insertion torque. Press-fit implants are inserted by a tapping action with a dedicated mallet instrument (Fig. 7.15a–d).

Final position and suturing

In many circumstances, the implant platform should be positioned such that the platform is flush to the ridge crest. Occasionally, the crest needs flattening or "tabling" for complete insertion of the implant. Some polished implant collars are designed to remain above the bone level. With anterior units, where bone damage is minimal and adjacent teeth have good gingival position, the implant platform should be positioned at the ridge crest or between 2.0 and 3.0 mm apical to the labial gingival line on the adjacent teeth. This positioning "hides" the metal implant and facilitates the achievement of good emergence profile and thus optimal gingival contour. The position of the platform should not be labial to an imaginary line between adjacent labial cervical line positions. An optimum result may be more achievable with immediate placement. Platform-switched implants may aid in marginal bone preservation and soft tissue height.

A cover screw or healing abutment is placed in the implant screw-hole, and flaps are sutured in place over the implant platform (in two-stage surgery), or around the projecting transmucosal collar or abutment (in one-stage surgery) (Fig. 7.16).

7.7 Implant surgical protocols

One-stage surgery

In one-stage surgery, an implant with an attached transmucosal healing abutment or with an integral transmucosal collar or abutment, is placed but is not covered by oral mucosa for healing (Fig. 7.17) (see Chapter 6).

Two-stage surgery

In two-stage surgery, an implant is placed with its platform at the ridge crest level, and is allowed to heal for between 3 and 6 months submucosally without loading. The implant is then uncovered and a transmucosal abutment is placed. Esposito et al. (2009a) have suggested that this technique may be more appropriate for edentulous cases, due to the risk of inadvertent loading during healing (see Chapter 6).

Implant placement variations

These placement variations include:

- Immediate placement into an extraction site (Enríquez-Sacristán et al. 2011)
- Early placement (or immediate-delayed) following soft tissue healing for 4–8 weeks after extraction
- Delayed placement following bony socket healing for 3–6 months
- Delayed placement after socket augmentation with alloplastic graft materials and healing for 3–6 months (Chen and Buser 2008)
- Delayed placement following healing for 6–9 months after ridge augmentation or ridge block grafting
- Implant placement in conjunction with bone augmentation, grafting, sinus lift (crestal access [indirect] or direct sinus lift) (Jensen and Katsuyama 2011)

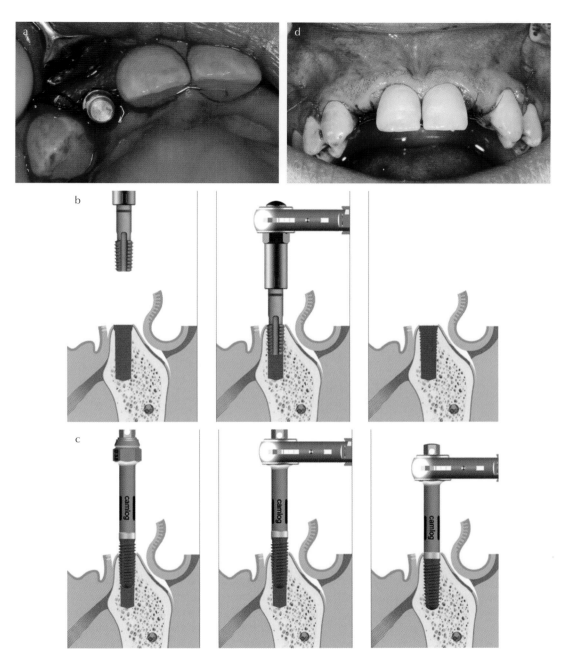

7.15. (a) Alignment pin or guide in pilot drill hole (courtesy Dr. S. Whitney). (b) Diagram of thread-forming the osteotomy (courtesy of CAMLOG). (c) Diagram of implant placement (courtesy of CAMLOG). (d) Sutured mucoperiosteal flaps (courtesy of Dr. A. Bradley).

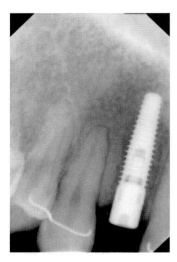

7.16. Stage 2 surgery abutment connection: baseline radiograph (courtesy of Dr. S. Whitney).

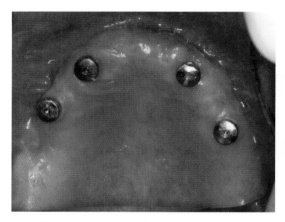

7.17. One-stage surgery with transmucosal healing and ITI implants (courtesy of Dr. T. Taylor).

Immediate placement

The possibility of immediate placement of implants following atraumatic extraction and socket curettage should be considered for patients based on their individual needs. Chen et al. (2004) and Lang et al. (2012) noted that survival rates and clinical outcomes of immediate and delayed implants, in the short term, were similar to those of implants placed in healed alveolar ridges. Sanz et al. (2012) suggested that immediate placement of implants may preserve both soft tissue and bone, when compared with delayed protocols. This would optimize aesthetics for the final restoration. However, a systematic review by Esposito et al. (2010b) showed insufficient evidence to determine possible advantages or disadvantages of immediate, immediate-delayed (early), or delayed implant placement. They caution that immediate and immediate-delayed implants may be at higher risk of implant failure and complications than delayed implants. Atieh et al. (2009) corroborated the higher risk of immediate placement versus the conventional surgical protocols. Hämmerle et al. (2012) noted the risk of mucosal recession in aesthetic zones and suggested that the immediate placement procedure may be more appropriate for nonaesthetic areas.

Aesthetic soft tissue management

Optimum aesthetics may be achievable when a healthy but damaged tooth needs to be extracted. In this situation, an implant can be placed immediately and allowed to heal with a transmucosal abutment or provisional crown. Recently, platform-switching has been promoted as a way of further optimizing bone retention and soft-tissue aesthetics. There is currently insufficient evidence available to validate the aesthetic benefit (Esposito et al. 2012). These factors are considered important for aesthetic soft tissue management:

- Maintenance or creation of an adequate band of attached gingiva
- Maintenance of interdental papillae when possible
- Tissue shaping to establish the optimal emergence profile of a crown and maintain soft tissue shape after restoration

- Platform-switching to retain bone and soft tissue.

Gingival grafting may be performed to recover soft tissue recession or to create an adequate band of attached gingiva.

Ridge preservation (socket augmentation) following extraction

Surgical protocols that use various grafting material and membranes have been used for alveolar preservation after tooth extraction. Ten Heggeler et al. (2011) and Vignoletti et al. (2012) reviewed this subject and found that adoption of such therapies demonstrated less vertical and horizontal contraction (bone loss) of the residual alveolar ridge.

Implant placement with simultaneous ridge augmentation or sinus lift

These variations are complex and require greater experience on the part of the implant treatment group both surgically and restoratively. Implant placement can be combined with various augmentation and sinus elevation procedures (see Chapter 11) (Fig. 7.18 and Fig. 7.19).

7.8 Solutions for insufficient bone volume at the implant site

Significant bone deficiency may be congenital, or the result of trauma, pathology, or long-term edentulism. Autogenous bone grafts have long been the standard for increasing edentulous ridge bone volume. However, given the morbidity of harvesting bone from remote sites, other less invasive bone augmentation techniques have become popular for increasing bone volume (Jokstad 2009; Froum 2010).

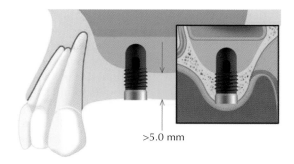

>5.0 mm

7.18. Diagram of indirect sinus lift procedure (courtesy of CAMLOG).

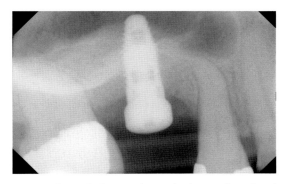

7.19. Radiograph showing the result of an implant placed using an indirect sinus lift procedure.

Augmentation may be strategically important in certain scenarios in order to achieve ideal aesthetic and biomechanical implant placement. In other cases, where implant length is an issue, shorter implants have been shown to provide a viable alternative to vertical ridge augmentation (Esposito et al. 2009b; Annibali et al. 2012).

Solutions for inadequate bone volume

- Use short implants and/or more implants
- Use horizontal and/or vertical ridge augmentation.

Types of ridge grafting/augmentation

- Horizontal and/or vertical ridge augmentation with block grafting and/or guided bone regeneration (GBR) techniques. Block autografts may be harvested from mandible, iliac crest, or tibia
- Indirect sinus lift/sinus augmentation using Summers osteotome technique (Davarpanah et al. 2001)
- Open sinus grafting or direct sinus lift (Caldwell–Luc procedure)
- Distraction osteogenesis
- Ridge splitting to expand the ridge width
- Mandibular nerve repositioning to allow for implant placement (Dibart and Dibart 2011) (see Chapter 11).

Types of graft materials and membranes

- Autograft: block or particulate host bone
- Allograft: bone derived from another human, usually from a cadaver. It may be freeze dried (FDBA) or decalcified and freeze dried (DFDBA).
- Xenograft: nonhuman bone such as bovine or porcine
- Alloplast: synthetic graft materials based on hydroxylapatite or $CaSO_4$
- Recombinant human bone morphogenetic growth factor (rhBGF) or platelet-derived growth factor (rhPDGF) along with a collagen or other support matrix
- Absorbable membranes (BAM)
- Nonabsorbable membranes (NAM) (see Chapter 11).

7.9   Implant selection

Implant selection is based on comprehensive diagnosis and restorative preplanning along with careful surgical site assessment during surgery. Implant systems present an array of diameters, lengths, shapes, and surface characteristics. The surgeon must balance all his knowledge and experience with company recommendations and decide on the best solution for the clinical situation. Guidelines have been developed empirically over the past thirty years. While scientific rationale is limited, factors such as the size and number of missing teeth and bone volume and quality are important.

Implant platform, diameter

Clinicians develop a preference for particular implant designs for different clinical situations, for example, parallel walled or tapered implants, or implants with machined, textured, or flared collars. An implant diameter should allow a satisfactory emergence profile of the final restoration. The required implant diameter can be loosely related to cervical tooth diameter measurements (Stanley and Nelson 2010). The following guidelines may be used:

- *Narrow or small diameter* (3.0–3.5 mm) for maxillary lateral incisors and mandibular incisors
- *Standard or regular diameter* (4.0–4.5 mm) for maxillary central incisors, canines and premolars. This size is also ideal for overdentures and hybrid dentures
- *Wide diameter* (>5.0 mm) for molars.

Implant length

Clinicians are cognizant of tooth length and the concept of crown-to-root ratio, and are comfortable duplicating these ratios with implants. Early Brånemark protocol expected engagement of both cortical plates in the anterior mandible regardless of implant length. As implant therapy was applied to other areas of the jaws, there was uncertainty about the desired implant length due to variations in bone height and density in other areas of the jaws. In general, it is currently acceptable to have an approximate implant length in the region of 10–15.0 mm regardless of the implant shape or diameter. Short implants may be regarded as less than 10.0 mm long. With immediate placement, the implant must engage bone in the apical portion of the socket or beyond, often making the implant longer than the tooth root it replaces. It has been suggested that placing shorter implants may be more desirable than complex ridge augmentation procedures that enable the use of longer implants (Esposito et al. 2011). There are no clear guidelines for the use of short implants, and limited data on their survival rates in different clinical scenarios. Van Assche et al. (2012) demonstrated excellent short-term results for short implants with maxillary overdentures. Romeo et al. (2010) also found no significant differences in survival rates for short and longer implants.

Implant number

When bone height dictates the use of short implants, the clinician should consider using additional implants (up to a maximum of one implant per premolar unit). Similarly, if small diameter implants must be used, then the number of implants should be increased.

Implant configuration

Certain implant companies promote implant designs for areas with minimal height and soft bone quality (e.g., Bicon, Nobel Active®). Evidence currently suggests that machined surfaces are less desirable than textured surfaces, especially in soft bone. Tapered screws achieve greater initial stability than cylindrical screws. Many press-fit implants have adopted threads to enhance initial stability. Platform-switched designs, with a textured surface extended to the implant platform, may offer the best prognosis

in areas of soft bone and in aesthetic zones (Atieh et al. 2010).

7.10 Provisional restorative options

The ultimate success of the implant restoration is of utmost importance to the patient, but having a provisional restoration may also be an important issue for some patients. Implant integration must not be compromised by inadvertent loading caused by a provisional restoration. It is important that the early stages of osseointegration are not disturbed by function. Provisional restorations can be inserted at the time of surgery or soon after. Postsurgical soft tissue swelling and pressure on healing tissue must be accounted for. Removable prostheses must provide generous relief over the implant site. Options include:

- No provisional restoration
- An acrylic partial or complete denture fabricated in advance. It may be modified clinically with soft materials
- A resin retained FDP fabricated in advance
- A provisional FDP supported by adjacent teeth
- An implant supported provisional restoration with no occlusal contact.

Immediate/early loading

Traditionally, implants are loaded after between 3 and 6 months of bone healing. The restorative dentist and surgeon may cooperate to carry out immediate loading with a provisional restoration, or place one at second-stage surgery to shape the tissue for a better aesthetic result.

The surgeon will have a view as to when the implants should be loaded depending on implant stability at the time of surgery.

Alternative loading protocols have been introduced in order to shorten treatment times and provide better interim aesthetics and function (Morton and Ganeles 2007; Wismeijer et al. 2010). With immediate loading, a temporary abutment is connected, and a provisional crown is placed at the time of implant insertion (see Chapter 12). This protocol requires that the implant be stable at an insertion torque force of >45 Ncm, which usually means that there is excellent bone quality (Type I or Type II). The provisional restoration is kept out of occlusion. Immediate loading may create an unnecessary risk to osseointegration, and it is advisable to refer patients demanding such treatments to a specialist implant group.

With the advent of shorter osseointegration times through the use of textured surfaces, it has become possible to functionally restore implants in as little as 6 weeks after surgery (Grütter and Belser 2009). More long-term studies are needed to validate early loading protocols.

7.11 Postoperative management and surgical review

The surgeon prescribes antibiotics and pain medication (NSAIDs or opiate preparations) as indicated by the particular case. Additionally, chlorhexidine or saline mouthwash may be prescribed. Certain minor problems may be anticipated depending on the case, such as minor bleeding, swelling and bruising, and transient paresthesia. The patient is given postoperative instructions for minor oral surgery. Most problems that may arise, such as wound opening and infection, while undesirable, are easily treated. Nonabsorbable sutures are removed after 10–14 days, and provisional procedures are then finalized. If there is ongoing infection, it may be necessary to remove a nonintegrating or mobile implant.

7.12 Second-stage surgery

After a healing period of 3–6 months, second-stage surgery is performed to uncover the implant. The waiting period is determined by the surgeon and is based on the surgeon's knowledge of the nuances of the surgical placement procedure, such as bone density and initial stability at the time of placement. The implant healing cap is located with a probe and either a flap is elevated, or a surgical punch is used to remove the overlying mucosa. The punch technique is not recommended when there is only a small band of attached mucosa. When feasible, the punch method is kinder to the patient as there is minimal discomfort. Maintenance of an adequate labial band of attached gingiva is paramount for hygiene measures, and occasionally an apically repositioned flap is indicated to recreate a band of attached gingiva. Labial soft tissue grafting may also be needed to fill out a bony depression depending on the circumstances. There are many surgical techniques for soft tissue manipulation, for the purpose of improving aesthetics. These are covered in textbooks on advanced implant topics.

Clinical indicators of osseointegration

- Absence of infection and mobility
- Lack of crestal bone loss (on radiograph)
- A radiograph that shows no radiolucency around the implant
- A ringing sound, indicating ankylosis, when tapping the implant with a metal instrument, for example, mirror handle.

A transmucosal healing abutment is selected, finger tightened to between 10 and 15 Ncm, and checked with a radiograph. Alternatively, an expanded healing abutment or provisional crown may be placed in order to create optimum soft tissue contour for the final restoration.

If implant movement is detected, or significant discomfort occurs while removing the cover screw or abutment, or tightening an abutment, then loss of integration may be suspected.

If the movement is minimal and painful, it may be possible to leave it in place and monitor the situation for infection or reintegration; no guidelines are currently available. Alternatively, the implant should be removed, the osteotomy site debrided, in-filled with particulate graft material, and allowed to heal for 6 months.

Implant stability testing

Primary implant stability at placement is subjective and related to the type of bone, type of implant and the implant placement technique. Insertion torque value gives a measure of initial stability (see Chapter 3).

Secondary implant stability is attributable to osseointegration, and has been assessed by several methods. Impact testing (Periotest®) and resonance frequency analysis (Osstell™) are noninvasive stability testing devices that show promise for future clinical use. Their clinical prognostic value has not been established at this time.

7.13   Complications

Complications related to surgery and healing

- Life-threatening problems with anesthesia and surgery
- Hemorrhage, infection, pain, swelling, and ecchymoses
- Failure of implant to osseointegrate
- Dehiscence and fenestration of alveolar plates of bone
- Damage to vital anatomic structures necessitating implant removal for example, perforation of the mandibular canal floor of nose or sinus
- Neurosensory problems
    - Trauma to mental nerve during flap retraction
    - Postoperative pressure on nerve due to hematoma or edema
    - Direct injury to mandibular nerve during osteotomy: trauma and transection
    - Pressure on nerve by implant
    - Transection of minor or accessory nerves in anterior mandible
- Wound dehiscence
- Poor position or angulation of implant.

References

AAOMS (2007) American Association of Oral and Maxillofacial Surgeons position paper on bisphosphonate-related osteonecrosis of the jaws. Advisory Task Force on Bisphosphonate-Related Ostenonecrosis of the Jaws, American Association of Oral and Maxillofacial Surgeons. *J Oral Maxillofac Surg.* 65(3):369–76.

Annibali S, Cristalli MP, Dell'Aquila D, Bignozzi I, La Monaca G, Pilloni A. (2012) Short dental implants: a systematic review. *J Dent Res.* 91(1):25–32.

Atieh MA, Payne AG, Duncan WJ, Cullinan MP. (2009) Immediate restoration/loading of immediately placed single implants: is it an effective bimodal approach? *Clin Oral Implants Res.* 20(7): 645–59.

Atieh MA, Ibrahim HM, Atieh AH. (2010) Platform-switching for marginal bone preservation around dental implants: a systematic review and meta-analysis. *J Periodontol.* 81(10):1350–66.

Baig MR, Rajan M. (2007) Effects of smoking on the outcome of implant treatment: a literature review. *Indian J Dent Res.* 18(4):190–5.

Block MS. (2011) *Color Atlas of Dental Implant Surgery,* 3rd ed. Saunders, St. Louis.

Cavalcanti R, Oreglia F, Manfredonia MF, Gianserra R, Esposito M. (2011) The influence of smoking on the survival of dental implants: a 5-year pragmatic multicentre retrospective cohort study of 1727 patients. *Eur J Oral Implantol.* 4(1):39–45.

Cavézian R, Pasquet G. (2012) [Cone Beam computerized tomography and implants]. *Rev Stomatol Chir Maxillofac.* 113(4):245–58. [in French].

Chen S, Buser D. (2008) *ITI Treatment Guide: Volume 3: Implant Placement in Post-Extraction Sites—Treatment Options.* (eds. D Buser, D Wismeijer, U Belser). Quintessence, Berlin.

Chen ST, Wilson TG Jr, Hämmerle CH. (2004) Immediate or early placement of implants following tooth extraction: review of biologic basis, clinical procedures, and outcomes. *Int J Oral Maxillofac Implants*. 19 Suppl:12–25.

Colella G, Cannavale R, Pentenero M, Gandolfo S. (2007) Oral implants in radiated patients: a systematic review. *Int J Oral Maxillofac Implants*. 22(4): 616–22.

Davarpanah M, Martinez H, Tecucianu JF, Hage G, Lazzara R. (2001) The modified osteotome technique. *Int J Periodontics Restorative Dent*. 21(6): 599–607.

Dibart S, Dibart J-P. (eds.) (2011) *Practical Osseous Surgery in Periodontics and Implant Dentistry*. Wiley-Blackwell, Ames.

Enríquez-Sacristán C, Barona-Dorado C, Calvo-Guirado JL, Leco-Berrocal I, Martínez-González JM. (2011) Immediate post-extraction implants subject to immediate loading: a meta-analytic study. *Med Oral Patol Oral Cir Bucal*. 16(7): e919–24.

Esposito M, Grusovin MG, Chew YS, Coulthard P, Worthington HV. (2009a) One-stage versus two-stage implant placement. A Cochrane systematic review of randomised controlled clinical trials. *Eur J Oral Implantol*. 2(2):91–9.

Esposito M, Grusovin MG, Felice P, Karatzopoulos G, Worthington HV, Coulthard P. (2009b) The efficacy of horizontal and vertical bone augmentation procedures for dental implants—a Cochrane systematic review. *Eur J Oral Implantol*. 2(3): 167–84.

Esposito M, Grusovin MG, Loli V, Coulthard P, Worthington HV. (2010a) Does antibiotic prophylaxis at implant placement decrease early implant failures? A Cochrane systematic review. *Eur J Oral Implantol*. 3(2):101–10.

Esposito M, Grusovin MG, Polyzos IP, Felice P, Worthington HV. (2010b) Timing of implant placement after tooth extraction: immediate, immediate-delayed or delayed implants? A Cochrane systematic review. *Eur J Oral Implantol*. 3(3):189–205.

Esposito M, Pellegrino G, Pistilli R, Felice P. (2011) Rehabilitation of posterior atrophic edentulous jaws: prostheses supported by 5 mm short implants or by longer implants in augmented bone? One-year results from a pilot randomised clinical trial. *Eur J Oral Implantol*. 4(1):21–30.

Esposito M, Maghaireh H, Grusovin MG, Ziounas I, Worthington HV. (2012) Soft tissue management for dental implants: what are the most effective techniques? A Cochrane systematic review. *Eur J Oral Implantol*. 5(3):221–38.

Fanning B. (2011) CBCT: the justification process, audit and review of the recent literature. *J Ir Dent Assoc*. 57(5):256–61.

Froum SJ. (ed.) (2010) *Dental Implant Complications: Etiology, Prevention, and Treatment*. Wiley-Blackwell, Ames.

Grütter L, Belser UC. (2009) Implant loading protocols for the partially edentulous esthetic zone. *Int J Oral Maxillofac Implants*. 24 Suppl:169–79.

Hämmerle CH, Araújo MG, Simion M; Osteology Consensus Group 2011. (2012) Evidence-based knowledge on the biology and treatment of extraction sockets. *Clin Oral Implants Res*. 23(Suppl 5): 80–2.

Heitz-Mayfield LJ. (2008) Peri-implant diseases: diagnosis and risk indicators. *J Clin Periodontol*. 35(8 Suppl):292–304.

Javed F, Romanos GE. (2009) Impact of diabetes mellitus and glycemic control on the osseointegration of dental implants: a systematic literature review. *J Periodontol*. 80(11):1719–30.

Javed F, Al-Hezaimi K, Al-Rasheed A, Almas K, Romanos GE. (2010) Implant survival rate after oral cancer therapy: a review. *Oral Oncol*. 46(12): 854–9.

Jensen S, Katsuyama H. (2011) *ITI Treatment Guide. Volume 5. Sinus Floor Elevation Procedures*. (eds. S Chen, D Buser, D Wismeijer). Quintessence, Berlin.

Jokstad A. (ed.) (2009) *Osseointegration and Dental Implants*. Wiley-Blackwell, Ames.

Lang NP, Pun L, Lau KY, Li KY, Wong MC. (2012) A systematic review on survival and success rates of implants placed immediately into fresh extraction sockets after at least 1 year. *Clin Oral Implants Res*. 23(Suppl 5):39–66.

Lekholm U, Zarb GA. (1985) Patient selection and preparation. In: P-I Brånemark, G Zarb, T Albrektsson (eds.), *Tissue-Integrated Prostheses: Osseointegration in Clinical Dentistry*. Quintessence, Chicago, pp. 199–209.

Lindhe J, Meyle J; Group D European Workshop on Periodontology Collaborators (13). (2008) Peri-implant diseases: Consensus Report of the Sixth European Workshop on Periodontology. *J Clin Periodontol*. 35(8 Suppl):282–5.

Madrid C, Sanz M. (2009a) What influence do anticoagulants have on oral implant therapy? A systematic review. *Clin Oral Implants Res*. 20(Suppl 4): 96–106.

Madrid C, Sanz M. (2009b) What impact do systemically administered bisphosphonates have on oral implant therapy? A systematic review. *Clin Oral Implants Res*. 20(Suppl 4):87–95.

Mellado-Valero A, Ferrer García JC, Herrera Ballester A, Labaig Rueda C. (2007) Effects of diabetes on the osseointegration of dental implants. *Med Oral Patol Oral Cir Bucal.* 12(1):E38–43.

Misch CE. (2007) *Contemporary Implant Dentistry*, 3rd ed. Mosby, St. Louis.

Mombelli A, Cionca N. (2006) Systemic diseases affecting osseointegration therapy. *Clin Oral Implants Res.* 17(Suppl 2):97–103.

Morton D, Ganeles J. (2007) *ITI Treatment Guide. Volume 2. Loading Protocols in Implant Dentistry: Partially Dentate Patients.* (eds. D Wismeijer, D Buser, U Belser). Quintessence, Berlin.

Romeo E, Bivio A, Mosca D, Scanferla M, Ghisolfi M, Storelli S. (2010) The use of short dental implants in clinical practice: literature review. *Minerva Stomatol.* 59(1–2):23–31.

Sanz I, Garcia-Gargallo M, Herrera D, Martin C, Figuero E, Sanz M. (2012) Surgical protocols for early implant placement in post-extraction sockets: a systematic review. *Clin Oral Implants Res.* 23(Suppl 5):67–79.

Scully C, Wolff A. (2002) Oral surgery in patients on anticoagulant therapy. *Oral Surg Oral Med Oral Pathol Oral Radiol Endod.* 94(1):57–64.

Sennerby L, Roos J. (1998) Surgical determinants of clinical success of osseointegrated oral implants: a review of the literature. *Int J Prosthodont.* 11(5): 408–20.

Shetty K, Achong R. (2005) Dental implants in the HIV-positive patient—case report and review of the literature. *Gen Dent.* 53(6):434–7, 446.

Stanley J, Nelson M. (2010) *Wheeler's Dental Anatomy, Physiology and Occlusion*, 9th ed. Saunders/Elsevier, St. Louis.

Tallgren A, Lang BR, Walker GF, Ash MM Jr. (1980) Roentgen cephalometric analysis of ridge resorption and changes in jaw and occlusal relationships in immediate complete denture wearers. *J Oral Rehabil.* 7(1):77–94.

Tan WL, Wong TL, Wong MC, Lang NP. (2012) A systematic review of post-extractional alveolar hard and soft tissue dimensional changes in humans. *Clin Oral Implants Res.* 23(Suppl 5):1–21.

Ten Heggeler JM, Slot DE, Van der Weijden GA. (2011) Effect of socket preservation therapies following tooth extraction in non-molar regions in humans: a systematic review. *Clin Oral Implants Res.* 22(8):779–88.

Tyndall DA, Price JB, Tetradis S, Ganz SD, Hildebolt C, Scarfe WC; American Academy of Oral and Maxillofacial Radiology. (2012) Position statement of the American Academy of Oral and Maxillofacial Radiology on selection criteria for the use of radiology in dental implantology with emphasis on cone beam computed tomography. *Oral Surg Oral Med Oral Pathol Oral Radiol.* 113(6): 817–26.

Van Assche N, Michels S, Quirynen M, Naert I. (2012) Extra short dental implants supporting an overdenture in the edentulous maxilla: a proof of concept. *Clin Oral Implants Res.* 23(5):567–76.

Vazquez L, Saulacic N, Belser U, Bernard JP. (2008) Efficacy of panoramic radiographs in the pre-operative planning of posterior mandibular implants: a prospective clinical study of 1527 consecutively treated patients. *Clin Oral Implants Res.* 19(1):81–5.

Vignoletti F, Matesanz P, Rodrigo D, Figuero E, Martin C, Sanz M. (2012) Surgical protocols for ridge preservation after tooth extraction. A systematic review. *Clin Oral Implants Res.* 23(Suppl 5): 22–38.

Wagenberg B, Froum SJ. (2006) A retrospective study of 1925 consecutively placed immediate implants from 1988 to 2004. *Int J Oral Maxillofac Implants.* 21(1):71–80.

Wismeijer D, Casentini P, Gallucci GO, Chiapasco M. (2010) *ITI Treatment Guide—Volume 4: Loading Protocols in Implant Dentistry—Edentulous Patients.* (eds. D Wismeijer, D Buser, U Belser) Quintessence, Berlin.

8

Single-Implant Crowns

8.1 Introduction

Single-implant crowns are the optimal and routine method of single tooth replacement in the majority of cases. Depending on the clinical situation, other options, such as orthodontics, traditional fixed bridgework, or even no treatment may be appropriate. The need for single-tooth replacement may arise congenitally, traumatically, or through caries or periodontal disease. While single units running from the canine posteriorly are relatively straightforward, implant supported incisors may present a formidable aesthetic challenge. In situations with significant ridge resorption, a high smile line, or intact adjacent teeth, it can be challenging to achieve a satisfactory aesthetic result. However, the single-implant crown may present a more conservative and durable option with a better aesthetic result than a conventional fixed dental prosthesis (FDP) (Salinas and Eckert 2007). Belser et al. (2007) have

presented an excellent guide for the treatment of single tooth replacement in the aesthetic zone. This chapter outlines some principles and procedures for single units.

8.2 Treatment options for single tooth absence

- No treatment
  - The patient does not desire treatment.
  - Second molar replacement is high risk due to the bone volume and quality, occlusal forces, and difficulty of access.
  - The space is unopposed or outside the aesthetic zone.
- Orthodontic treatment to close a space with no restoration needed
- Implant crown planned, implant placed but not restored, with or without interim RPD
  - The implant maintains the alveolar bone.

Fundamentals of Implant Dentistry, First Edition. Gerard Byrne.
© 2014 John Wiley & Sons, Inc. Published 2014 by John Wiley & Sons, Inc.
Companion website: www.wiley.com/go/byrne/implants

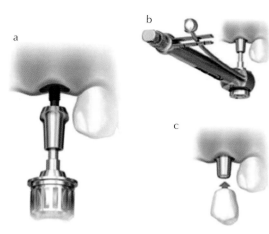

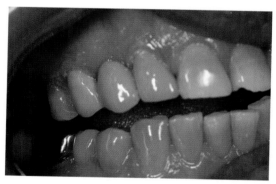

8.1. Diagram showing abutment placement (a, b) and crown cementation (c) (courtesy of Nobel Biocare).

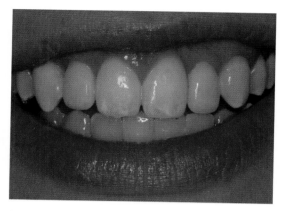

8.2. Congenitally missing lateral incisors replaced by single implant crowns (courtesy of Dr. S. Whitney).

- Implant supported crown (Fig. 8.1 and Fig. 8.2)
- Conventional FDP
  - Conventional three-unit FDP (Fig. 8.3)
  - Cantilever two-unit bridge (canine + lateral)
  - Resin-retained FDP (Maryland).
- Removable partial denture
  - Orthodontic Hawley-type retainer for the growing patient
  - Conventional interim resin RPD.

8.3. Canine replacement with a conventional three-unit FDP.

8.3 Advantages and disadvantages of various treatments

Implant single crown

(+) Maintains alveolar bone
(+) Avoids destruction of natural teeth (as with conventional FDP)
(+) Proven longevity
(+) Patient satisfaction
(−) Length of treatment process
(−) Expense.

Conventional FDP

(+) Simplicity of treatment
(+) Expense
(+) Patient satisfaction
(−) Tooth destruction
(−) Continuing alveolar resorption
(−) Longevity.

Removable prosthesis

(+) Diagnostic value as mock-up of final appearance
(+) Can be modified to use as surgical guide or radiographic guide (drill guide holes)

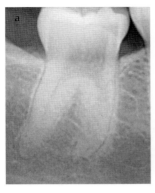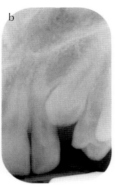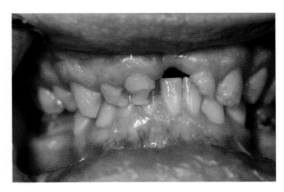

8.4. (a) Invasive cervical resorption may lead to tooth extraction (courtesy Dr. F. AlSaleeh). (b) Canine impaction may lead to extraction.

8.5. Ridge atrophy 6 months after extraction creates an aesthetic restorative dilemma.

(+) Space maintenance (Hawley orthodontic retainer)
(+) Simplicity
(+) Gives patient time to consider options
(−) Resorption promoted
(−) Patient satisfaction.

8.4 The implant site

In situations in which the tooth is still present, a decision must be made as to whether the tooth is restorable or maintainable with a reasonable 10-year prognosis, or whether extraction and an implant crown provide the better long-term prognosis. Fugazzotto (2009) discusses when to extract and when to retain a tooth based on the best available evidence. The reader is also referred to Schwartz et al. (2010) for a review of invasive cervical resorption and its management and prognosis. (Fig. 8.4a)

The nature of, and the time since tooth loss determines the residual edentulous ridge volume. In cases of *congenital absence* of a tooth, there is a relative lack of ridge width development. The reasons for tooth loss or potential tooth loss such as trauma, caries, and periodontal disease, give valuable information on bone volume and socket health. When it is

determined that a tooth needs to be extracted, it becomes the most favorable situation for implant treatment, as the alveolar bone may have not yet resorbed (Fig. 8.4b). The presence of unrestorable teeth with healthy roots and bone, but that are deemed unrestorable in a traditional manner also make good implant sites. With *traumatic tooth loss*, there may be resultant damage to the socket. Endodontic problems may present with apical pathology and bone resorption. Periodontal bone loss may also complicate implant treatment.

Residual bone volume

The tooth to be replaced and the residual ridge configuration will determine the diameter and length of implant that can be placed. These factors will also have a major bearing on the aesthetic outcome. A recent extraction site may have minimal bone volume change. A long-standing edentulous space will have substantial loss of ridge height and width (Van der Weijden et al. 2009; Tan et al. 2012). In the maxilla, significant facial bone resorption occurs in the first 6 months after extraction (Fig. 8.5). Damaged ridges may require augmentation in the aesthetic zone. Facial resorption creates a problem in that either the implant must be placed more lingually, or the ridge must be grafted facially, in order to give optimum aesthetics. Reduced ridge volume may also be related to periodontitis, pulpal infection, or socket damage from (surgical) extraction. Bone volume of an edentulous space can be best assessed by *ridge mapping* with a calibrated probe and local anesthetic, or with a CBCT scan. These tests may be delayed until the surgical consult.

Evaluating the aesthetic zone

If the gingival line is visible when the patient smiles, the case becomes advanced in terms of difficulty, rather than straightforward (Dawson and Chen 2009) (Fig. 8.6a,b). The gingiva frames the teeth and creates an aesthetic balance. When this balance is pleasing, it must be maintained. When an asymmetrical balance is present, this must be demonstrated to the patient, and a compromise worked out. Photographs and study models are invaluable for patient education and treatment planning. The smile line can be marked on study models.

A slightly inadequate implant crown may still be preferable to a three-unit conventional bridge over a long period, especially for a young patient. Bone loss can only get worse with time and hence successive bridges become more challenging (Fig. 8.7a,b and Fig. 8.8a,b).

Gingival biotype and the width of the band of attached mucosa (gingiva)

Cases with a fine gingival biotype are considered more complex (see Chapter 5, Fig. 5.14a,b). These patients must be forewarned about the risk of gingival recession or papilla loss or "black triangle" effect with anterior implant crowns. The problem is more severe in cases with a high smile line. The patient should be warned in advance and offered alternatives

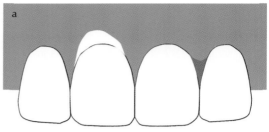
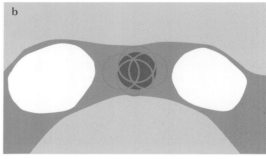

8.6. (a) Diagram showing potential for aesthetic problems in a case with a thin labial plate, a thin gingival biotype, and a high smile line. Unsightly labial recession (white area #8) or papilla loss (#9 and #10) can occur (courtesy of H. Byrne). (b) Diagram showing ideal centered *(gray)* and nonideal off-center *(green circles)* positioning of an implant in the residual ridge (courtesy of H. Byrne).

before commencing treatment. Thick gingival biotypes with blunted papillae are less of a problem.

A band of attached mucosa should surround an implant or implant abutment. Although the presence or absence of attached mucosa may not directly affect implant prognosis, implant hygiene is easier. By facilitating plaque control, the long-term prognosis of the implant is enhanced. Soft tissue grafting may have to be considered in the aesthetic zone.

Vertical and mesio-distal space for a crown

Supereruption of opposing teeth can create a spatial problem for implant crowns. Study models and diagnostic mock-ups are the best

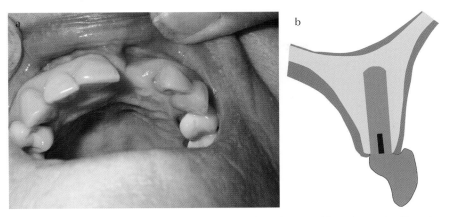

8.7. (a) Ridge resorption from the labial aspect creates a potential aesthetic problem due to the lingual positioning of the implant (courtesy of T. George). (b) Diagram of lingual implant placement (sagittal section) potentially leading to an unsatisfactory ridge-lap situation (courtesy of H. Byrne).

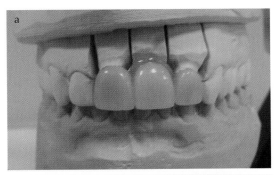

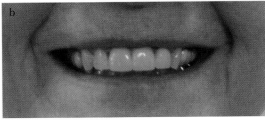

8.8. (a) Ridge atrophy with FDP replacement of tooth #9: pink porcelain is used to replace ridge deficiency. (b) FDP in place with favorable smile line and aesthetic result (courtesy of T. George).

way to make such spatial assessments. A vertical space of between 5.0 and 7.0 mm is desirable for fixed prostheses. Less space necessitates the use of cemented crowns. Vertical space is often limited when deciduous teeth are retained and then lost, due to superuption of opposing teeth. Class II incisor relationships do not restrict crown space, but create an unfavorable force situation.

There should be a space of between 1.0 and 2.0 mm mesially and distally between adjacent teeth to accommodate surgical access, interdental papillae, proximal bone, and access for cleaning and good crown emergence profile.

8.5   Implant surgery

Several surgical protocols (see Chapter 7) should be considered based on the clinical presentation. The surgeon will discuss these options with the patient and the referring dentist. Immediate placement into a socket shortens the treatment time, but has greater risk. This may be feasible in cases with healthy extraction sites and low aesthetic risk (Sanz et al. 2012). The clinician must weigh up risks and benefits in each case. Immediate or early loading adds further risk. Platform-switching implants should be considered in the aesthetic zone as they may be beneficial for marginal bone preservation (Atieh et al. 2010; Cumbo et al. 2013).

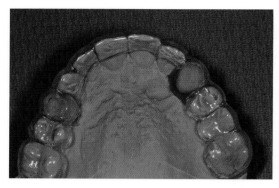

8.9. Surgical guide for single implants, retaining proposed crown outlines and providing access for surgical pilot drills.

The surgical guide

A surgical guide is a helpful way of communicating to the surgeon the proposed crown and implant location and angulation (Fig. 8.9). Following diagnostic mock-up, the position of the crown may be readily duplicated in vacuum-formed resin. A discussion with the surgeon ensures a serviceable guide. The important factor is the reproduction of the proposed tooth position for the surgeon, and noninterference with surgical access and flaps. Some complex guides determine drill angulation and depth, whereas simpler guides represent the final crown position and thus the approximate implant position relative to the proposed crown. A radiographic guide is indicated if a CBCT scan will be recorded. This stent uses radio-opaque teeth or a radio-opaque filler in an implant guide hole.

8.6   Provisional restoration

Provisional restoration requirements depend on the needs of the individual patient and the clinical situation. In younger patients, a provisional restoration may be needed for space maintenance. In many nonaesthetic areas, no provisional restoration may be required. In aesthetic areas, a provisional restoration is often required during implant osseointegration. A resin-retained FDP will give good short-term function; a resin interim RPD could also suffice. An RPD should only be worn for appearance and not function. It is also possible to place an *immediate provisional crown* at the time of surgery.

At second-stage surgery, an implant supported provisional crown can be placed. It may also be used to contour the soft tissue shape that will accommodate the final emergence contour of the crown. As the implant shape is different to that of a natural root, the emergence profile of the restoration must be customized to simulate natural tooth emergence through the gingiva. This is best achieved by using a screw-retained custom resin crown. Alternatively, a custom resin abutment with a cemented provisional crown can be fabricated, or the final abutment (stock or custom) may be screwed into place and surmounted by a provisional crown in order to confirm final contours and tissue levels before completing the final crown. When properly executed, the final gingival contour can be achieved before the final crown is delivered.

Provisional options include the following (Fig. 8.10a,b and Fig. 8.11):

- No provisional restoration
- Resin RPD, Hawley retainer, or other orthodontic retainer
- Resin-retained FDP
- Implant-supported provisional crown. This may be immediate or delayed, screw-retained (one piece) or cement retained (two piece)
- Definitive abutment with provisional crown
- Prefabricated resin protective caps for stock abutments, for example, Nobel Biocare Multi-unit and Snappy® abutment caps.

Immediate provisional crowns

It is possible to place a provisional crown at the time of implant surgery. This is considered

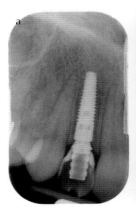
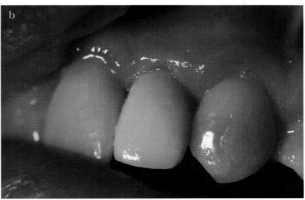

8.10. (a) Radiograph of a screw-retained provisional crown. (b) Cemented provisional lateral incisor crown.

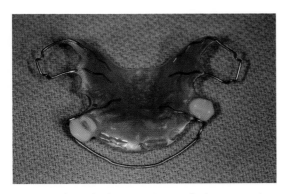

8.11. Hawley orthodontic retainer replacing two teeth.

immediate loading even if there is no functional occlusal contact. A temporary abutment is connected, and a provisional crown is either screwed or cemented in place. The current protocol requires that the implant be stable at an insertion torque force of 45 Ncm. The technique is cumbersome at the time of surgery especially when cement is used.

NB: When a prefabricated abutment is used, and a provisional crown made using a vacuum-formed template and resin, there is a high risk of the resin "locking" *in place on the rigid implant structure between adjacent teeth.*

8.7 Implant crown fabrication

If there was an infection or integration problem at second-stage surgery, it will have been dealt with by the surgeon and appropriate action taken. When the patient presents for the permanent crown, it is necessary to assess the implant clinically and radiographically. Radiographs should clearly show thread detail, but cannot rule out a fibrous "union."

It is necessary to remove a provisional crown or healing abutment prior to impression taking. The implant site is irrigated, dried, and probed gently for signs of infection and bone loss (Fig. 8.12a). It may also be necessary to commence tissue shaping prior to impression taking, using contoured abutments or custom provisional crowns.

Indicators of implant health

- Tapping on the implant abutment with a mirror handle should give a "ringing" sound. The ringing sound indicates some osseointegration or ankylosis but does not rule out bone loss, a poor quality of integration, or a failing implant.

- There should be no pain during abutment removal or seating with finger torque. If an implant is not integrated, it will have a tendency to unscrew during removal of the healing abutment causing pain.
- There should be no suppuration during gentle probing.
- A peri-apical radiograph should show no bone loss or peri-implant radiolucency.

Tissue shaping

In the aesthetic zone, a shaped healing abutment, a custom final abutment, or provisional crown may be used to change the soft tissue shape prior to the impression and restoration. Tissue shaping using special expanded healing abutments may be used in advance of provisional fabrication to simplify the procedure.

Implant level impression taking

- Insert an implant matching impression coping into the implant and tighten with a finger driver (Fig. 8.12b,c).
- Take a peri-apical radiograph to confirm complete seating of the coping.
- Syringe an appropriate impression material around the coping and adjacent teeth.
- Use a custom or stock impression tray. An occlusal hole may be needed for longer impression copings (Fig. 8.13a–c).

Laboratory steps (master cast, implant analogs)

- The impression coping is reseated in the impression and sent to the laboratory.
- A matching implant analog is connected to the impression coping *in situ*.

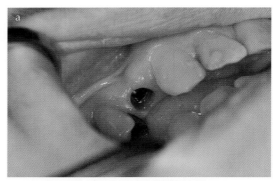
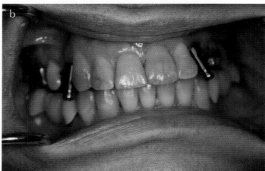
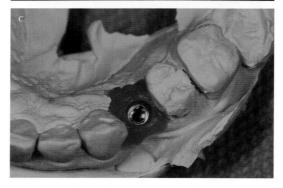

8.12. (a) Healing abutment removed. (b) Impression copings in position for closed-tray impression. (c) Implant master cast with silicone soft tissue "mask" and implant analog.

- The master cast is poured along with soft tissue duplication using a pink silicone material, also called a tissue mask (Fig. 8.12c).
- The implant analog is incorporated in the master cast surrounded by a soft silicone representing the gingival.

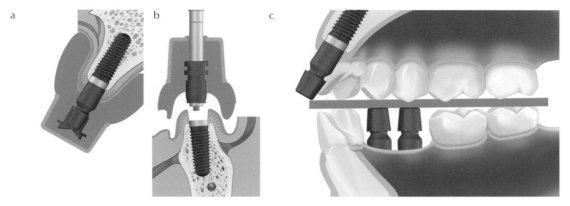

8.13. Diagrams of impression procedure and records: (a) closed tray impression (courtesy of CAMLOG); (b) open tray impression (courtesy of CAMLOG); and (c) copings in place for interocclusal records in more complex cases (courtesy of CAMLOG).

Restorative abutments for laboratory fabrication

Prefabricated abutments for cemented crowns

Prefabricated ZrO_2 and Ti abutments may be used when implant position and angulation favors their use (Fig. 8.14a,b). Some of these abutments may be modified or customized for height and finish-line location, while others such as the Nobel Biocare Snappy® are not meant to be modified.

UCLA customizable abutments for cemented or screw-retained crowns

These are standard templates for waxing and casting custom alloy abutments. The final abutment may take the form of a tooth preparation for a cemented crown, a coping for porcelain application, or a gold crown.

CAD/CAM custom ceramic or Ti abutments for cemented or screw-retained crowns

These are custom fabricated by the laboratory by scanning the master cast and by

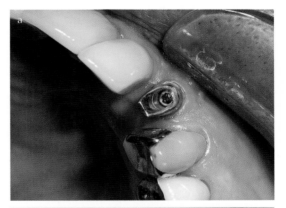

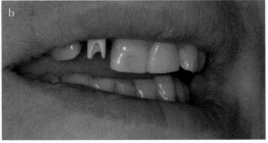

8.14. (a) Titanium custom abutment (courtesy Dr. S. Whitney). (b) Zirconia custom abutment (courtesy Dr. S. Whitney).

computer-designing and machining a custom ceramic or Ti coping. Despite the undoubted laboratory measured strength of Zirconia abutments, there is a risk of spontaneous ceramic fracture during screw torquing.

8.8 Crown adjustment and delivery

Cement-retained crown (abutment and separate crown)

Cement-retained crowns are cemented onto pre-fabricated or custom abutments, which resemble a traditional tooth preparation (Fig. 8.15a–c). The retention and resistance form of the abutment "preparation" must loosely follow tooth preparation guidelines for length and taper. A minimum preparation height of 4.0 mm is recommended. The abutments are torque-screwed into the implant, and the crown is tried-in in the conventional manner. The abutment screw-hole may be filled with cotton only, a silicone material, or cotton and a soft or hard resin material, as the screw must be readily accessible should the crown fail or need to be removed. Visible finish lines should be placed approximately 1.0–2.0 mm subgingivally. This is more critical with metal abutments.

Cemented crowns have certain advantages over screw-retained crowns:

- They are usually required in the anterior maxilla due to the unfavorable angle of the crown relative to the implant.
- They are used when the abutment screw would penetrate a cusp tip or side-wall of a crown.
- They are favored by dentists due to ease of try-in and adjustment of proximal contacts, especially with posterior crowns.
- There is no unsightly occlusal screw-hole to be restored.

Crown fit should be passive, with good marginal adaptation to minimize the sub-gingival

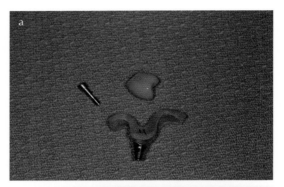

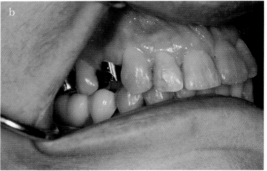

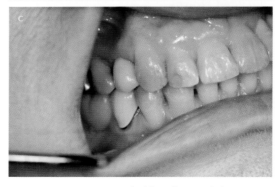

8.15. (a) Resin "try-in jig" holding the metal abutment in correct orientation for clinical try-in. (b) Custom CAD/CAM abutment torqued into position. (c) Cemented maxillary first premolar metal-ceramic crown.

plaque retention. Tissue shaping should precede cementation. It can be difficult to seat a crown fully when there is back-pressure from the stretched gingiva; cementation seating may thus be incomplete. It may be wise to provisionalize over the abutment and only complete the

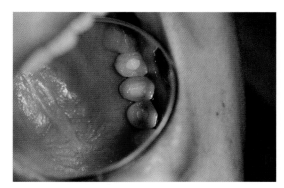

8.16. Screw-retained implant crowns: access holes filled with composite resin.

final cementation when one is satisfied that the gingival position is stable.

Screw-retained crown

The screw-retained crown is a combined abutment–crown with a screw-hole for retention (Fig. 8.16). It is an *implant-level* crown in that it connects directly to the implant. It often comprises of a UCLA sleeve onto which alloy is cast and porcelain applied. The combination abutment-crown may also be fabricated entirely from a ceramic material. It should be noted that seating such a crown often distends the gingival tissue, which blanches initially and then recovers in 15–30 minutes.

Screw-retained crowns have certain advantages:

* It is a simple technique with no subgingival cement clean-up.
* The crown is retrievable should something fail.
* They may be used routinely posteriorly, due to the long axis alignment of implant and crown.
* They can be used when there is limited crown height space. A minimum crown preparation height of 4.0 mm is desirable for cemented crowns.

* Tissue is forcibly reshaped by the crown. If the gingival line recedes, the aesthetic effect is negligible due to the subgingival extension of porcelain. Subgingival porcelain or Ti is compatible with soft tissue.
* There is no subgingival cement line, thus there is no cement clean-up and plaque retention is reduced.

Crown try-in and proximal adjustment

Positive proximal contact is important in order to prevent food impaction with its consequent risk of interproximal mucositis and peri-implantitis. It is more challenging to adjust contact with an implant crown due the fact that there is no implant movement; a natural tooth can move slightly to accommodate a "heavy" contact. A resin *try-in jig* fabricated by the laboratory is often useful to help orient an abutment to its correct clinical position; a crown's orientation should be self-evident. The complete seating of abutments or implant-level crowns must be confirmed at try-in with a peri-apical radiograph. This radiograph also records a crestal bone level baseline for future diagnosis of bone loss (Lang and Berglundh 2011). The type of implant-abutment connection has a bearing on the ease of try-in and adjustment. Internal connections allow for easier positioning into/onto subgingival implants as compared with external connections, because of the potential for soft tissue interference with the latter. Parallel-sided internal connections give a very positive seating position, as with the Nobel Biocare Tri-channel™ connection. However, it is possible for the abutment internal connection parallel post to "bind" as it seats when a proximal contact is tight, making it difficult to remove the abutment crown, and risking implant damage. Conversely, it can be difficult to know when an external hex or internal conical abutment–crown is fully seated during try-in.

Torquing the abutment screw in this situation could lead to stress on the implant collar and risk cracking the implant; this is known as *hoop stress.*

Generally, it is easier to place an abutment as a separate procedure, followed by crown adjustment and cementation. For the combination crown, the screw must be finger tightened for each proximal adjustment. A separate abutment and crown can be treated in the manner of a conventional crown.

Occlusal adjustment

Occlusion should be adjusted to the patient's maximum intercuspation (MI) position in forceful biting contact, and eccentric glides, to ensure harmonious contact in normal habitual contact and forceful biting. In habitual intercuspation and eccentric glides, shimstock (of 5-μm thickness) should pull through without tearing, except when canine rise is maintained on a canine implant crown. The crown may be just out of contact in light habitual maximum intercuspation contact. Canine guidance on an implant crown may possibly be converted to group function in order to lessen lateral loads. Accommodation will occur over time for both proximal and occlusal contacts, as adjacent and opposing natural teeth move imperceptibly through function. In his review, Carlsson (2009) discusses occlusal principles for implants (see Chapter 6).

Torquing and cementation

Screw retention

For screw retention, familiarity must be gained with the action of torque drivers. It is vital that the screwdriver head is properly engaged in the screw-head. Torque is applied as stated in the specific manufacturer's instructions; this is usually between 20 and 35 Ncm. Incorrect use of a torque driver can damage the screw or the implant. Torque tightening should be repeated a second time to ensure correct tightening. For convenience and safety, the screw should be carried to the implant within the crown or abutment and finger tightened initially. It is sometimes difficult to engage the driver into deeply set screws, especially on posterior crowns. As a consequence, the novice may believe that the screw has been torqued when it has not. Verify screw tightening by attempting to loosen the screw with a finger driver.

Cementation

Cementation is the same as with conventional crowns. Some clinicians have advocated using temporary cements, whereas others see no advantage. It is likely that whichever cement is used, the loosening of an abutment screw will necessitate cutting through the crown or sectioning the crown in order to reach the abutment screw. Supragingival posterior units are straightforward for cementation. However, anterior subgingival margins require more attention to detail. If tissue shaping is not achieved prior to abutment connection, then the future gingival line is unpredictable on account of the pressure exerted on the soft tissue by the abutment and crown. It can be difficult to do an aesthetic try-in or to cement a crown due to tissue back-pressure. It is wise to place the crown margin 1.0–2.0 mm subgingivally labially to ensure a balance between access for cement removal and masking of the abutment metal (if used); the use of ceramic abutments helps eliminate the risk of metal exposure. Cement removal is a priority in order to avoid peri-implant soft tissue complications (see Chapter 13).

Postdelivery checks and advice

- Recheck proximal and occlusal contacts.
- Proximal contact may change following torque-driving of crowns.
- Recheck for cement debris.

- Fabricate a protective orthotic device for patients with parafunction.
- Advise light function for 3–6 months.
- Provide maintenance advice and a recall schedule.

8.9 Clinical notes on single-implant crowns

Use the correct size and shape impression coping

Soft tissue can interfere with complete seating of impression copings and abutments. One must be certain that the anti-rotation device engages, thus allowing accurate final position of the abutment. Incomplete seating of an impression coping leads to a short final crown in infraocclusion. Failure to completely seat a final abutment or abutment-crown will lead to supraocclusion, fistula formation, and/or crown movement or rotation

Proximal contacts

Implants, unlike natural teeth, are immobile and proximal adjustments are more challenging. Dentists are more familiar with adjusting cemented crowns than screw-retained crowns. It can be challenging to adjust proximal and occlusal contact on screw-retained crowns, as finger tightening of screws is necessary for each check. Finger tightening may also not produce complete seating. When a crown is finally torqued into place, there can be a change in proximal contact pressure as the crown may shift slightly depending on the precision of the implant-abutment connection. Torquing of an incompletely seated abutment leads to stress on the implant and risks implant damage.

When an internal connection abutment-crown "binds" or "locks" in place during proximal adjustment, one should check for complete seating with a radiograph. If seating is complete, proceed to adjustment occlusion. When occlusion is satisfactory, loosen the abutment screw without removal, and recheck if the crown can now be removed. If the crown is still "locked," finger-tighten the screw, seal with cotton and temporary cement, and leave for 1 week. At that time, the crown can be loosened and removed, and adjustments can be made prior to final torquing.

Occlusal contact

If occlusion is adjusted in the manner of a conventional crown, forces will be relatively heavier on the implant crown since the implant crown has negligible movement in function compared with natural teeth. This may not be a significant problem as it is not clear whether these fine adjustments have any bearing on outcomes. It is probable that functional occlusal equilibrium is reached via natural tooth movement. Screw-retained crowns must have occlusion rechecked after sealing the occlusal screw-hole with resin composite.

Aesthetic deficit

It is inevitable that there is some loss of bone and soft tissue height following extraction. This renders the achievement of ideal gingival contour around anterior implant crowns challenging.

After cementation and an initial period of service, it is possible that the gingival margin recedes and/or the papillae become more blunted. This effect may be mitigated somewhat by *tissue shaping* in advance of cementation. Smile line is very important and potential aesthetic complications must be explained to the patient before treatment. Metal components may cause a gray color to show through the gingiva. Although ceramic abutments are more likely to fracture, there are less aesthetic problems with their usage.

Soft tissue distension

With screw-retained crowns, gingival blanching often occurs, which can be disconcerting for the patient during an aesthetic try-in, even though it disappears quickly.

Soft tissue resistance is also a problem for cementable crowns unless adequate tissue shaping has been achieved. The crown tends to "spring back" or "push-back" during both aesthetic try-in and cementation, making both operations more challenging. It is unwise to be in a situation where the tissue must be forced out of the way to make space for cementing the crown. The final crown cementation should take place in the presence of healthy gingival tissues that have been shaped to receive the bulk of the crown.

8.10 Complications

When problems arise, it is likely that they may be retrospectively traced back to diagnosis and treatment planning. Problems may be aesthetic, biologic or mechanical. Careful diagnosis and treatment planning will minimize postoperative problems and assure positive treatment outcomes (see Chapter 13). The cumulative complication rate is relatively high for single-implant crowns (see Table 13.1). Generally, if a crown feels loose to the patient, it is probably the abutment or crown that is loose and not the implant. This problem can usually be resolved.

References

Atieh MA, Ibrahim HM, Atieh AH. (2010) Platform-switching for marginal bone preservation around dental implants: a systematic review and meta-analysis. *J Periodontol.* 81(10):1350–66.

Belser U, Martin W, Jung R, Hammerle C, Schmid B, Morton D, Buser D. (2007) *ITI Treatment Guide: Volume 1: Implant Therapy in the Esthetic Zone for Single-Tooth Replacements.* (eds. D Buser, U Belser, D Wismeijer) Quintessence, Berlin.

Carlsson GE. (2009) Dental occlusion: modern concepts and their application in implant prosthodontics. *Odontology.* 97(1):8–17.

Cumbo C, Marigo L, Somma F, La Torre G, Minciacchi I, D'Addona A. (2013) Implant platform-switching concept: a literature review. *Eur Rev Med Pharmacol Sci.* 17(3):392–7.

Dawson A, Chen S. (eds.) (2009) *The SAC Classification in Implant Dentistry.* Quintessence, Chicago.

Fugazzotto PA. (2009) Evidence-based decision making: replacement of the single missing tooth. *Dent Clin North Am.* 53(1):97–129.

Lang NP, Berglundh T; Working Group 4 of Seventh European Workshop on Periodontology. (2011) Peri-implant diseases: where are we now?: Consensus of the Seventh European Workshop on Periodontology. *J Clin Periodontol.* 38(Suppl 11): 178–81.

Salinas TJ, Eckert SE. (2007) In patients requiring single-tooth replacement, what are the outcomes of implant- as compared to tooth-supported restorations? *Int J Oral Maxillofac Implants.* 22(Suppl): 71–95.

Sanz I, Garcia-Gargallo M, Herrera D, Martin C, Figuero E, Sanz M. (2012) Surgical protocols for early implant placement in post-extraction sockets: a systematic review. *Clin Oral Implants Res.* 23(Suppl 5):67–79.

Schwartz RS, Robbins JW, Rindler E. (2010) Management of invasive cervical resorption: observations from three private practices and a report of three cases. *J Endod.* 36(10):1721–30.

Tan WL, Wong TL, Wong MC, Lang NP. (2012) A systematic review of post-extractional alveolar hard and soft tissue dimensional changes in humans. *Clin Oral Implants Res.* 23(Suppl 5):1–21.

Van der Weijden F, Dell'Acqua F, Slot DE. (2009) Alveolar bone dimensional changes of post-extraction sockets in humans: a systematic review. *J Clin Periodontol.* 36(12):1048–58.

9 Multi-Unit Implant Fixed Prostheses

9.1   Introduction

Multi-unit fixed implant restorations comprise fixed dental prostheses (FDPs) supported by two or more implants. Two- to four-unit FDPs fall within the purview of the novice implant clinician, provided case selection and treatment planning are rigorous. Treatment planning is more complex than with single-unit cases; there are many possibilities to be considered. Conventional bridges and removable partial dentures have been the traditional treatment options. These are good options, are well understood by dentists and can be accomplished quickly. Implant bridges take longer but provide an elegant and potentially more durable long-term solution for the same clinical problem.

A scenario that commonly arises in general practice and that requires a multi-unit implant restoration, is the failure of a conventional FDP with one, two, or even three pontics, and two or more natural tooth abutments. Often one or more abutments are unrestorable, and the ridge is deficient in the pontic area(s). A decision must be made as to the viability of a new conventional FDP, a removable dental prosthesis (RPD), or an implant FDP. Photographs and diagnostic mock-ups are invaluable for assessment, patient education, and treatment planning. A diagnostic mock-up will help determine potential aesthetics, the need for bone grafting, or soft tissue colored restorative materials.

The implant multi-unit prosthesis often restores significant occlusal function, and as

Fundamentals of Implant Dentistry, First Edition. Gerard Byrne.
© 2014 John Wiley & Sons, Inc. Published 2014 by John Wiley & Sons, Inc.
Companion website: www.wiley.com/go/byrne/implants

such requires careful biomechanical planning. It may be screw or cement retained. Wittneben and Weber (2013) have presented a useful treatment guide.

9.2   Treatment options for multiple tooth loss

- No implant treatment:
  - ○ Patient declines implant treatment.
  - ○ A shortened dental arch is acceptable to the patient. It may not be necessary or wise to replace first or second molars. Adequate function may be provided by 20 (up to the second premolars) or 24 (up to the first molars) tooth occlusion (Carlsson 2009).
  - ○ There is inadequate bone volume and density for implantation with risk to vital anatomic structures.
- Implant fixed dental prosthesis (FDP): two or more units supported by two or more implants (Fig. 9.1)
- Conventional fixed dental prosthesis (FDP): conventional ≥4-unit bridge
- Removable prosthesis: a metal RPD or an interim resin RPD

9.3   Advantages and disadvantages of various treatments

Implant FDP

(+) Retains alveolar bone
(+) Avoids preparation of natural tooth abutments
(+) Prosthesis failure does not compromise adjacent healthy teeth
(+) Proven longevity
(+) Patient satisfaction and acceptance
(−) Length of treatment process
(−) Expense
(−) Complexity.

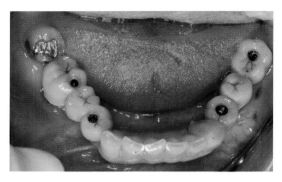

9.1. Three-unit screw-retained implant FDP during try-in (#28,29,30) with two terminal abutments and one pontic (courtesy of Dr. B. Kim).

Conventional FDP

(+) Simplicity
(+) Short length of treatment process
(+) Patient satisfaction and acceptance
(−) More pontics means greater risk of failure as span-length increases
(−) Natural tooth destruction with endodontic risk
(−) Crown margins promote plaque retention with risk of caries and periodontal disease
(−) Continuing alveolar resorption.

Removable resin partial prosthesis

(+) Simplicity
(+) Allows patient time to contemplate implant treatment
(+) Useful as diagnostic guide for potential implant prosthesis
(−) Ridge resorption promoted
(−) Plaque control hampered
(−) Poor function
(−) Patient satisfaction and acceptance.

Removable metal partial prosthesis

(+) Simplicity
(+) Versatile treatment for many problems or situations
(+) Inexpensive

(+) Can be an interim treatment

(−) Plaque control hampered

(−) Poor function unless fully tooth-supported

(−) Patient satisfaction and acceptance

(−) "Removable" has a negative connotation for many patients.

9.4   Clinical assessment

There are many possible treatment variations with multiple missing teeth, but the diagnostic and treatment planning principles are the same as with single-unit implants (see Chapters 5–8).

9.5   Examination of the implant site and surgical consultation

General factors

The situation with multiple tooth loss is more complex than with single tooth loss; additional factors are involved (see Chapters 5–8). In some cases, there is no preexisting prosthesis; in other cases, there may be a failed FDP and abutments may need to be extracted. Force factors become important with multi-unit prostheses, as in many cases a significant fraction of the occlusal table or occlusal function is being restored.

The residual ridge bone volume will determine the number, length and diameter of implants that can be placed. An approximate assessment can be made using palpation, routine radiographs, and study models. The ridge volume can be accurately assessed using a CBCT scan. This is often delayed until the surgical consultation, when a *radiographic guide* can be provided for the scan. A radiographic guide provides radio-opaque references (gutta-percha insert, radio-opaque teeth) for proposed implant positions based on a diagnostic mock-up. With longstanding tooth loss, substantial ridge resorption takes place, making the need for grafting more likely, especially as vital anatomic structures come into the proximity to potential osteotomies. The extent of lateral and vertical resorption, as well as the extent of supereruption of opposing teeth can readily be examined and explained to patients using articulator-mounted study casts and CBCT images. With the help of diagnostic mock-ups, interim RPD restorations, and the input of the surgeon, the patient will be given the implant options and must choose between grafting and nongrafting, and various other conventional restorative options (Wittneben and Weber 2013).

Mesio-distal spacing

The mesio-distal dimension of the edentulous space determines how many implants can be placed and their spacing. A minimum gap of 3.0 mm is recommended between two adjacent implants to decrease the risk of bone loss between implants and ensure an accessible cervical embrasure for plaque control. The same guides for implant diameter apply to single- and multi-unit implant prostheses. The number, length, and diameter of implants needed to support the prosthesis are based on bone volume and the functional demands of the case, and are determined by the dentist in consultation with the surgeon. Appropriate mesio-distal implant positioning is important for the aesthetics and biomechanical support of the final restoration. A surgical guide is fabricated in preparation for surgery (Fig. 9.2). More implants should be used when bone volume limits implant diameter and length.

Vertical space/alignment with opposing teeth

Supereruption of opposing teeth is often a factor with bridgework, even when a prior fixed prosthesis has been in place. Space for a

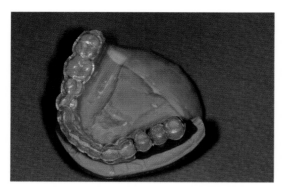

9.2. Diagnostic mock-up for distal extension tooth loss plus a surgical guide.

new implant restoration may thus be compromised. Diagnostic mock-ups are essential to planning decisions.

Opposing arch and force factors (see Chapter 3)

Surgical consultation

The main factors for the surgeon to consider in multi-unit cases are:

- The volume and quality of bone available, which will determine the number, size and diameter of implant to be used
- The need for ridge or sinus augmentation procedures
- The need for one- or two-stage surgery, and immediate or delayed implant placement.

9.6   Diagnosis and treatment planning

It is absolutely imperative that a diagnostic mock-up is made for multi-unit cases, and that a surgical guide is made for examination by the surgeon at the consultation stage. The surgeon and dentist can then decide whether a radiographic guide is indicated. This can be used during the CBCT scan and helps the surgeon

with deciding on implant position and the need for grafting. The surgeon can virtually plan the implant position in bone, relative to the clinical crown position (radio-opaque marker), using interactive computer software (see Chapters 5 and 8).

In many presenting cases, a traditional tooth-borne FDP will have failed with the demise of one or several abutment teeth. Abutment extraction, if necessary, will usually leave a good implant site, so that if both abutments are lost, there will be two good implant sites. If one abutment is to be lost and grafting of the edentulous ridge is not an option, it may be practical to place short (<10.0 mm) or narrow platform (3.0 mm) implants in the pontic area. From a biomechanical perspective, it is not advisable to use an implant and a natural tooth abutment to support a fixed prosthesis (see Chapter 3).

When there is no preexisting FDP and when two adjacent teeth are being replaced, each tooth usually needs individual implant support. Occasionally, a single canine or central incisor implant can support a lateral incisor pontic. When replacing three adjacent missing teeth, two implants, one at either end may be adequate. When four teeth are being replaced, it may be prudent to use at least three implants or even four depending on the clinical situation. If in doubt, or if narrow or short implants must be used, it is best to use one implant per tooth (Fig. 9.2). Do not compromise the longevity of the restoration by using too few implants. Mandibular incisor replacement is exceptional, in that two narrow platform implants may be used to support a four incisor FDP.

Key treatment planning factors

The treatment plan must take into account the health of the dentition and the patient's requirement for function and aesthetics. It is important at the outset to inform the patient of risks and potential future problems with preexisting

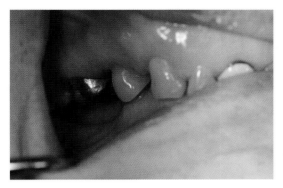

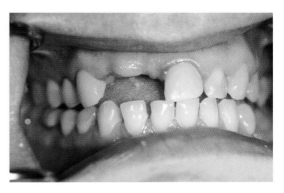

9.3. Partially edentulous case with supereruption, bruxism wear, and increased vertical overlap (referral).

9.5. Failed long-standing anterior FDP, with loss of lateral incisor, presents the possiblility of bone grafting and implant replacement

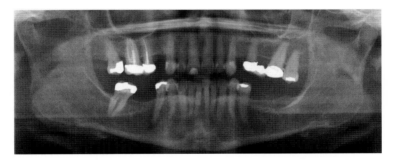

9.4. Radiograph of case with good residual bone volume, but wear and supereruption (referral).

restorations and active oral disease conditions (Fig. 9.3 and Fig. 9.4). Key treatment factors include:

- Medical conditions
- Condition of dentition
- Patient expectations
- Ridge bone volume (Fig. 9.5)
- Aesthetic challenge
- Implant positioning for function and aesthetics
- Whether occlusion is favorable: vertical overlap, super-eruption, and parafunction (Fig. 9.3 and Fig. 9.4)
- Condition of adjacent teeth and the opposing dentition
- Percentage of occlusal function being replaced

- Whether second molars should be replaced
- Finances
- Compliance.

Nonaesthetic zone

Provided adequate bone volume is available, the primary decision to be made is how many implants are required and can be placed safely. This judgment will be based primarily on functional requirements. The default number of implants is one per tooth space. The clearest indication for an implant multi-unit FDP is the loss or absence of both premolars and molars in one quadrant. Traditionally, the only treatment option for this was an RPD. A three-unit implant FDP (three premolar units or two

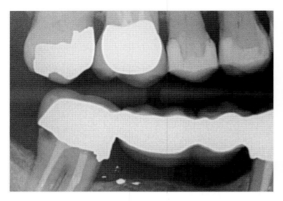

9.6. Failing conventional FDP due to caries; it may be possible to replace pontic spaces with implants, and abutments could be recrowned.

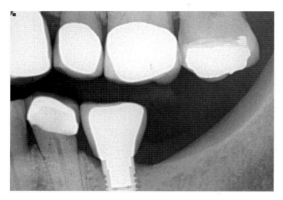

9.7. Multiple tooth loss in one quadrant with a "shortened arch" solution, that is, first molar only replacement.

premolar units and a molar unit) provides an elegant solution when adequate bone volume is available. Alternatively, a shortened arch solution may be appropriate (Fig. 9.6 and Fig. 9.7).

Aesthetic zone

When a conventional anterior three-unit FDP and abutments have failed, and are being replaced by an implant prosthesis, a two-implant three-unit FDP is an excellent solution. The implant FDP will have a similar appearance and function.

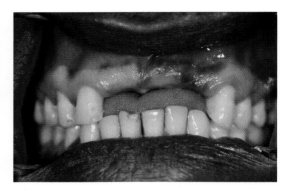

9.8. A complex case with a large anterior edentulous space with some vertical and horizontal ridge atrophy and supereruption of opposing teeth.

Two missing maxillary incisors create a unique aesthetic problem, in that it is almost impossible to recreate the interproximal soft tissue when two implant supports are used. Joining the two porcelain units with interproximal pink porcelain fill-in is often necessary, but not entirely satisfactory. However, other restorative solutions are not necessarily better.

When multiple tooth loss is long standing with subsequent ridge resorption, ridge augmentation may be used to correct the deficiency (Fig. 9.5 and Fig. 9.8). Alternatively, tissue colored porcelain or resin is needed as with conventional bridgework and RPDs. The ridge defect may be quite large and an interim RPD gives valuable diagnostic information about the prosthetic solution. This can be modified to create a radiographic guide for a CBCT, and subsequently used as a surgical guide. The aesthetic compromise will work when it is acceptable to the patient, or when a low smile line is present. The clinician must be satisfied that the patient's expectations can be met.

Number, diameter, and position of implants

The reader is referred to Misch (2007) for further discussion on implant locations under implant FDPs.

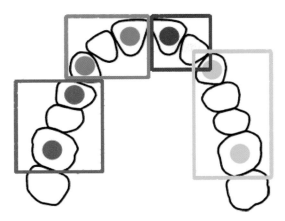

9.9. Diagram of FDP design possibilities outlined by colored rectangles; implants indicated by colored dots. In all cases, more implants could be used. Single-unit cantilevers may be acceptable in certain circumstances (courtesy of H. Byrne).

Here are some guidelines (Fig. 9.9):

- Canines or first molars involved in FDPs should have direct implant support.
- Terminal implant abutments should be used.
- Two missing teeth should generally have two implant supports.
- Three missing teeth should have two or three implant supports.
- Four missing teeth should have three or four implant supports, unless opposed by movable dentures, in which case, two terminal implants may suffice.
- When a canine and lateral incisor are missing, it may be reasonable to cantilever the lateral incisor unit from a canine implant, depending on the occlusion.
- If three maxillary incisors are missing, two terminal implants would be recommended; occasionally a cantilever may be used depending on bone volume
- If implants are placed side by side, there will be difficulty in creating an aesthetic result.

- Wide or extra wide diameter implants are recommended for molar units
- Regular or standard diameter implants are recommended for premolars, canines, and maxillary central incisors. Narrow or small diameter implants are recommended for maxillary laterals and mandibular incisors.

Financial constraints

The cost of placing 2, 3, or 4 implants, followed by the fixed prosthesis is significant and is increased further when ridge augmentation surgery is indicated. The outlay does not necessarily guarantee aesthetic success, but may raise expectations. The benefits of implant treatment over traditional treatments must be adequately explained to patients.

9.7 Patient education, expectations, and consent

The patient must be made aware of the added complexity of implant multi-unit prostheses (see Chapter 5). Additional expenses can be incurred when provisional restorations are involved in the treatment. Ridge grafting makes treatment quite complex and may be unacceptable to some patients. Alternatives must be presented.

The treatment plan options should be clearly explained and presented in written form with projected fees so as to avoid confusion later. A customized *consent form* is signed by the patient before proceeding to implant surgery.

9.8 Implant surgery

Prior to surgery, the restorative dentist will have discussed the tentative technical design of the final prosthesis with the surgeon and laboratory technician (see Chapter 7).

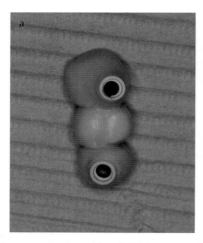

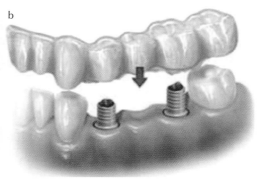

9.10. (a) Screw-retained provisional FDP (courtesy of Dr. B. Kim). (b) Diagram of fabrication of screw-retained provisional restoration using temporary abutments (abutment screw-holes blocked-out with cotton), an acetate template, and resin (courtesy of Nobel Biocare).

The surgical guide and radiographic guide

An interim resin prosthesis is often a vital component in determining implant placement and the need for bone grafting and soft tissue correction, especially in the aesthetic zone. This will give the surgeon a better understanding of the demands to be placed on the implants and the importance of accurate placement. It can be used to fabricate a surgical guide or a radiographic guide if a CBCT is planned. Implants must be placed in alignment with restorative units in a favorable 3D position to meet functional and aesthetic requirements.

Solutions for insufficient bone volume at the implant site

- Short implants, narrow diameter implants, and/or more implants
- Vertical or horizontal ridge augmentation

- Indirect sinus lift using osteotomes (Summers' osteotome technique)
- Direct or open sinus lift technique (a Caldwell–Luc procedure)
- Block autografts
- Distraction osteogenesis
- Ridge splitting (see Chapters 7 and 11).

9.9   Provisional restorations

The need for a provisional restoration will depend on the needs of the individual patient and the clinical situation. It is more problematic in more complex cases. In many nonaesthetic areas, no provisional restoration will be required. In the aesthetic zone, a provisional restoration will be required during implant osseointegration and while the permanent prosthesis is being fabricated. A resin RPD works quite well. The main disadvantage of an RPD is the risk of pressure on healing implants. At second-stage surgery, a screw-retained resin provisional FDP may be fabricated if the patient desires this option (Fig. 9.10a,b).

Summary of provisional options

- No provisional
- Resin RPD
- Provisional FDP after osseointegration, either screw-in or cementable
- Final abutments with provisional FDP
- Protective caps for certain abutments for example, Nobel Biocare Multi-unit and Snappy® abutments.

Tissue shaping

A provisional implant FDP enables tissue shaping prior to the final FDP impression (see Chapter 8). Tissue shaping is an option on most posterior cases, but may be essential on anterior ones. Shaped healing abutments or provisional implant crowns can be used to change the peri-implant soft tissue shape. The clinician may also choose to place the final abutments and a provisional FDP before finalizing the definitive FDP (Fig. 9.11a,b).

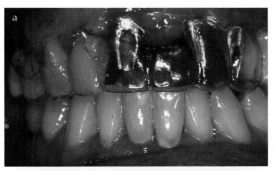
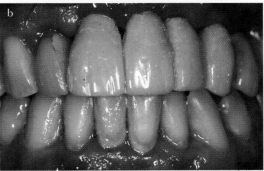

9.11. (a) Fabrication of cement-retained provisional FDP over custom implant abutments using a clear template and methacrylate resin (courtesy of Dr. E. Kim). (b) Provisional FDP cemented in position (courtesy of Dr. E. Kim).

9.10 Implant multi-unit FDP design

When the patient presents for final restoration, it is necessary to assess the implants clinically and radiographically. Appropriate impression copings are placed with a finger driver, checked radiographically, and an implant-level impression is recorded. A master cast is poured with implant analogs and a tissue mask. A final decision is made on the technical design of the prosthesis (see Chapter 8).

Designs for implant FDPs

Several FDP designs are available and will have been discussed with the patient at the treatment planning stage. The dentist will have a certain bias, as will the patient. In each case, the prosthesis is fabricated by conventional means or by computer-aided design/computer-aided manufacturing (CAD/CAM). CAD/CAM should give the best possible fit, provided that the impression transfer to the master cast is accurate.

An implant FDP may be fabricated as a *one-stage or two-stage* process. A one-stage FDP is screwed directly to the implants with abutment screws. A two-stage FDP is attached to intermediary abutments and is either cemented over the abutments or retained by small *prosthetic screws*.

Some clinicians favor the retrievability of screw-retained prostheses, while others favor the traditional approach of cementation, which should ensure a passive fit. With cemented prostheses, there is a risk that if abutment screws come loose, sectioning of the FDP would be required to access the abutment screws for retorquing. Similarly, porcelain fracture would usually necessitate cutting off a cemented prosthesis. Retrievable screw-retained *two-stage prostheses* may be favored in molar areas, where risk of overload is highest or in patients with bruxing habits. However, prosthetic screws are very small and difficult to handle at the back of the mouth.

One-stage screw-retained FDP

When implants are *aligned optimally*, it is possible to fabricate a *one-stage* screw-retained prosthesis incorporating UCLA abutments (as with single units) into the FDP framework. A custom Ti or ceramic FDP framework may also be fabricated by scanning the master cast and using a CAD/CAM technique. The final prosthesis is torqued into place with abutment screws. With the evolution of computer technology, the CAD/CAM one-stage or direct screw-retained prosthesis may be the optimal bridge solution (Fig. 9.12a,b).

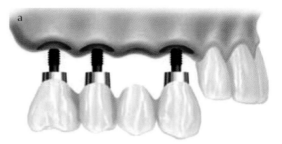

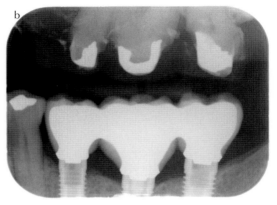

9.12. (a) Diagram of one-stage screw-retained FDP (courtesy of Nobel Biocare). (b) One-stage screw-retained FDP at try-in stage.

Two-stage FDP using abutments and a cemented prosthesis

With anterior bridges, cementation is the obvious choice given the adverse angle of the implants and the location of potential screw holes.

Prefabricated or stock abutments may be selected on the master cast, and the FDP fabricated in traditional fashion, for cementation. Prefabricated abutments can be modified to correct alignment. Custom abutments can be fabricated using UCLA abutments and also with CAD/CAM. The final prosthesis is cemented over the torque-tightened abutments (Fig. 9.13a–c).

Two-stage FDP multi-unit abutments and a screw-retained prosthesis

This is a very conservative option that allows for retrieval of both the prosthesis and abutments. Standard or conical pre-fabricated "multi-unit" abutments are chosen on the master cast. The FDP is fabricated using UCLA abutment sleeves or by CAD/CAM. The multi-unit abutments are torqued into position, followed by the FDP which is retained by small prosthetic screws. The original Brånemark fixed full-arch "hybrid" prosthesis was of this design. This is a useful technique for cases in which there is severe bone damage and soft tissue loss following trauma or ablative surgery (Fig. 9.14a,b).

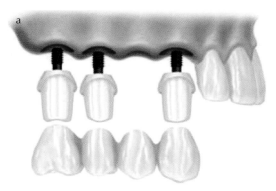

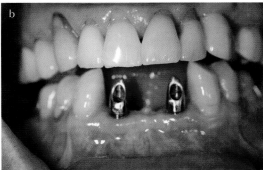

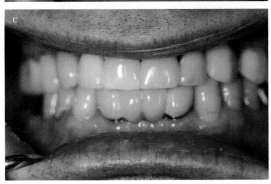

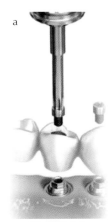

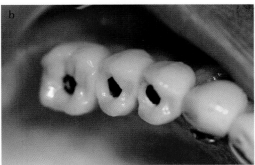

9.14. (a) Diagram of two-stage screw-retained FDP using multi-unit abutments (courtesy of Nobel Biocare). (b) Two-stage screw-retained three-unit FDP at try-in (courtesy of Dr. E. Kim).

9.13. (a) Diagram of two-stage cemented FDP (courtesy of Nobel Biocare). (b) Abutments torqued in place for cemented FDP. (c) Cemented FDP.

Advantages and disadvantages of screw-retained and cemented FDPs

Each design has its benefits (+) and shortcomings (−) and each will have its proponents and detractors.

Screw-retained FDP

(+) Are easily retrievable if problems arise, for example, peri-implantitis.

(+) Avoid inconvenience of sub-gingival margins and cement clean-up.

(+) Can be suitable for cases with limited vertical space.

(−) It is difficult to assess the fit of abutments to implants sub-gingivally.

(−) Screw holes can be unsightly.

(−) Screw-retention is impractical if screws would exit labially or through cusps or incisal edges.

Cemented FDP

(+) The machine-fit between abutments and implants is guaranteed.

(+) It is easy to seat and remove the FDP for try-in adjustments.

(+) There are no occlusal access holes.

(−) Sub-gingival cement removal can be challenging.

(−) The FDP must be cut off if problems arise.

9.11 Biomechanical factors

From a biomechanical standpoint, one implant per tooth satisfies most treatment goals. Sometimes, it is feasible to fabricate implant FDPs with a middle pontic or a cantilevered pontic. Cantilevers present a risk due to the potential for overloading the screw connections to the implants (see Chapter 3).

Individual units versus joined units

Although there is no clinical evidence to support the concept, implant units may be splinted together with a view to distributing biting forces over two or more implants. Conversely, misfit of joined units may create resting strain in the implant–bone system; this is difficult to assess. Additionally, it is challenging to manage proximal contacts on adjacent immobile single-implant crowns.

Cantilevers

Moment forces occur when the functional force is offset from the implant axis; the greater the offset, the greater the moment of force. Cantilevered pontics act as force multipliers, create moment forces on the implant FDP, and should be avoided.

Implants combined with natural teeth

Retrospective studies suggest some relative success of FDPs supported by combinations of implants and natural teeth (Lang et al. 2004; Pjetursson et al. 2004a, 2004b; Jokstad 2009) (see Table 13.1). However, the procedure is not recommended biomechanically, as the entire load is borne by the implant or implant abutment screw. It may be an acceptable procedure on older patients with relatively immobile teeth, such as canines and molars.

9.12 FDP procedures, provisionals, adjustment, and delivery

Impression and master cast

Implant level impression is currently the standard technique, although digital scanning or electronic imaging is becoming popular. A closed impression tray with impression copings is simplest. An alternative technique using an open tray, in which the impression copings remain in the impression, is still favored by some clinicians (see Chapter 8).

It is also possible to take abutment level impressions after selecting abutments, but this should generally not be necessary, as it is easier to select abutments on an implant level master cast.

FDP try-in-fit, proximal contact, occlusion

A resin try-in jig fabricated in the laboratory is often useful to orient separate abutments for a cementable FDP to their correct clinical position (see Chapter 8). The complete seating of abutments or implant bridges must be confirmed with a peri-apical radiograph. The abutments are torqued into place, followed by adjustment and cementation of the prosthesis. The FDP should have good marginal adaptation and good proximal contacts (see Chapter 8).

FDP fit must be passive, whether screw-in or cemented, and abutments must seat passively onto or into the implants. Failure to achieve passive fit will cause resting strain within the bone–implant–prosthesis system. It easier to achieve passive fit when using a two-stage cemented FDP.

It is more difficult to verify the seating of bridge abutments to the implants of one-stage screw-retained FDPs. Some clinicians favor installing one screw while checking the misfit of other units radiographically (Fig. 9.12b). Other clinicians use a silicone medium. It is more problematic to adjust proximal contacts while using screws for retention.

For occlusal adjustment refer to Chapters 3 and 8.

Torquing screws and cementation

Torque is applied to screws as stated in the specific manufacturer's instructions. Abutment and prosthetic screws are quite different, and one must be careful to apply the correct and recommended torque. Cementation follows the same protocol as for traditional crown and bridgework (see Chapter 8).

Postdelivery checks/advice (See Chapters 6, 8)

Protective orthotic occlusal devices

An orthotic occlusal guard is planned for patients with parafunction in order to mitigate excessive nonfunctional forces (Carlsson 2009). This may work well for patients who comply and whose parafunction is predictable. However, protection from prosthesis overload and mechanical failure cannot be guaranteed, and there is a high risk of mechanical failure of implant bridges in these patients. Such parafunction issues will have been diagnosed and discussed in advance of implant treatment. Patients will have been warned about the higher risk of complications and additional expenses (Jokstad 2009).

NB: One should suspect a parafunctional habit and consequential excessive forces in any patient with extensive and failing crown and bridgework. These patients are often brachiofacial with well-developed masseter muscles.

9.13 Clinical notes on implant FDPs

- Use the correct size and shape of impression coping, based on the implant data, and the size and shape of the healing abutment.
- The correct torque driver and torque values must be used.
- Torquing should be checked twice.
- Proximal contacts are difficult to adjust on screw-retained bridges.
- It is difficult to assess the quality of fit of one-stage screw-retained bridges.
- Soft tissue resistance may complicate try-in and cementation.

9.14 Maintenance and complications

FDPs perform a significant amount of occlusal function. Hence, it must be emphasized to the patient that function of the FDP should be curtailed for the first 6 months (see Chapters 6, 8, and 13). This is recommended to allow an initial functional remodeling of the bone in line with Brånemark's original guidelines. Although the implant has osseointegrated, the strength of the bone–implant connection increases with functional loading (Brånemark et al. 1985).

As our knowledge is still limited regarding the etiology of peri-implant infection, it is better to prevent than to recover the situation when bone loss has already occurred and implant threads have been exposed. Cases of peri-implantitis should be referred to the surgeon or periodontist of record. Peri-implantitis evaluation and treatment may involve removal of the prosthesis (see Chapter 13).

References

Brånemark P-I, Zarb G, Albrektsson T. (1985) *Tissue-Integrated Prostheses: Osseointegration in Clinical Dentistry*. Quintessence, Chicago.

Carlsson GE. (2009) Dental occlusion: modern concepts and their application in implant prosthodontics. *Odontology*. 97(1):8–17.

Jokstad A. (2009) *Osseointegration and Dental Implants*. Wiley-Blackwell, Ames.

Lang NP, Pjetursson BE, Tan K, Brägger U, Egger M, Zwahlen M. (2004) A systematic review of the survival and complication rates of fixed partial dentures (FDPs) after an observation period of at least 5 years. II: combined tooth-implant supported FDPs. *Clin Oral Implants Res*. 15(6):643–53.

Misch CE. (2007) *Contemporary Implant Dentistry*, 3rd ed. Mosby, St. Louis.

Pjetursson BE, Tan K, Lang NP, Brägger U, Egger M, Zwahlen M. (2004a) A systematic review of the survival and complication rates of fixed partial dentures (FDPs) after an observation period of at least 5 years. I: implant supported FDPs. *Clin Oral Implants Res*. 15(6):625–42.

Pjetursson BE, Tan K, Lang NP, Brägger U, Egger M, Zwahlen M. (2004b) A systematic review of the survival and complication rates of fixed partial dentures (FDPs) after an observation period of at least 5 years. IV: cantilever FPDs. *Clin Oral Implants Res*. 15(6):667–76.

Wittneben JG, Weber HP. (2013) *ITI Treatment Guide-Volume 6: Extended Edentulous Spaces in the Esthetic Zone*. (eds. D Wismeijer, S Chen, D Buser). Quintessence, Berlin.

10 Mandibular Implant Overdentures

10.1 Introduction

The loss of natural teeth and the wearing of complete (full) dentures, results in chronic resorption of residual alveolar ridges over time (Tallgren 1972). The mandibular implant-supported, also termed implant-stabilized and implant-retained, overdenture, using two implants in the anterior mandible, has become a popular treatment modality for the edentulous patient (Fig. 10.1, Fig. 10.2, and Fig. 10.3). It is a great treatment option to be able to offer a patient, either one who is failing to adapt to new complete dentures, or one with a long, negative denture experience that is not improving. It is a procedure that falls comfortably within the skill-set of the general dentist. Other implant treatment modalities, such as full-arch fixed implant prostheses and maxillary overdentures, are available for edentulous patients, but are not considered a good starting point for the novice implant practitioner, and will be discussed in advanced topics (see Chapters 11 and 12).

The *mandibular implant overdenture* is one of the most beneficial applications for dental implant therapy. It has been proposed by leading experts in the field that this form of treatment should be considered the "standard of care" for an edentulous patient (Feine et al. 2002; Feine and Carlsson 2003; Taylor 2003). It is a relatively simple procedure that imparts a major improvement in oral function and quality of life for the complete denture patient or dental invalid. There is relatively little surgical risk, reasonable expense, a high implant survival rate, and high prosthetic success rate and

Fundamentals of Implant Dentistry, First Edition. Gerard Byrne.
© 2014 John Wiley & Sons, Inc. Published 2014 by John Wiley & Sons, Inc.
Companion website: www.wiley.com/go/byrne/implants

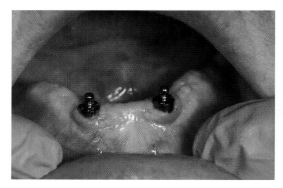

10.1. Nobel Biocare ball abutments for a mandibular implant overdenture.

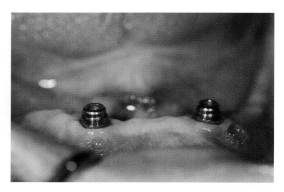

10.3. Zest Locator® abutments for mandibular implant overdenture.

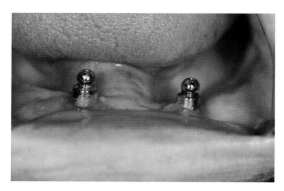

10.2. Large ball abutments for rubber "O" ring retention.

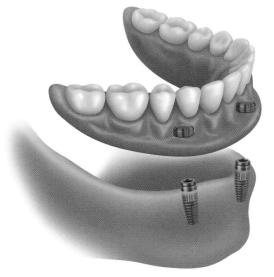

10.4. Diagram of Zest Locator® supported overdenture using two implants (courtesy of Zest Anchors).

patient satisfaction (Davarpanah 2003; MacEntee et al. 2005; Vercruyssen et al. 2010). While it imparts a marked improvement in retention, stability, and function of the denture, it also limits resorption of the mandibular ridge by providing significant vertical and horizontal resistance to denture movement.

In most cases, a satisfactory maxillary complete denture can be fabricated and the patient will accept its limitations, whereas the outcome of a conventional mandibular complete denture is far less predictable even in expert hands. With the inevitable increased popularity of implants, and declining costs of research, development, and manufacture, implant overdenture treatment will become more widespread (Fig. 10.4 and Fig. 10.5). As life expectancy rises in the world, so also the number of edentulous patients requesting implant treatment continues to increase (Feine et al. 2002; Mojon 2003).

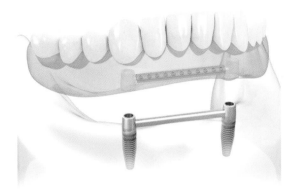

10.5. Diagram of bar-retained overdenture (courtesy of Nobel Biocare).

10.2   Patient education, expectations, and consent

The loss of natural teeth is devastating psychologically and functionally, and the clinician needs to be empathetic and understanding. Dentate patients sometimes wrongly assume that dentures are the solution to all their dental troubles, They are also unlikely to understand the limitations of the implant overdenture when compared with natural teeth. This latter situation is more likely when the patient has transitioned from natural teeth to a complete upper denture and a lower implant overdenture without having worn complete dentures for an interim period. Experienced dentists know that the expectations of "denture patients" are notoriously unpredictable. In general, it is easier to deal with an edentulous patient who is an existing patient of your practice than a new patient. An implant overdenture may be a less satisfactory solution than a fixed full-arch implant prosthesis for a patient who is just about to lose natural teeth, than for a patient who has worn complete dentures for many years. Tooth loss and transition to complete dentures must be managed carefully such that the patient understands realistic outcomes.

Home care and regular implant maintenance visits must be emphasized for overdenture patients, especially those who have had no natural teeth for some time. It is easy to forget implants hidden under a denture base. It is easier to prevent peri-implantitis than to recover the situation when bone loss has occurred and implant threads have been exposed. When the advantages, limitations, and costs of overdenture and alternative treatments have been explained, written consent must be obtained (see Chapter 5).

NB: Manage expectations prior to treatment not afterwards.

10.3   Medical assessment

As with any surgical procedure, it is necessary to assess medical risk in advance. With overdenture patients, the clinician is usually dealing with an older demographic with a higher prevalence of chronic illness and reliance on prescription medications. It is necessary to keep abreast of developments in the medical field with regard to pharmacologic and surgical risk. Careful assessment must be made of the relative risk compared with the potential benefit for the patient. The medical conditions, which may predominate in the older overdenture group of patients, must be assessed in concert with the patient's physician, and include (see Chapter 7):

- Blood clotting problems
- Chronic cardiovascular disease
- Uncontrolled diabetes
- Antiresorptive medications such as bisphosphonates
- Joint replacements
- Jaw or neck irradiation cancer treatment
- Long-term medications, e.g. steroids, chemotherapy.

Implants may be *contraindicated* if it is determined that a patient cannot cope with the rigors of the procedures, or if they are unable to cope with implant maintenance because of dexterity or other problems. Each patient has their unique set of circumstances and must not be prejudged.

10.4 Clinical assessment and surgical consultation

General aspects of the clinical examination and surgical consultation are covered in Chapters 5, 6, and 7. Rehabilitation of edentulousness is unique in dentistry and certain factors must be considered.

Volume of bone available for implants

Resorption (atrophy) of the mandibular alveolar bone ranges from minor to severe. Some patients may have minimal bone resorption due to recent tooth loss and no history of periodontal disease. Other patients may have severe resorption from long-time denture wearing, with prominent genial tubercles, and minimal bone volume and sulcus depth (Fig. 10.6). The atrophic residual ridge may provide little lateral resistance to denture movement, placing more force on the retentive implant anchors. In many cases, there is severe resorption of the posterior mandible with minimal anterior resorption due to the late retention of anterior teeth. Some cases may require ridge reduction or flattening/tabling during implant surgery. The bone configuration will determine the diameter and length of implant that can be placed.

Intermaxillary space

One must carefully assess the vertical space or vertical dimension available for the implant prosthesis inclusive of implant abutments and retentive components. A space of at least 10.0 mm from the implant platform or bony ridge crest to the occlusal plane or occlusal contact is desirable in order to fabricate an

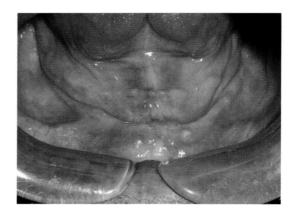

10.6. Severe mandibular ridge atrophy with a small band of attached gingiva.

implant overdenture. Cases that have limited vertical space, as with recent extractions or little or no bone loss, may require ridge reduction prior to implant placement. Fabrication of satisfactory replacement complete dentures can be diagnostic in this regard, and this step is a good prequel to implant placement as it enables a thorough assessment of vertical space for implant attachment components and denture base material.

Width of the band of attached mucosa

An implant or implant abutment should ideally be surrounded by a band of attached mucosa. Although the presence or absence of attached mucosa may not directly affect implant prognosis, implant hygiene is facilitated. By facilitating implant maintenance, the long-term prognosis of the implant is enhanced. During surgical flap reflection, the attached band may be split evenly labio-lingually to give the optimum result. This can be quite challenging in cases of severe ridge resorption (Fig. 10.6).

Skeletal jaw relationships

Severe skeletal class II and III jaw relationships present formidable clinical biomechanical

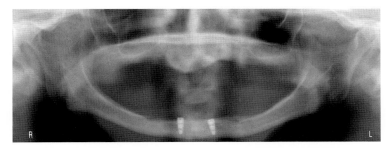

10.7. Panoramic radiograph of mandible with severe alveolar atrophy and two 8.0 mm implants.

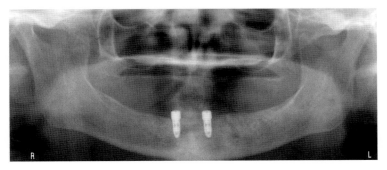

10.8. Panoramic radiograph of mandible with little alveolar atrophy and two 10.0 mm implants.

challenges in edentulous patients. It may be wise for the general dentist to refer cases that show extreme skeletal variation from normal.

Quality of existing complete dentures

The clinician must make an assessment of existing dentures in terms of extension, tooth position, vertical dimension, centric relation, occlusion, aesthetics, and phonation. It must be determined whether existing dentures are satisfactory, or whether they should be remade before providing implant treatment.

NB: *In all cases, the assessment of the patient's existing dentures and concerns must be reconciled before proceeding to implant treatment.*

Radiographs

A panoramic radiograph is the standard diagnostic film (Fig. 10.7 and Fig. 10.8). Other radiography may be required, and should be chosen by the surgeon, for the assessment of the cross-sectional bone configuration. A *lateral skull film* may prove useful to the surgeon for assessment of the mandibular cross-sectional dimensions, particularly if CBCT is unavailable. *Computed tomography (CBCT)* is becoming widely available. It provides an accurate 3D rendering of bone configuration at the proposed implant sites and shows features such as the extent of a "knife edge" bony ridge, sublingual concavities, and accessory lingual canals (Fig. 10.9 and Fig. 10.10).

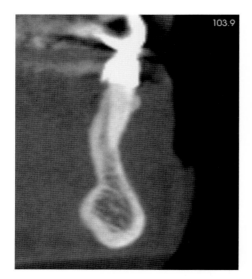

10.9. CBCT; cross-sectional image of dentate anterior mandible showing narrow alveolar process and lingual indentation (courtesy of Dr. S. Gonzalez).

10.10. CBCT; cross sectional image of edentulous mandible in the mental canal area (courtesy Dr. S. Gonzalez).

10.5   Treatment options for the edentulous patient

Conventional complete dentures

Conventional complete dentures are an acceptable and economically viable option for many patients. This treatment provides good aesthetics, but relatively poor function. To date, there is no compelling evidence that a combination of an upper complete denture and an implant supported mandibular overdenture gives a more successful outcome than conventional complete dentures for edentulous patients.

Mandibular implant overdenture opposing maxillary complete denture

In most cases, a satisfactory stable and retentive maxillary complete denture can be fabricated. However, the circumstances are very different for the mandibular complete denture

and some patients cope poorly, or not at all. The mandibular implant overdenture can overcome the difficulties with a lower denture in a relatively simple and economical way. It is also possible to provide a similar implant overdenture treatment in the maxilla with two or more implants, but implant position is more problematic in terms of bone availability (both quantity and quality), ridge angulation, and mechanical stability of the denture. Long-term studies have documented the success of implant-retained mandibular overdentures (Gotfredsen and Holm 2000; Rutkunas et al. 2008). There may be an increased long-term risk of anterior maxillary resorption when a maxillary complete denture opposes an implant overdenture.

Fixed full-arch prostheses

Fixed implant prostheses in both arches are arguably the optimum prosthetic treatment for the edentulous patient. It is a very challenging undertaking and is discussed at length in specialist textbooks (see Chapter 12).

10.6   Treatment planning factors

At the outset, it is important to inform patients that an implant-supported prosthesis is a good replacement for an existing prosthesis, but *not a substitute for a natural dentition*. The following suggestions may be useful in terms of case selection.

The need to fabricate new complete dentures

According to some expert clinicians (Feine et al. 2002), the dentist should fabricate a satisfactory set of *new complete dentures* for the patient, incorporating all the basic prosthodontics principles, prior to implant treatment. Implants should not be expected to compensate for poorly made complete dentures.

Adapting to complete dentures

It seems reasonable that a patient should try to adapt to a good set of complete dentures prior to the provision of implants. This will enable the patient to appreciate the quantum leap in comfort and function when implants are added to the equation, thereby avoiding potential disappointment with the outcome.

Transitioning to full dentures

In general, transitional partial dentures are a desirable prelude to edentulism and complete dentures. It is difficult for a patient to cope following extraction of all remaining teeth and the provision of new complete dentures in one treatment sequence. Similarly, a patient who transitions from natural teeth to implant-supported dentures is less likely to appreciate the impact of implant support. It is not uncommon for patients who have had implants placed immediately after extraction to complain that the function of the new implant overdenture is not comparable with that of the lost natural teeth.

Immediate implant placement

The possibility of immediate placement of implants should be considered for a patient based on their individual needs and desires. The patient should be informed of a higher risk of implant complications in comparison with conventional placement, based on current evidence (Esposito et al. 2009). However, it is not unreasonable for patients to request extractions and implant placement at the same surgical appointment. Such an approach could work well where planning is good and the extent of ridge reduction required is predicted in advance of surgery. In such cases, an existing partial denture may be modified to replace anterior teeth after extraction, or a new interim denture provided. The implants are placed appropriately after ridge reduction osteotomy. A new overdenture is fabricated later.

Immediate and early loading

The early loading technique was popularized by ITI (Payne et al. 2003a, 2003b). It involves the placement of four implants in the anterior mandible that are immediately connected by a rigid bar. The bar stabilizes the implants for immediate or early loading. Very slightly reduced implant survival rates have been reported by Chiapasco and Gatti (2003) and Alsabeeha et al. (2010). Ma and Payne (2010) reviewed the literature and suggested that long-term data are as yet very limited for immediate loading of two overdenture implants.

Severely atrophic mandible

In most cases, it is possible to place implants in a severely resorbed mandible. Stellingsma et al. (2013) have demonstrated that success can be achieved with short implants (<10.0 mm) in the severely atrophic mandible. However, due to the lack of posterior ridge height and support, more stress will be transmitted to the implants and small retentive components. As a result, there will be a regular need for component replacement resulting in a relatively unsatisfactory situation for the patient. This aspect needs to be discussed in advance with the patient. Such cases may be more suited to multiple implants and bars, or fixed full-arch prostheses.

Referrals

Referral to a restorative specialist is rarely the wrong decision in more difficult cases as follows:

- High patient expectations that you feel you cannot meet, communication issues or a patient who demands fixed prostheses
- Psychological issues
- Drug abuse
- Severely resorbed mandible ≤10.0 mm bone height
- "Combination syndrome," involving a severely resorbed anterior maxilla with remaining mandibular anterior teeth, which will be extracted
- Mandibular denture opposing maxillary natural teeth
- Severe class II or class III skeletal base relationships
- Mandibular dyskenesia in a patient who has worn ill-fitting dentures for a long time.

10.7 Mandibular overdenture protocols

Mandibular overdenture with two independent implants

Mandibular overdentures utilizing natural canine roots are a satisfactory and well-established prosthetic treatment. Implant overdentures are a variation on this theme. Two independent implants are placed in the lateral incisor or canine regions with *resilient attachments* to support and retain the denture, while allowing some denture movement. The female retentive devices, also termed *matrices*, are incorporated into the resin denture base. This technique requires the least space within the denture base for retentive components, and is the simplest and least expensive to fabricate. The retentive devices allow for some denture movement. The residual ridge provides some vertical and lateral resistance in the posterior region. The denture functions normally, but has the additional support and retention afforded by two solid implants. An opposing well-fabricated complete denture provides a balanced treatment solution for complete edentulousness.

Because it was traditional to use mandibular canines as overdenture abutments, it became popular to place implants in the canine position. However, the current trend is to place implants in the lateral incisor position, or the space between the lateral and canine. This places the implants as far forward as possible, thus limiting anteroposterior rotational movement of the denture, while still affording lateral stability.

Mandibular overdenture with two implants joined by a bar

Another popular option for mandibular overdentures is the use of two implants with a joining cast bar and a retentive matrix or clip.

This type of anchor is also considered *resilient*, allowing for some denture movement. This is a little more complex and expensive to fabricate as it involves laboratory casting and soldering, or CAD/CAM. The presence of a bar component makes plaque control more difficult for the patient, but it may be better than individual attachments in terms of function and longevity (Wismeijer and Stoker 2003). There is currently no evidence that a joining bar improves the prognosis of the implant-supported overdenture. A minimum space of >10.0 mm is recommended between implants to accommodate the retentive devices. Bars may be needed when implants are poorly aligned.

Mandibular overdenture with three or more implants with or without joining bars

Clinicians will often use three or four implants in the anterior mandible. This is a good option for cases of *severe mandibular resorption*, as it improves denture stability. However, there is a risk of an undesirable "rocking" anterior–posterior action that may lead to early loss of retention or damage to retentive matrices. When the implants are spread out anteriorly and posteriorly, the denture essentially becomes wholly implant-supported. Cantilevered bars may be incorporated in order to extend denture support posteriorly. This overdenture design has the advantage of being removable by the patient for hygiene while being almost as stable as a fixed prosthesis. As with two implants, bars can be used to overcome the problem of badly aligned implants.

Bar constructions are more popular for maxillary overdentures (see Chapter 12). They are particularly useful where the bone quantity and quality can severely limit implant positioning and angulation. It may be possible for bars to create supportive cantilevers where there is

no implant, with the resultant load being shared by several widely spaced implants.

ITI have researched and promoted a protocol using four implants joined by bars, supporting an overdenture where loading is immediate (Babbush et al. 1986).

Mandibular overdenture with a single implant

In certain situations, it may be a viable option to place a single implant to support a mandibular overdenture. Information on this clinical technique is currently minimal (Feine and Carlsson 2003; Alsabeeha et al. 2009).

Mandibular and maxillary implant supported overdentures or combinations with fixed implant prostheses

These are complex cases requiring experience and skill. When considering wholly implant-borne full-arch prostheses and combination cases (implant arches opposing natural dental arches), there are issues with interarch space and biting forces, and it may be prudent to refer these cases.

10.8 Planning phase and case preparation

A reasoned, unhurried approach gives the dentist the option of referring the case if potential problems are encountered during assessment, planning, or treatment. The following steps summarize the planning process:

- Discuss the rationale for implant overdentures. Explain the advantages and disadvantages, and give other treatment options.
- Educate the patient about the process and fabrication sequence.

- Present the costs, timeline of the process, and follow-up maintenance program.
- Refer the patient to the surgeon for consultation, and liaise with the surgeon on the treatment proposal. Discuss implant placement and ridge height reduction if anticipated.
- Liaise with the dental laboratory regarding their current implant capability.
- Fabricate new complete dentures as needed.
- Review the case for implants with the patient as you progress.
- Review the adaptation of the patient to the denture over 3–6 months, and decide whether to proceed with implant therapy.
- Present the patient with a complete estimate of costs.
- Have the patient sign consent forms and appoint the patient for surgery.
- Liaise with the surgeon and provide a surgical guide. Discuss the implant number, location, diameter, length, and parallelism.

NB: It is better to anticipate potential complications and inform the patient in advance rather than offer explanations after the event.

10.9   The surgical guide

A surgical guide is a helpful way to communicate the proposed implant location and angulation to the surgeon (Fig. 10.11). The usual method of guide fabrication is to duplicate the patient's existing satisfactory mandibular denture using a duplicating flask and alginate. The resultant denture void is filled with a clear self-curing acrylic resin. This can be done either by the laboratory or by the dentist. The anterior lingual flange is removed, and the labial flange is reduced, while leaving the labial and occlusal outline of the anterior teeth intact. This allows the surgeon good access for flap management and guidance for implant positioning. Alternatively, guide holes may be drilled to indicate implant positioning. The guide is cold-sterilized for surgery.

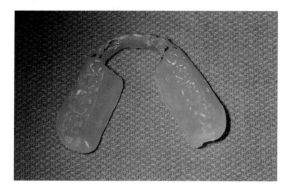

10.11. Surgical guide for mandibular overdenture implants with flanges removed in area of surgical flaps with second-stage abutments (courtesy of C. Filbert).

10.10   Implant surgery

One- or two-stage surgery

A choice must be made between one-stage or two-stage implant surgery. It has been shown that both are successful, although two-stage surgery is favored in edentulous cases due to the risk of inadvertent loading during integration (Esposito et al. 2009) (Fig. 10.12). In a one-stage surgery technique, the implant or its attached healing abutment, extends through the mucosa and is visible intraorally. This is efficient surgically and may be appropriate for elderly or medically compromised patients.

Implant position

From a prosthetic perspective, implants should be placed symmetrically relative to the midline, parallel to each other, at the same occlusal height, and perpendicular to the occlusal plane. There should be a minimum space of 10.0 mm between the implant platform and the occlusal plane of the mandibular denture. Implants are placed in the lateral incisor/canine position rather than canine position, and approximately 10.0 mm apart. Positioning of implants as described facilitates the additional placement

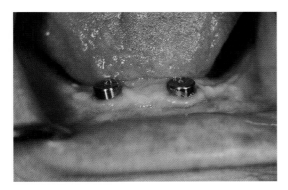

10.12. Healing abutments in position following second-stage surgery.

of implants in the midline and distally, should the patient choose to have a fixed mandibular prosthesis (with 5 implants) at a later date. Placement of implants in the canine area creates a scenario in which there may be tendency toward anteroposterior "rocking."

Implant diameter and length

Regular or standard 4.0 mm implants are favored. It would seem ideal if the residual ridge height would accommodate two 10.0 mm long implants. However, shorter implants have been shown to be successful.

Ridge modification

Ridge height reduction or ridge contouring may be needed in cases with sharp narrow ridge crests, and in cases where sufficient alveolar resorption has not yet occurred. Narrow ridge crests increase the risk of peri-implant bone loss with dehiscence and thread exposure. A minimum bucco-lingual ridge width of 6.0 mm is required for a 4.0 mm implant. Ridge height reduction is almost always required when implants are placed immediately following extractions.

Immediate implant placement

Following extractions, it is traditional to allow bone healing prior to implant placement. However, immediate implant placement into extraction sites is feasible and may be preferable in cases that indicate a minimum number of surgical procedures. The reported success rate for this technique is comparable to placing implants in a healed ridge (Esposito et al. 2009).

Implant loading and osseointegration

The implant integration period should be 3–6 months or as determined by the attending surgeon. The surgeon will have a view, based on clinical experience, as to when the implants should be loaded. Protocols have been developed for *immediate* and *early loading* (within 2–4 weeks) (Payne et al. 2003a; Kawai and Taylor 2007; Alsabeeha et al. 2010).

Surgical summary

- Reduce ridge height as needed where there is limited mandibular resorption or when implants are being placed at the time of extraction.
- Eliminate sharp or narrow ridge crests.
- Place parallel implants at least 10.0 mm apart and perpendicular to the occlusal plane.
- Ensure a minimum occlusal clearance of 10.0 mm.
- Use standard postsurgical hygiene with chlorhexidine 0.2% antibacterial mouthwash; this is especially important with one-stage implants.
- The mandibular denture should not be used for 7–10 days postsurgery.
- Modify the denture base with a soft liner and repeat as necessary.
- Follow-up as necessary for 3–6 months. Reline as necessary.

- At second-stage surgery, place healing abutments.
- Modify the denture base with a soft liner to accommodate healing tissue and healing abutments.

10.11 Prosthetic phase

Choice of anchor or attachment system

There are many commercially available anchorage possibilities for implant overdentures (Felton 2009). These include Nobel Biocare ball attachments (Nobel Biocare website, http://www.nobelbiocare.com/), Zest Locator® and "O-ring" attachments (Zest Anchors website, http://www.zestanchors.com), Sterngold ERA® attachments (Sterngold 1996) and various magnetic and bar attachments (Cendres Métaux website, http://www.cmsa.ch/en/dental/Pages/). Implant companies provide technical guidance for their own systems. The Zest Locator and ERA systems have the smallest height requirements. The choice of attachment is a matter of personal preference. When multiple implants and bars are used and the denture is fully or almost fully implant-borne,

it is necessary to consider a metal reinforcement, such as a cast metal framework within the overdenture base.

Selecting implant abutments chairside

The healing abutments are placed at second-stage surgery. After 1–2 weeks, the healing abutments are removed and appropriate anchor abutments are chosen based on clinical measurements of the peri-implant tissues. A periodontal probe is used to measure the height of soft tissue cuff occlusal to the implant platform. Abutments are selected that match the implant diameter, and whose cylindrical, nonretentive section extends 1.0–2.0 mm above the soft tissue. The abutment's retentive features will extend still further above the soft tissue. These abutments are inserted and a final denture impression recorded (Fig. 10.13, Fig. 10.14, and Fig. 10.15).

Selecting abutments at the laboratory

When provided with detailed instructions about your preferences, the laboratory

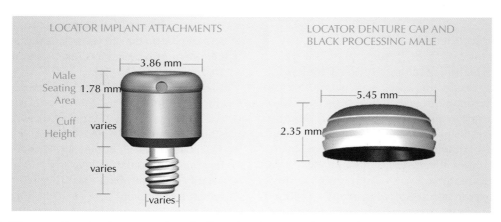

10.13. Diagram of Locator abutment and matrix dimensions (courtesy of Zest Anchors).

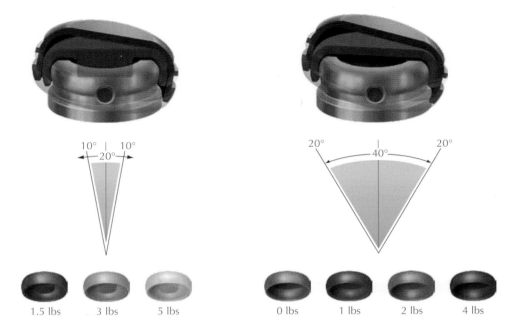

10°	10°		20°	40°	20°

| 1.5 lbs | 3 lbs | 5 lbs | 0 lbs | 1 lbs | 2 lbs | 4 lbs |

10.14. Color-coded Locator attachment retention inserts and angulation tolerance (courtesy of Zest Anchors).

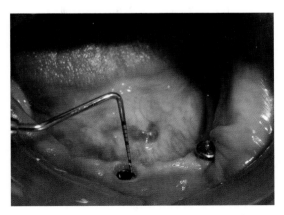

10.15. Periodontal probe to measure height of soft tissue cuff around implant

technician may select and supply the final abutments, as they are familiar with the components and may keep them in stock. A preliminary diagnostic alginate implant-level impression, with impression abutments, is sent to the laboratory. The technician selects appropriate sized anchor abutments and returns them to the dentist along with a custom tray for a final *abutment-level* denture impression. Alternatively, an *implant-level* final denture impression is made. This is achieved using standard impression abutments attached to the implants. The technician then selects anchor abutments using measurements from the master cast with its implant analogs.

Selecting bar abutments

When a bar attachment is used, an implant level final impression is recorded. The technician selects the appropriate height abutments on the master cast that will allow room for soldering a bar. The implant-borne bar substructure is returned as one piece for clinical try-in and fit verification prior to denture processing. Bars may be round or oval with suitable

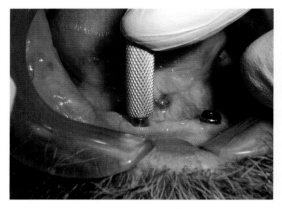

10.16. Finger tightening a Locator abutment.

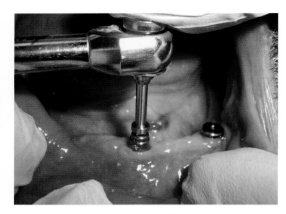

10.17. Torque driving a Locator abutment.

retentive clips. Ackermann®, Hader®, and Dolder® Bars are popular in prosthodontic reconstructions. CAD/CAM-fabricated bars are becoming more popular.

Seating anchor abutments

Healing abutments are removed one at a time, and the selected anchor abutment is quickly inserted with finger tightening. This is necessary due to the tendency for the surrounding soft tissue to collapse over the implant, making it more likely to pinch tissue when inserting an abutment if there is any delay. The male anchor abutments are checked with a radiograph to verify complete seating, and torqued into place at the recommended torque (usually between 15 and 20 Ncm). The denture is then modified and relined with a soft liner to accommodate the new abutments. It is important not to select abutments that are too long, as this makes it more challenging to accommodate them within the normal confines of the denture base, resulting in bulky denture bases or base fractures (Fig. 10.16 and Fig. 10.17).

10.12 Overdenture protocol 1: retrofit implant attachments to the definitive mandibular complete denture

Following implant surgery, the mandibular denture is left out for 1–2 weeks and then relieved and relined with a soft liner over the implant sites. At second-stage surgery, following a 3–6 month integration interval, implants are uncovered and healing abutments are placed. After 1–2 weeks' healing, the dentist can proceed with anchor abutment selection and placement. The anchor abutments are torqued into place and the denture is *hollow-ground* to accommodate them. This is done using a silicone material such as Exabite™ or Fit-Checker™ to confirm abutment noncontact with the resin base. A soft lining may be used to improve stability.

Indirect technique

A localized reline impression is made of an already well-adapted denture base, with a high viscosity impression material, such as a

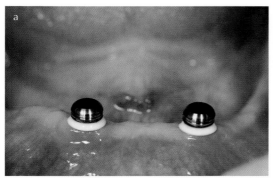

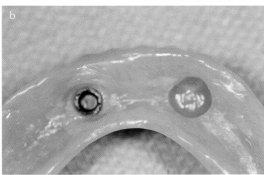

10.18. (a) Direct technique for "pick-up" of locator matrices seated on abutments; teflon washers in place to prevent resin locking around the abutments. (b) Intaglio of denture showing one locator matrix in position with black vinyl processing blank, and a hollowed out space to accommodate the second matrix.

polyether or silicone (Fig. 10.18a,b). The technician processes the retentive female matrices into the denture base and returns the denture for insertion. Retentive nylon inserts are placed chairside (Zest Locator), or checked for activation (Nobel Biocare Ball).

Direct technique

A common alternative to the indirect method is to directly fit the matrices chairside. The denture is *hollow-ground* to accommodate the matrices, and the matrices are "picked-up" by

the denture base using a cold-cure resin. This can work well for locator matrices and save on laboratory expense. This technique is not recommended for ball anchors due to the risk of locking the pick-up resin around the implant abutments.

10.13 Overdenture protocol 2: fabricate a new mandibular denture over implants

The dentist may opt to use an interim denture during the surgical phase and fabricate a new mandibular denture when the implants have osseointegrated. In this protocol, after 3–6 months integration, new complete dentures are fabricated over the newly placed implant abutments. Impression copings are placed over the abutments and a border-moulded final impression is recorded (Fig 10.19a). This is an *abutment-level impression*, and abutment analogs are incorporated into the master cast. The presence of the anchor abutments at the records and try-in phases of denture construction will greatly improve the stability of the lower base during these procedures. When the denture is returned from the laboratory for final insertion it will have the retentive matrices processed into the denture base.

10.14 Overdenture delivery

When the denture is returned from the laboratory with the processed retentive matrices, it is tried-in and checked for fit and occlusion. For dentures using locator attachments, the blank black vinyl processing inserts are left in place until fit and occlusion have been verified. These processing inserts are then replaced with appropriate retentive nylon inserts (Fig. 10.19b,c). Color-coded nylon locator inserts of varied retentive value are available, as are special inserts for off-axis implants. With Nobel Biocare

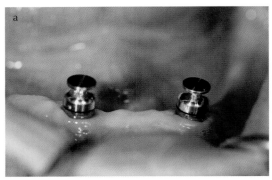

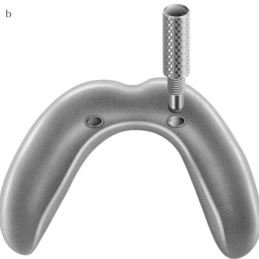

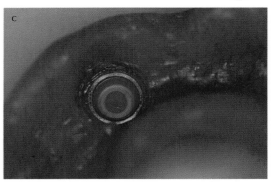

10.19. (a) Indirect technique; impression copings *in situ* prior to final denture impression. (b) Black processing inserts are removed and replaced with definitive blue nylon retentive inserts at delivery (courtesy of Zest Anchors). (c) Zest Anchor blue retentive nylon insert in denture base.

ball attachments, the matrices are adjusted for retention.

With retentive inserts in place, or ball matrices activated, or with slightly misaligned implants, the denture can be very retentive and difficult for the patient to remove. The clinician may choose to postpone nylon insert placement or ball matrix activation until the 1-week follow-up visit.

NB: It is important that the patient can easily remove and reinsert the denture, prior to dismissal.

10.15 Clinical notes

Locator matrices/direct technique

The direct placement of matrices chairside is a relatively straightforward option for locator attachments and a definitive denture (Fig. 10.18a,b). Following insertion of the chosen locator abutments, the intaglio of the denture base is *hollow-ground* to accommodate the abutment. A nylon spacer is placed over the abutment followed by the female matrix. Self-curing acrylic resin such as ERA® PickUp™ (Sterngold) resin is placed inside the relevant denture base areas and the denture is seated with the patient closing lightly into MI. After setting for 3–4 minutes, the denture is removed and excess resin is ground away (Fig. 10.19c). One attachment is completed at a time. Appropriate retentive inserts are placed.

Locator retentive nylon inserts

In cases of implant abutments with good parallelism, there are standard nylon retentive inserts of varied retentive values. Nonparallel abutments require specific modified inserts. A special Locator tool is available for nylon insert placement and removal (Fig. 10.14 and 10.19b).

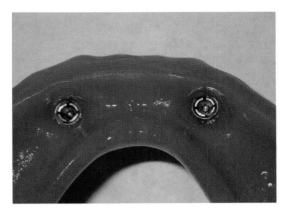

10.20. Denture base with ball retentive matrices in position.

Nobel Biocare ball attachments and the indirect technique

With Nobel Biocare ball attachments, it is best to use an indirect technique with an *abutment-level* impression, and have the laboratory technician set the retentive matrices into the denture base. With a direct technique, it can be challenging to pick up ball matrices clinically, and there is a risk of getting resin locked around the abutments and inside the matrices. It is traumatic for the patient if the denture gets locked onto the implants and has to be cut free (Fig. 10.20).

Altering retention of ball matrices

When the denture is returned from the laboratory, the matrices should be passive, or minimally active. A specialized screwdriver is used to increase or decrease the amount of retention of the ball matrices. Retention is adjusted in one-quarter turn steps, plus or minus.

10.16 Maintenance considerations

Peri-implant health (see Chapter 6)

Prosthetic stability

The mandibular overdenture and its opposing complete denture need to maintain good tissue adaptation due to ongoing ridge atrophy. Occlusal change with loss of posterior contact is a key indicator of ridge atrophy. The quality of denture base adaptation should be checked periodically and relined as necessary. Tissue adaptation can be checked by making a trial silicone impression without adhesive. Failure to reline the denture as needed would lead to denture base instability, occlusal instability, and damage to retentive components. For ball attachments, it is possible for both abutments and matrices to wear out and they may have to be replaced periodically. For Locator attachments, only the nylon inserts will wear and need to be replaced. Bar and ball matrices may need to be changed or reactivated.

Maintenance problems

Difficulties arise in cases when a patient's dexterity or vision becomes impaired, and when a patient's living circumstances change dramatically, for example, confinement to bed, rest homes, or hospitals. In these situations, detailed instructions must be given to carers for implant and denture care.

Overdenture complications

The complication rate is relatively high, in the region of 30%, for implant overdentures (Goodacre et al. 2003) (see chapter 13). Many problems are minor, but repetitive. Problems that may occur include:

- Plaque and calculus accumulation with peri-implant mucositis and soft tissue hyperplasia
- Peri-implantitis bone loss around implants
- Soft tissue recession and bone loss with implant thread exposure
- Perforation or fracture of the denture base around the retentive matrices
- Abutment wear or loosening
- Matrix wear or loosening
- Denture movement such as "rocking"
- Debris in retentive components.

Careful treatment planning and management of patient expectations will minimize postoperative problems and assure positive treatment outcomes.

References

Alsabeeha N, Payne AG, De Silva RK, Swain MV. (2009) Mandibular single-implant overdentures: a review with surgical and prosthodontic perspectives of a novel approach. *Clin Oral Implants Res.* 20(4):356–65.

Alsabeeha N, Atieh M, Payne AG. (2010) Loading protocols for mandibular implant overdentures: a systematic review with meta-analysis. *Clin Implant Dent Relat Res.* 12(Suppl 1):e28–38.

Babbush CA, Kent JN, Misiek DJ. (1986) Titanium plasma-sprayed (TPS) screw implants for the reconstruction of the edentulous mandible. *J Oral Maxillofac Surg.* 44(4):274–82.

Chiapasco M, Gatti C. (2003) Implant-retained mandibular overdentures with immediate loading: a 3- to 8-year prospective study on 328 implants. *Clin Implant Dent Relat Res.* 5(1):29–38.

Davarpanah MMD. (ed.) (2003) *Clinical Manual of Implant Dentistry.* Quintessence, London.

Esposito M, Grusovin MG, Chew YS, Coulthard P, Worthington HV. (2009) One-stage versus two-stage implant placement. A Cochrane systematic review of randomized controlled clinical trials. *Eur J Oral Implantol.* 2(2):91–9.

Feine JS, Carlsson GE. (2003) *Implant Overdentures: The Standard of Care for Edentulous Patients.* Quintessence, Chicago.

Feine JS, Carlsson GE, Awad MA, Chehade A, Duncan WJ, Gizani S, Head T, Lund JP, MacEntee M, Mericske-Stern R, Mojon P, Morais J, Naert I, Payne AG, Penrod J, Stoker GT, Tawse-Smith A, Taylor TD, Thomason JM, Thomson WM, Wismeijer D. (2002) The McGill consensus statement on overdentures. Mandibular two-implant overdentures as first choice standard of care for edentulous patients. Montreal, Quebec, May 24–25, 2002. *Int J Oral Maxillofac Implants.* 17(4):601–2.

Felton DA. (2009) Treatment of edentulous maxilla and mandible with implant retained overdentures. In: A Jokstad (ed.), *Osseointegration and Dental Implants.* Wiley-Blackwell, Ames, pp. 27–32.

Goodacre CJ, Bernal G, Rungcharassaeng K, Kan JY. (2003) Clinical complications with implants and implant prostheses. *J Prosthet Dent.* 90(2): 121–32.

Gotfredsen K, Holm B. (2000) Implant-supported mandibular overdentures retained with ball or bar attachments: a randomized prospective 5-year study. *Int J Prosthodont.* 13(2):125–30.

Kawai Y, Taylor JA. (2007) Effect of loading time on the success of complete mandibular titanium implant retained overdentures: a systematic review. *Clin Oral Implants Res.* 18(4):399–408.

Ma S, Payne AG. (2010) Marginal bone loss with mandibular two-implant overdentures using different loading protocols: a systematic literature review. *Int J Prosthodont.* 23(2):117–26.

MacEntee MI, Walton JN, Glick N. (2005) A clinical trial of patient satisfaction and prosthodontic needs with ball and bar attachments for implant-retained complete overdentures: three-year results. *J Prosthet Dent.* 93(1):28–37.

Mojon P. (2003) The world without teeth: demographic trends. In: JS Feine, GE Carlsson (eds.), *Implant Overdentures;The Standard of Care for Edentulous Patients.* Quintessence, Chicago, pp. 3–13.

Payne AG, Tawse-Smith A, Thompson WM, Kumara R. (2003b) Early functional loading of unsplinted roughened surface implants with mandibular overdentures 2 weeks after surgery. *Clin Implant Dent Relat Res.* 5(3):143–53.

Payne AGT, Tawse-Smith A, Thomson WM, Duncan WJ. (2003a) Loading strategies for mandibular implant overdentures. In: JS Feine, GE Carlsson (eds.), *Implant Overdentures: The Standard of Care for Edentulous Patients.* Quintessence, Chicago, pp. 111–28.

Rutkunas V, Mizutani H, Peciuliene V, Bendinskaite R, Linkevicius T. (2008) Maxillary complete denture outcome with two-implant supported mandibular overdentures. A systematic review. *Stomatologija Balt Dent Maxillofac J.* 10(1):10–5.

Stellingsma K, Raghoebar GM, Visser A, Vissink A, Meijer HJ. (2013) The extremely resorbed mandible, 10-year results of a randomized controlled trial on 3 treatment strategies. *Clin Oral Implants Res.* doi: 10.1111/clr.12184; [Epub ahead of print].

Sterngold (1996) http://www.sterngoldrestorative systems.com/Sterngold/Docs/Era.pdf (last accessed January 7, 2014).

Tallgren A. (1972) The continuing reduction of the residual alveolar ridges in complete denture wearers: a mixed-longitudinal study covering 25 years. *J Prosthet Dent.* 27:120–32.

Taylor TD. (2003) Indications and treatment planning for mandibular implant overdentures. In: JS Feine, GE Carlsson (eds.), *Implant Overdentures; The Standard of Care for Edentulous Patients.* Quintessence, Chicago, pp. 71–82.

Vercruyssen M, Marcelis K, Coucke W, Naert I, Quirynen M. (2010) Long-term, retrospective evaluation (implant and patient-centred outcome) of the two-implants-supported overdenture in the mandible. Part 1: survival rate. *Clin Oral Implants Res.* 21(4):357–65.

Wismeijer D, Stoker GT. (2003) Comparison of treatment strategies for implant overdentures. In: JS Feine, GE Carlsson (eds.), *Implant Overdentures; The Standard of Care for Edentulous Patients.* Quintessence, Chicago, pp. 61–70.

11

Advanced Topics: Surgery

11.1	Introduction	11.5	Ridge augmentation/guided bone regeneration
11.2	Surgical complexity	11.6	Block autografts
11.3	Immediate and early implant placement	11.7	Sinus-lift/sinus augmentation
11.4	Graft materials, osteogenic materials, and scaffolds/matrices	11.8	Other surgical techniques
		11.9	Virtual treatment planning and guided surgery

11.1 Introduction

What makes an implant case challenging? Complexity may be of a surgical or restorative nature, or both. As one becomes more experienced in implant treatments, it is reasonable to undertake more challenging cases. From a simplistic point of view, more challenging cases may mean more units of restorative dentistry. From a technical surgical perspective, a case may be considered complex when there is inadequate bone volume and where implant placement would impinge on vital anatomic structures. Restorative complexity relates to aesthetic and biomechanical limitations where the desired outcome cannot be realistically achieved. For example, the patient may be very demanding with unrealistic expectations with respect to a single tooth space in the aesthetic zone with a high smile line and severe alveolar atrophy.

Modern imaging technology has greatly helped the visualization of bone volume and configuration for implant placement and the relative position of vital structures and projected restorations. Nonetheless, when the boundaries of technical difficulty are pushed, surgical cases become more complex and the complication risk increases.

11.2 Surgical complexity

The ITI group (Dawson and Chen 2009) has presented some guidelines to define the degree of difficulty for implant cases as follows: straightforward, advanced, or complex (SAC classification) based on certain criteria (see Chapters 5 and 7). More complex protocols carry greater risk.

The prominent factors which render surgery complex include:

Fundamentals of Implant Dentistry, First Edition. Gerard Byrne.
© 2014 John Wiley & Sons, Inc. Published 2014 by John Wiley & Sons, Inc.
Companion website: www.wiley.com/go/byrne/implants

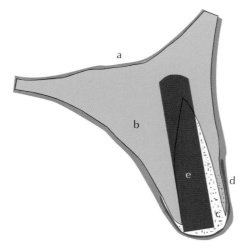

11.1. Diagram of immediate placement in a socket with a thin labial plate: (a) sinus space; (b) bone; (c) graft material; (d) membrane (blue line); (e) implant (courtesy of H. Byrne).

- Compromised bone volume and quality
- Anterior cases with high aesthetic demands; cases with thin tissue biotype are at greater risk of soft tissue recession
- Immediate placement, guided bone regeneration, grafting procedures and early loading protocols
- Medical conditions affecting bone healing or osseointegration, for example, immunodeficiency, jaw irradiation, and IV biphosphonate medication
- General medical conditions carrying risk for oral surgery, for example, chronic cardiaovascular disease.

11.3 Immediate and early implant placement

Several modern surgical protocols have been developed and described for implant placement (Dibart and Dibart 2011; Hämmerle et al. 2004) (Fig. 11.1).

Placement protocols

Type I, *immediate placement*: simultaneous extraction and implant placement.

Type II, *early placement*: implant placement, after 4 to 8 weeks, when there is complete soft tissue coverage of the socket.

Type III, *early placement with partial bone healing*: implant placement, after 12–16 weeks, when there is substantial bone fill of the socket.

Type IV, *late placement*: implant placement, after 4–6 months, into the healed site.

Immediate placement

The immediate placement of implants into extraction sites has become a popular treatment modility in an effort to preserve bone and soft tissue and reduce treatment times. It may be considered a higher risk strategy than late placement, except in experienced hands (Beagle 2006; Evans and Chen 2008). Esposito et al. (2010a) in a systematic review found insufficient evidence to give a positive recommendation for the procedure. With immediate placement, the patient should be informed of a higher risk of implant complications in comparison with conventional placement. Experience in case selection and implant surgery should lead to satisfactory outcomes (Schropp and Isidor 2008). The clinician must weigh the risks of failure against the desired expedience. The concept aims to extract a tooth and place the implant in the socket in one operation. Implant selection in terms of length, diameter, and collar design are all important. The procedure is more suited to a single-root tooth and a tooth with a healthy residual root with little or no bone loss and no peri-radicular pathology. Extraction sites with infection or apical pathology or labial socket damage may be augmented, if deemed necessary, using guided bone regeneration techniques, and allowed to heal for 3–6 months. Immediate placement in multi-rooted

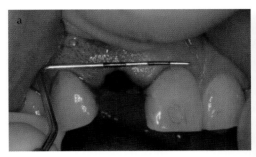
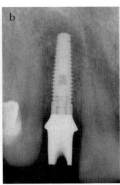

11.2. (a) Immediate implant placement: visualizing implant depth and adjacent cervical lines (courtesy of Dr. S. Whitney). (b) Implant with definitive abutment (courtesy of Dr. S. Whitney).

sockets is more complex and has been reviewed by Smith and Tarnow (2013).

The implant must be kept to the lingual aspect of a maxillary anterior socket in order to avoid thinning of labial bone with risk of dehiscence and fenestration. Anatomically, there is more bone to the lingual of the incisor root apices. The labial cortical plate is often less than 1.0 mm thick. The osteotomy may need to be extended 4.0–5.0 mm apical to the socket to achieve initial implant stabilization. Tapered implants such as the Dentsply Frialit® may be preferred by some clinicians for their initial fit and stability in the socket site. If primary stability cannot be achieved, then the implant placement should be delayed until socket healing has occurred. Usually, socket anatomy leads to voids remaining around the implant. These may be in-filled with autogenous bone from the osteotomy preparation, or an alloplastic material. There should be primary flap closure with or without a membrane, or alternatively suturing of tissue around a transmucosal healing abutment as with one-stage surgery (Fig. 11.1).

It has been noted that some ridge resorption still occurs in these cases, but may have less clinical significance than the resorption that occurs rapidly when an extraction socket is allowed to heal normally (Schropp et al. 2003) (Fig. 11.2a,b).

Summary of criteria for immediate placement:

- An healthy oral environment
- A thick gingival biotype, and healthy bone
- No infection or radicular pathology
- An atraumatic extraction with no flap, if possible
- No loss of socket wall before or during extraction
- Sufficient bone apical to the root to enable initial implant stability.

There are certain pitfalls to be avoided:

- The buccal plate of bone is often less than 1.0 mm thick and is easily fractured during extraction. A labial muco-periosteal flap would further compromise the labial plate.
- The osteotomy needs to be directed palatally on maxillary incisors to avoid proximity to the labial bony plate, and to engage new bone.
- The sinus invaginates between roots of multi-rooted teeth risking antral perforation.
- Socket outlines and interradicular bony septa may misdirect drills.
- The implant platform must be positioned 2.0–3.0 mm apically with the expectation of some bone resorption of the bony socket margins.

11.4 Graft materials, osteogenic materials, and scaffolds/matrices

Traditionally autogenous/autologous (host) bone grafts have been used to replace deficient bone. Bone can be harvested from osteotomy sites, or in block sections from other parts of the bony anatomy. More recently, surgical techniques have evolved that use allografts, xenografts, and alloplastic particulate graft materials along with gels, membranes, and titanium mesh stents, to confine the graft materials in position. The alloplastic materials and collagen gel matrices act as fillers and scaffolds that are replaced by new bone growth. Matrices/scaffolds/gels can be used in combination with growth factors to stimulate new bone formation. Allografts/xenografts/alloplasts may have lower performance than autogenous bone but they also have a lower risk of infections. Barrier membranes, either absorbable (BAM) or nonabsorbable (NAM), are used to cover the grafted site completing the technique known as guided bone regeneration (GBR). Barrier membranes prevent the ingrowth of epithelium and connective tissue while new bone growth occurs.

Graft materials

- *Autograft or autogenous (host bone) graft* is the traditional and most predictable graft material. A second operation is needed to harvest bone from the mandible, tibia or ilium.
- *Allograft (bone from another human):* Cadaveric bone is available from a bone bank, for example, freeze-dried bone allograft (FDBA) and demineralized freeze-dried bone allograft (DFDBA). Demineralized bone matrix (DBM) contains collagen, proteins, and growth factors from allograft bone. There is a slight risk of disease transmission from these products.
- *Xenograft (nonhuman bone):* This is sterilized nonorganic material from animal bones,

for example, bovine or porcine (CPB) derivatives.

- *Alloplastic graft materials (alloplasts):* Inorganic materials, often synthetic, are used as a bone substitute. These materials can be treated with growth factors. Alloplasts are comprised of a variety of products derived from: hydroxyapatite (HA), bioactive glass (BG), $CaSO_4$, $CaCO_3$, $Ca_3(PO_4)_2$, porous ceramics, and coralline hydroxyapatite (CHA).
- *Growth factors:* Recombinant human bone morphogenetic protein (rhBMP) and platelet-derived growth factor (PDGF) or rhPDGF.
- *Carrier scaffolds or matrices made from collagen:* Absorbable collagen sponge (ACS), for example, polylactide-polyglycolide acid sponge, synthetic polymers, and hyaluronic gels.
- *Barrier membranes* are used for guided bone regeneration (GBR) often with the concomitant use of graft materials. Ingrowth of connective tissue is prevented while new bone growth occurs. They are *bio-absorbable* (BAM) and *nonabsorbable* (NAM) *membranes*, for example, polytetrafluoroethylene (PTFE) (Jokstad 2009; Froum 2010; Dibart and Dibart 2011).

Tissue engineering and osteoconduction

Active tissue engineering involves the use of growth factors in extracellular matrices combined with membranes. Growth factors are introduced to the bone defect site within a carrier matrix or delivery system of collagen foam or gel, synthetic polymer, hyaluronic gels, or a host of particulate graft materials, such as demineralized bone matrix (DBM), calcium phosphate preparations (e.g., hydroxyapatite and coralline hydroxyapatite), and Bioglass.

During osseointegration, numerous cell types (marrow stomal cells, osteoblasts, platelets, etc.) release various growth factors (BMP,

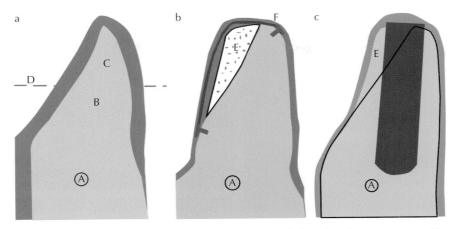

11.3. Ridge augmentation/guided bone regeneration. (a) Atrophic mandibular ridge: The narrow crest of bone (C) above line (D) must be flattened for implant placement in suitable bone (B). The mandibular canal (A) is at risk (courtesy of H. Byrne). (b) Guided bone regeneration with graft material (E) without ridge reduction will increase working volume of ridge. Membrane (F) (blue line) covers the addition (courtesy of H. Byrne). (c) New bone formation (E) and implant placed above the mandibular canal (A) (courtesy of H. Byrne).

PDGF, IGF, FGF, etc.) (Dibart and Dibart 2011). These factors act on target mediator cells to carry out the complex biochemical mechanisms of tissue healing, including cell chemotaxis, differentiation, stimulation, and proliferation (Devescovi et al. 2008). As such, growth factors play an important role in cascade reactions for defect granulation, callus formation, bone repair, remodeling, or regeneration. The availability of recombinant DNA-derived growth factors has enabled their use for skeletal repair and bone augmentation procedures. Examples of recombinant DNA-derived materials are recombinant human bone morphogenetic proteins (rhBMPs), recombinant human platelet derived growth factor (rhPDGF), and fibroblast growth factor (FGF) (Dibart and Dibart 2011). Research is ongoing and aims to expand the use of recombinant DNA derived growth factors. Research has shown some promising results in periodontics, (Fiorellini and Nevins 2003) but, as yet, this field is in its infancy (Scheyer 2009).

11.5 Ridge augmentation and guided bone regeneration (GBR)

Surgical grafting has long been associated with the morbidity of the autogenous graft donor site. This is a major disadvantage for most patients. Advances are being made in tissue engineering in areas such as skin grafting and bone grafting. Similar methods using barrier membranes, growth factors, matrices, and alloplasts have been used in periodontal surgery for guided tissue regeneration (GTR) for some time (Karring and Warrer 1992; Fiorellini and Nevins 2003; Wang et al. 2005; Camelo et al. 2012). McGuire and Scheyer (2006) have shown evidence of periodontal regeneration using rhPDGF + BetaTCP (tricalcium phosphate) with a collagen membrane. It is a logical progression that such materials and techniques should be applied to guided bone regeneration (GBR) at implant sites in order to increase bone volume (ridge height and width) or to recover peri-implantitis cases (Fig. 11.3a–c).

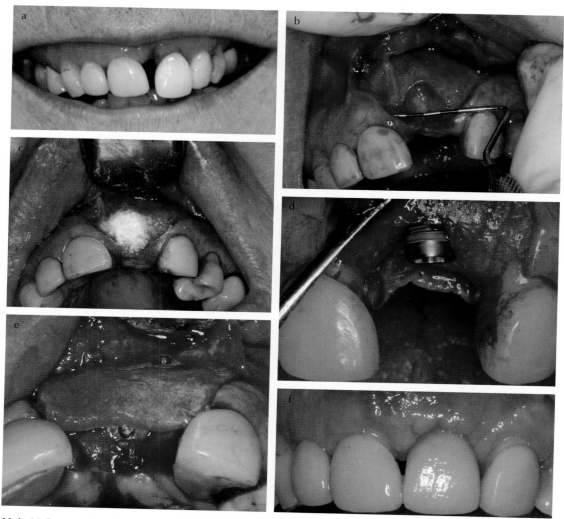

11.4. (a) Preoperative photograph of periodontally compromized left central incisor. (b) Mucoperiosteal flap raised showing extraction site with bone loss. (c) Socket and defect filled with particulate alloplastic graft material. (d) Healed bone site after 6 months. Implant placed, but still some bony defect present. (e) Collagen sponge placed prior to flap closure. (f) Final implant crown (courtesy of Dr. S. Whitney).

Many techniques, graft materials, and membranes are available for GBR. The technique may be applied to correct ridge deficiencies, both vertical and horizontal. It has also been used to regenerate bone in extraction sites, or in the maxillary sinus. It is becoming more popular as a method to correct peri-implant complications such as bony dehiscence, and to treat peri-implant bone loss (Schwarz and Becker 2010) (Fig. 11.4a–e). It may be combined successfully with immediate implant placement (Dawson and Chen 2009). Systematic reviews by Ten Heggeler et al. (2011) and Vignoletti et al. (2012) have demonstrated a positive effect of GBR on ridge preservation techniques following extraction.

Aghaloo and Moy (2007) reviewed bone augmentation techniques and found that sinus augmentation has been well documented. Long-term implant survival (>5 years), regardless of graft material(s) used, compares favorably with survival of implants placed conventionally with no grafting procedure. Conversely, they found that alveolar ridge augmentation may be more technique and operator sensitive, and that implant survival may be more a function of the native bone than of the regenerated bone. Tonetti and Hämmerle (2008) suggest a cautionary approach to GBR, based on higher complication rates and reduced long-term implant survival rates.

Dibart and Dibart (2011) have illustrated a ridge augmentation technique for using rhBMP-2 carried by an absorbable collagen sponge (ACS), and a shaped titanium mesh for maintaining the ridge shape. The blood supply and the distribution of the growth factor within a suitable carrier matrix is considered critical to success. This field will continue to expand and may make grafting of deficient ridges prior to implantation a routine procedure (Fig. 11.5a–c).

11.6 Block autografts

Blocks of autogenous bone harvested from the ramus or mentalis region of the mandible, or alternatively from the iliac crest or tibia, may be shaped and fitted to areas of severe bone loss. The cortical plate of the receptor site is perforated with a small round bur to improve the vascular supply of the graft bed. The graft is usually immobilized by being screwed into position, and allowed to heal for between 6 and 12 months before placement of implants (Fig. 11.6). Tension-free primary flap closure is performed. Harvesting autogenous bone blocks is a fairly significant surgical procedure and

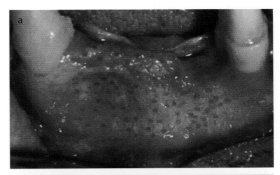
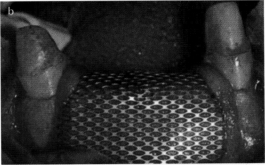
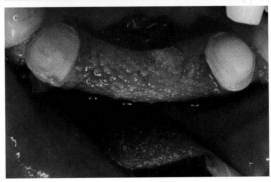

11.5. Ridge augmentation series: (a) Host site cortical bone perforation. (b) Titanium retaining mesh over collagen sponge (absorbable collagen sponge) impregnated with rhBMP-2. (c) Regenerated bone upon reentry after 7 months (courtesy of Dibart and Dibart 2011).

tends to be reserved for the more extreme atrophy cases following extensive jaw bone loss such as with jaw tumor surgery. The most common complications with block grafting are suture line wound dehiscence and infection.

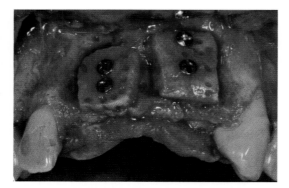

11.6. Autogenous block bone grafts (courtesy of Dibart and Dibart 2011).

11.7 Sinus-lift/sinus augmentation

There are two well-known sinus-lift or sinus augmentation techniques that provide new bone for maxillary implants, *direct and indirect sinus-lift* (Jensen and Katsuyama 2011). These surgical techniques have revolutionized the accessibility of the posterior maxilla for dental implants. The indirect method has become quite routine and is less complicated than the direct lateral wall approach (Esposito et al. 2010b). The posterior maxilla is a unique area of the dental anatomy that suffers from both internal resorption (expansion of the sinus) and external resorption (alveolar bone loss) when teeth are extracted. This resorption has been referred to as *centrifugal* and *centripetal* resorption. As a consequence, bone height is often of the order of 5.0 mm or less. This bone is also of low density (Type IV), and without augmentation is not accessible for conventional implant placement. The success of sinus augmentation has been enhanced by the use of textured, as distinct from smooth, implant surfaces, and by the use of alloplastic materials instead of autogenous bone (Wallace and Froum 2003; Del Fabbro et al. 2004, 2008). The cumulative survival rate of implants placed with these sinus-lift techniques is in the region of 95% (Emmerich et al. 2005) (Fig. 11.7).

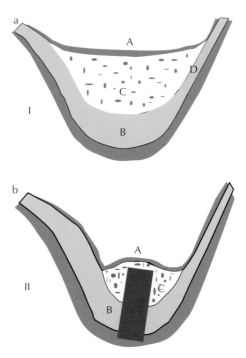

11.7. Diagram of sinus lift procedures: sinus (A), bone (B), and alloplast (C). (a) Diagram I: direct technique using lateral sinus window (D) (courtesy of H. Byrne). (b) Diagram II: indirect technique with access through the implant osteotomy and immediate implant placement (courtesy of H. Byrne).

Indirect sinus lift/internal bone core sinus elevation/transcrestal

The indirect sinus-lift or transcrestal approach was introduced by Summers (1994) and involves the use of osteotomes during the osteotomy preparation to forcibly push back and raise the sinus membrane along with a small amount of attached bone. The space created is filled with a graft material, which will gradually convert to host bone. Computed tomography may be used to determine the sinus configuration, for example, location of bony antral septa. The implant is placed into the osteotomy and extends into the graft material without penetrating the Schneiderian or sinus membrane. Numerous studies have

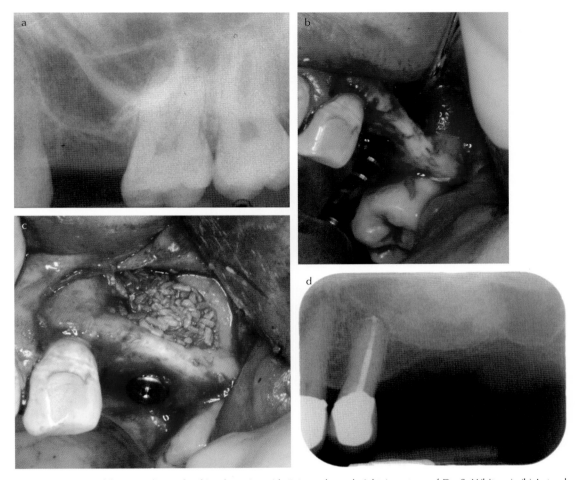

11.8. Direct sinus lift: (a) Radiograph of implant site with 5.0 mm bone height (courtesy of Dr. S. Whitney). (b) Lateral sinus window opened, sinus lining elevated, and osteotomy prepared (courtesy of Dr. S. Whitney). (c) Implant placed, sinus space packed with alloplast and ready for flap suturing (courtesy of Dr. S. Whitney). (d) A postoperative of radiograph of sinus in-fill after a direct sinus lift showing sinus radio-opacity in second premolar/first molar region (courtesy of Dr A. Bradley).

documented the success of this surgical approach (Wallace and Froum 2003; Boyne et al 2005; Emmerich et al. 2005).

Procedure requirements:

- A minimum of 5.0 mm of residual bone height
- Initial osteotomy should be undersized and just short of the sinus wall
- Alloplastic graft material
- Avoid early loading.

Direct sinus lift (Caldwell–Luc access)

This technique uses the traditional Caldwell–Luc lateral, direct sinus approach to access the maxillary sinus space for grafting (Fig. 11.8a–d) (Jokstad 2009; Wallace 2010). The surgical approach was described by Boyne and James (1980) using autogenous bone.

A window is opened in the bone of the lateral maxilla, allowing access to the sinus

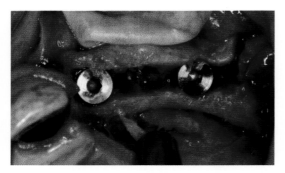

11.9. Ridge splitting tecnique used to create space for implants in narrow ridges with softer flexible bone (courtesy of Dibart and Dibart 2011).

membrane. This membrane is carefully elevated from its surrounding bone, creating a space for grafting material in the antrum. Traditionally, this space was filled with autogenous blocks or bone chips, but recently other particulate graft materials (i.e. allograft, alloplast, and xenograft) and osteogenic matrices have proven equally, and in some cases more effective than autograft (Wheeler 1997; Wallace et al. 2005; Aghaloo and Moy 2007). The bony window is sometimes covered with a barrier membrane before being allowed to heal for 6–12 months. Some clinicians favor immediate placement of the implants into the grafted site, while others favor a prolonged healing period of 6 months prior to placing implants.

11.8   Other surgical techniques

Ridge splitting

Simion et al. (1992) developed a ridge splitting technique for creating new bone volume in narrow ridges. Following the creation of a vertical split in the ridge, the bony plates are separated and infilled with grafting material. In many cases, the implants can be placed at the same time (Fig. 11.9).

Distraction osteogenesis

Chin (1998) presented distraction osteogenesis as a method of increasing vertical bone height to accommodate dental implants. The technique involves the separation of a section or block of bone from its base and gradual forcible movement occlusally with an *expansion screw*, similar to the device in orthodontic palatal expansion. This is complex surgery that is most often applied to the anterior maxilla.

Onlay horseshoe grafting

Onlay horsehoe grafting of the resorbed maxillary arch with autogenous iliac-derived bone blocks was proposed by Brånemark for atrophic maxillae with simultaneous implant placement to retain the graft (Brånemark et al. 1985). Keller et al. (1987) have proposed a LeFort I osteotomy in conjunction with an autogenous sandwich block graft for extremely resorbed maxillae.

11.9   Virtual treatment planning and guided surgery

The ITI 4th Consensus Conference identified two applications of computer technology to surgical implant dentistry (Wismeijer et al. 2010):

- *Computer-guided (static) surgery:* A static surgical template guides the surgeon. CT scan technology and computer guided surgery provide the clinician with the tools to achieve consistently accurate surgical implantation (Van Steenberghe et al. 2005). Immediate restoration is also a possibility in these cases. The same method has been applied to the design and implementation of digitally engineered bone augmentation prior to implantation (Pikos and Mattia 2009).

- *Computer navigated (dynamic) surgery:* A computerized surgical navigation system that allows for intraoperative changes in implant position. This technique has not yet gained popularity in dentistry.

Rationale for guided surgery

The impetus for guided surgery systems is efficient flapless surgery and immediate restoration. The prosthesis is made in advance and inserted at the time of surgery. Although the planning process is quite arduous, the benefit lies in less invasive surgery, reduced surgical and restorative clinical time, and immediate function (Moy et al. 2008; Froum 2010; Dibart and Dibart 2011).

Background of computer-guided surgery planning

Medical CT technology was initially adopted by dentistry to create accurate transparencies of facial bone cross sections. This was a great improvement on distorted 2-D images such as the orthopantomogram, but it was cumbersome, expensive and not interactive. In 1994, Simplant® produced the first dental implant interactive software for a personal computer that could utilize CT data for user manipulation. The cross-sectional and panoramic views could be overlapped with virtual implants (Jokstad 2009; Dibart and Dibart 2011).

More recently, smaller, in-office cone-beam computer tomography (CBCT) machines were introduced that reduce radiation dosage and give greater detail, while bringing tomography technology to a wider audience. Interactive computer programs have developed simultaneously for the manipulation of these 3-D images, virtual implant treatment planning, and ultimately guided surgery and computer-aided design/computer-aided manufacturing

(CAD/CAM) of a prosthesis in advance of implant placement (Fig. 11.10a–c).

NobelGuide™ system

Textured surface implants allow more rapid osseointegration, and more effective immediate loading protocols. These implants, combined with computer interactive technology to manipulate CT images, culminated in the introduction by Nobel Biocare of the *NobelGuide™* system. This system combined CT scanning with interactive planning software for virtual implant positioning and fabrication of custom stereolithographic surgical guides. The system allowed for accurate guided placement of implants, and immediate restoration of edentulous arches and spaces (Procera® CAD/CAM). This early computer-based planning system was marketed with the logo *"Teeth-in-a-Day™."* A previous attempt at immediate implantation and restoration by Nobel Biocare was termed "All-On-4™" (Moy et al. 2008).

Computer technology and surgery

With all computer technology, systems evolve and upgrade and will continue to do so; something that is state of the art today will be passé tomorrow. Currently, there are several software systems available, for example, Nobel-Clinician™, Anatomage™, and Simplant. The software and support systems allow for virtual implant planning and placement using interactive software and fabrication of computer-generated custom surgical guides. With such software design systems, there is a steep learning curve. Adherance to precise calibration is paramount in order to avoid major implant placement errors. Calibration of the CT machine, and precise fit and alignment of treatment guides, are crucial to surgical accuracy. They are a good educational tool for patients,

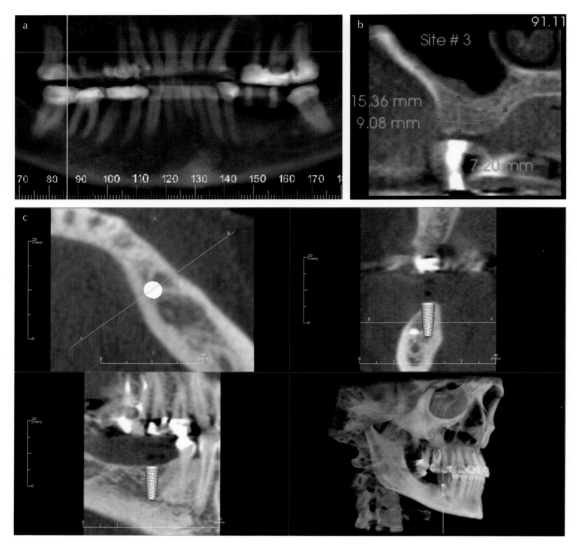

11.10. (a) Reformatted CBCT panoramic image showing radiographic guides with gutta-percha markers corresponding to teeth #3, 4, 19, and 20 (courtesy of Dr. O. Ahmad). (b) Cross-sectional image of right maxillary ridge with measurements beneath an opaque guide marker for tooth #3 (courtesy of Dr. O. Ahmad). (c) Anatomage™ software using CBCT data for with virtual implant placement in the mandibular second premolar/first molar area. Note the apical and buccal position of the mandibular canal and mental foramen relative to the proposed 10.0 × 4.3 mm Nobel Biocare implant (courtesy of Dr. O. Ahmad).

presenting a precise 3D rendering of the clinical situation.

Custom surgical guide

Proprietary software systems combine two CT image databases, a CT scan of the jawbone with a prosthodontic planning stent in place, and a scan of the prosthodontic stent on its own. The stent incorporates up to six radio-opaque reference markers for 3D orientation. Radio-opaque markers, such as barium-impregnated denture teeth or gutta-percha-filled implant guide holes, create a diagnostic radiographic guide for implant positioning.

These systems allow the clinician to manipulate computer images in order to determine bone volume, location of vital anatomic structures, and the potential size and location of implants. They enable the fabrication of a stereolithographic custom surgical guide for accurate 3D implant placement (Fig. 11.11a–d).

Guided surgery problems

Surgical guides encroach on the surgeon's ability to control the operating field especially with regard to flap design, flattening the ridge crest, irrigation, and drill control. Failure to calibrate the CBCT machine accurately, and failure to locate radiographic and surgical guides accurately, can lead to serious errors and damage to vital structures. Small inaccuracies can be expected even in ideal circumstances (Fitzgerald et al. 2010; D'haese et al. 2012). Immediate loading in concert with guided surgery has not been sufficiently validated at this time.

An ITI Consensus statement (Wismeijer et al. 2010) noted that the rapid development of undocumented technology, in a commercially driven process, has led to unrealistic expectations regarding the efficacy and ease of use of current computer technologies. It was further noted that there is no current evidence to indicate that survival or success of implants and prostheses placed using computer guided surgery are better than traditional methods (Fig. 11.12a,b).

Guided surgery summary

- Calibrate CBCT machine with a 3D reference model.
- Create an accurately fitting clinical mock-up and guide of the final restorative case, for example, FDP or denture with radio-opaque reference markers.
- Take a CBCT scan of guide.
- Take a CBCT scan of jawbones and guide.
- Use interactive software to determine the bone volume and the position of vital anatomic structures.
- Determine the implant size and position.
- Send data to the laboratory for fabrication of a stereolithographic custom surgical guide.
- No surgical flap is raised; punch access or occasionally miniflaps are used.
- Fix the surgical guide into position with guided pins.
- A specialized surgical kit with drills and guide sleeves is required.
- There is a predetermined drill sequence for osteotomy preparation.
- Implants are guided into their final 3D position by the surgical guide.
- An immediate interim or fixed restoration is optional.

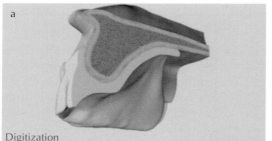

a

Digitization
A double-scan protocol of the patient and the radiographic guide is made using (CB)CT scanners. The scans are fused by the NobelClinician Software.

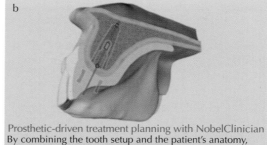

b

Prosthetic-driven treatment planning with NobelClinician
By combining the tooth setup and the patient's anatomy, implant locations are defined according to clinical, anatomical and prosthetic needs.

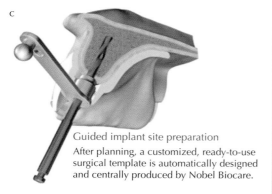

c

Guided implant site preparation
After planning, a customized, ready-to-use surgical template is automatically designed and centrally produced by Nobel Biocare.

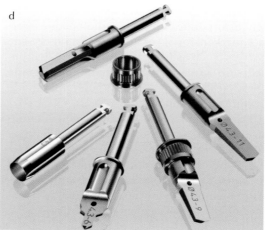

d

11.11. Nobel Clinician software for virtual treatment planning. (a) Digitization process (courtesy of Nobel Biocare). (b) Virtual implant placement (courtesy of Nobel Biocare). (c) Surgical guide guides the 3D implant placement (courtesy of Nobel Biocare). (d) Tissue punch, drills, and sleeves for guided surgery (courtesy of CAMLOG).

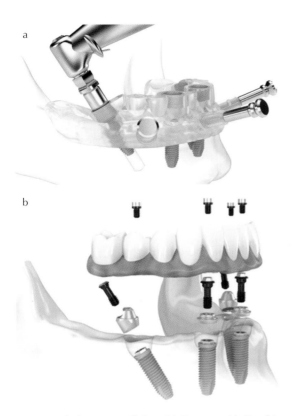

a

b

11.12. Nobel Biocare All-On-4™ Concept: (a) Graphic illustration of surgical guide, drilling, and implant placement (courtesy of Nobel Biocare). (b) Graphic illustration of immediate two-stage fixed restoration with the Nobel Biocare All-On-4™ concept (courtesy of Nobel Biocare).

References

Aghaloo TL, Moy PK. (2007) Which hard tissue augmentation techniques are the most successful in furnishing bony support for implant placement? *Int J Oral Maxillofac Implants.* 22 Suppl:49–70.

Beagle JR. (2006) The immediate placement of endosseous dental implants in fresh extraction sites. *Dent Clin N Am.* 50(3):375–89.

Boyne PJ, James RA. (1980) Grafting of the maxillary sinus floor with autogenous marrow and bone. *J Oral Surg.* 38(8):613–6.

Boyne PJ, Lilly LC, Marx RE, Moy PK, Nevins M, Spagnoli DB, Triplett RG. (2005) De novo bone induction by recombinant human bone morphogenetic protein-2 (rhBMP-2) in maxillary sinus floor augmentation. *J Oral Maxillofac Surg.* 63(12):1693–707.

Brånemark P-I, Zarb GA, Albrektsson T. (1985) *Tissue-Integrated Prostheses: Osseointegration in Clinical Dentistry.* Quintessence, Berlin.

Camelo M, Nevins M, Nevins ML, Schupbach P, Kim DM. (2012) Treatment of gingival recession defects with xenogenic collagen matrix: a histologic report. *Int J Periodontics Restorative Dent.* 32(2):167–73.

Chin M. (1998) The role of distraction osteogenesis in oral and maxillofacial surgery. *J Oral Maxillofac Surg.* 56(6):805–6.

Dawson A, Chen S. (eds.) (2009) *The SAC Classification in Implant Dentistry.* Quintessence, Berlin.

Del Fabbro M, Testori T, Francetti L, Weinstein R. (2004) Systematic review of survival rates for implants placed in the grafted maxillary sinus. *Int J Periodontics Restorative Dent.* 24(6):565–77.

Del Fabbro M, Rosano G, Taschieri S. (2008) Implant survival rates after maxillary sinus augmentation. *Eur J Oral Sci.* 116(6):497–506.

Devescovi V, Leonardi E, Ciapetti G, Cenni E. (2008) Growth factors in bone repair. *Chir Organi Mov.* 92(3):161–8.

D'haese J, Van De Velde T, Komiyama A, Hultin M, De Bruyn H. (2012) Accuracy and complications using computer-designed stereolithographic surgical guides for oral rehabilitation by means of dental implants: a review of the literature. *Clin Implant Dent Relat Res.* 14(3):321–35.

Dibart S, Dibart J-P. (2011) *Practical Osseous Surgery in Periodontics and Implant Dentistry.* Wiley-Blackwell, Ames.

Emmerich D, Att W, Stappert C. (2005) Sinus floor elevation using osteotomes: a systematic review and meta-analysis. *J Periodontol.* 76(8): 1237–51.

Esposito M, Grusovin MG, Polyzos IP, Felice P, Worthington HV. (2010a) Interventions for replacing missing teeth: dental implants in fresh extraction sockets (immediate, immediate-delayed and delayed implants). *Cochrane Database Syst Rev.* (9):CD005968.

Esposito M, Grusovin MG, Rees J, Karasoulos D, Felice P, Alissa R, Worthington HV, Coulthard P. (2010b) Effectiveness of sinus lift procedures for dental implant rehabilitation: a Cochrane systematic review. *Eur J Oral Implantol.* 3(1):7–26.

Evans CD, Chen ST. (2008) Esthetic outcomes of immediate implant placements. *Clin Oral Implants Res.* 19(1):73–80.

Fiorellini JP, Nevins ML. (2003) Localized ridge augmentation/preservation. A systematic review. *Ann Periodontol.* 8(1):321–7.

Fitzgerald M, O'Sullivan M, O'Connell B, Houston F. (2010) Accuracy of bone mapping and guided flapless implant placement in human cadavers using a model-based planning procedure. *Int J Oral Maxillofac Implants.* 25(5):999–1006.

Froum SJ. (2010) *Dental Implant Complications: Etiology, Prevention, and Treatment.* Wiley-Blackwell, Ames.

Hämmerle CH, Chen ST, Wilson TG Jr. (2004) Consensus statements and recommended clinical procedures regarding the placement of implants in extraction sockets. *Int J Oral Maxillofac Implants.* 19 Suppl:26–8.

Jensen S, Katsuyama H. (2011) In: S Chen, D Buser, D Wismeijer (eds.), *ITI Treatment Guide. Volume 5. Sinus Floor Elevation Procedures.* Quintessence, Berlin.

Jokstad A. (2009) *Osseointegration and Dental Implants.* Wiley-Blackwell, Ames.

Karring T, Warrer K. (1992) Development of the principle of guided tissue regeneration. *Alpha Omegan.* 85(4):19–24.

Keller EE, Van Roekel NB, Desjardins RP, Tolman DE. (1987) Prosthetic-surgical reconstruction of the severely resorbed maxilla with iliac bone grafting and tissue-integrated prostheses. *Int J Oral Maxillofac Implants.* 2(3):155–65.

McGuire MK, Scheyer ET. (2006) Comparison of recombinant human platelet-derived growth factor-BB plus beta tricalcium phosphate and a collagen membrane to subepithelial connective tissue grafting for the treatment of recession defects: a case series. *Int J Periodontics Restorative Dent.* 26(2):127–33.

Moy P, Palacci P, Ericsson I. (eds.) (2008) *Immediate Function and Esthetics in Implant Dentistry.* Quintessence, London.

Pikos MA, Mattia AH. (2009) Three-dimensional reverse tissue engineering for optimal dental implant reconstruction. In: A Jokstad (ed.), *Osseointegration and Dental Implants.* Wiley-Blackwell, Ames, pp. 197–204.

Scheyer ET. (2009) Pre-implant surgical interventions tissue engineering solutions. In: A Jokstad (ed.), *Osseointegration and Dental Implants.* Wiley-Blackwell, Ames, pp. 125–9.

Schropp L, Isidor F. (2008) Timing of implant placement relative to tooth extraction. *J Oral Rehabil.* 35 Suppl 1:33–43.

Schropp L, Wenzel A, Kostopoulos L, Karring T. (2003) Bone healing and soft tissue contour changes following single-tooth extraction: a clinical and radiographic 12-month prospective study. *Int J Periodontics Restorative Dent.* 23(4):313–23.

Schwarz F, Becker J. (2010) *Peri-implant Infection: Etiology, Diagnosis and Treatment.* Quintessence, London.

Simion M, Baldoni M, Zaffe D. (1992) Jawbone enlargement using immediate implant placement associated with a split-crest technique and guided tissue regeneration. *Int J Periodontics Restorative Dent.* 12(6):462–73.

Smith RB, Tarnow DP. (2013) Classification of molar extraction sites for immediate dental implant placement: technical note. *Int J Oral Maxillofac Implants.* 28(3):911–6.

Summers RB. (1994) A new concept in maxillary implant surgery: the osteotome technique. *Compendium.* 15(2):152, 154–6, 158.

Ten Heggeler JM, Slot DE, Van der Weijden GA. (2011) Effect of socket preservation therapies following tooth extraction in non-molar regions in humans: a systematic review. *Clin Oral Implants Res.* 22(8):779–88.

Tonetti MS, Hämmerle CH, European Workshop on Periodontology Group C. (2008) Advances in bone augmentation to enable dental implant placement: consensus Report of the Sixth European Workshop on Periodontology. *J Clin Periodontol.* 35(8 Suppl):168–72.

Van Steenberghe D, Glauser R, Blombäck U, Andersson M, Schutyser F, Pettersson A, Wendelhag I. (2005) A computed tomographic scan-derived customized surgical template and fixed prosthesis for flapless surgery and immediate loading of implants in fully edentulous maxillae: a prospective multicenter study. *Clin Implant Dent Relat Res.* 7 Suppl 1:S111–20.

Vignoletti F, Matesanz P, Rodrigo D, Figuero E, Martin C, Sanz M. (2012) Surgical protocols for ridge preservation after tooth extraction. A systematic review. *Clin Oral Implants Res.* 23 Suppl 5: 22–38.

Wallace SS. (2010) Complications in lateral window sinus elevation surgery. In: SJ Froum (ed.), *Dental Implant Complications: Etiology, Prevention, and Treatment.* Wiley-Blackwell, Ames, pp. 284–307.

Wallace SS, Froum SJ. (2003) Effect of maxillary sinus augmentation on the survival of endosseous dental implants. A systematic review. *Ann Periodontol.* 8(1):328–43.

Wallace SS, Froum SJ, Cho SC, Elian N, Monteiro D, Kim BS, Tarnow DP. (2005) Sinus augmentation utilizing anorganic bovine bone (Bio-Oss) with absorbable and nonabsorbable membranes placed over the lateral window: histomorphometric and clinical analyses. *Int J Periodontics Restorative Dent.* 25(6):551–9.

Wang HL, Greenwell H, Fiorellini J, Giannobile W, Offenbacher S, Salkin L, Townsend C, Sheridan P, Genco RJ, Research, Science and Therapy Committee. (2005) Periodontal regeneration. *J Periodontol.* 76(9):1601–22.

Wheeler SL. (1997) Sinus augmentation for dental implants: the use of alloplastic materials. *J Oral Maxillofac Surg.* 55(11):1287–93.

Wismeijer D, Casentini P, Gallucci GO, Chiapasco M. (2010) In: D Wismeijer, D Buser, U Belser (eds.), *ITI Treatment Guide—Volume 4: Loading Protocols in Implant Dentistry—Edentulous Patients.* Quintessence, Berlin.

12 Advanced Topics: Prosthetics

12.1 Introduction

Restorative scenarios present with different levels of complexity and risk for aesthetic and technical complications. Cases may be considered complex when the outcome is not readily visualized, or when a technique or clinical approach is not validated by clinical research. Fixed mandibular full-arch cases have been validated but are still considered complex or challenging cases. With complex cases, there is often a need to reassess and alter the treatment plan during treatment, which may increase the risk for complications. Cases may be considered complex or challenging for one or more of the following reasons:

- *Inadequate bone volume* as occurs when teeth have been missing for some time, where teeth are congenitally absent, with cleft palate cases, following jaw or facial surgery for example, after cancer surgery (Fig. 12.1)

- *High patient expectations for aesthetics* particularly when there is a high smile line, severe ridge atrophy, or there are two or more missing adjacent maxillary incisors.
- The patient has *a bruxing or clenching habit*.
- There is *functional occlusal compromise*, such as in cases in which the occlusion is unfavorable (severe Class III and Class II divisions 1 and 2) or where there is significant arch disruption due to drifting and supereruption.
- The patient requires fixed full-arch maxillary or mandibular restorations.

12.2 Prosthetic cases with high aesthetic risk

There is no doubt that aesthetics is important in implant dentistry. Difficulties arise in implant treatment when attempting to retain or reproduce soft tissue contour and crown emergence profile in the aesthetic zone. The degree of

Fundamentals of Implant Dentistry, First Edition. Gerard Byrne.
© 2014 John Wiley & Sons, Inc. Published 2014 by John Wiley & Sons, Inc.
Companion website: www.wiley.com/go/byrne/implants

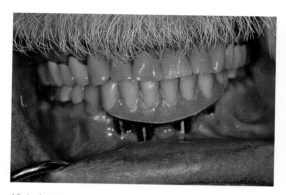

12.1. Large anterior mandibular ridge defect restored by screw-retained FDP with extensive pink acrylic.

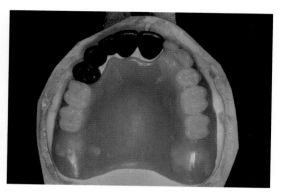

12.2. Diagnostic mock-up for provisional FDP and interim RPD (courtesy of Dr. B. Kim).

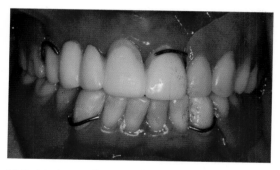

12.3. Interim prostheses in place for diagnostic purposes (courtesy of Dr. B. Kim).

difficulty relates to high smile lines, bone and soft tissue loss, and the number of missing teeth. In many clinical cases, the lack of alveolar bone is significant and long standing. Such cases are very demanding in terms of implant placement and restorative aesthetics. However, given the current state of the art, implant therapy provides the optimum treatment (Dawson and Chen 2009; Wittneben and Webber 2013).

As an example of high aesthetic risk, a presenting case might be a failing three- to six-unit maxillary anterior fixed dental prosthesis (FDP), which is often related to traumatic loss of incisors and the prior unavailability of implants. In such cases, the alveolar ridge will have resorbed significantly, both horizontally and vertically. The final solution requires both tooth and soft tissue elements. Ridge augmentation and/or gingival porcelain extensions are required to mimic natural aesthetics. Such a case requires thorough evaluation to establish bone volume and relative aesthetic tooth position. A diagnostic mock-up followed by an interim denture or provisional bridge can be used to demonstrate the limitations of the aesthetic situation to the patient and to transfer diagnostic information to the surgeon. The interim prosthesis, a removable dental prosthesis (RPD), can be modified for use as a radiographic guide or surgical guide (Fig. 12.2 and Fig. 12.3).

A similar situation arises when adjacent maxillary incisor implants are contemplated, regardless of the extent of bone and soft tissue loss. It is particularly difficult to reconstitute interdental papillae between two adjacent implants (Tarnow et al. 2010).

These are complex treatment decisions and must be represented as such to the patient prior to commencing implant treatment. Many restorative aesthetic difficulties are preempted by careful interdisciplinary planning (see Chapter 13).

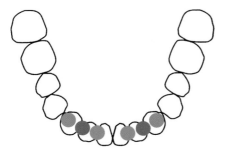

12.4. Diagram of desired mandibular implant locations: red dots indicate locations for placement of two overdenture implants; green dots show placement for four additional implants for a fixed hybrid prosthesis (courtesy of H. Byrne).

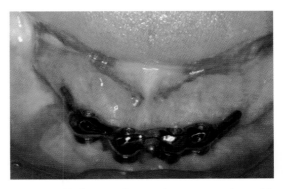

12.5. Mandibular overdenture bar construction with distal cantilevers supported by four implants (courtesy of Dr. J. Marshall).

12.3   Mandibular full-arch implant prostheses

Various options are available for full-arch mandibular restorations, as follows (Wismeijer et al. 2010) (Fig. 12.4):

* *Overdenture*: Two anterior free-standing implants with retentive prosthetic abutments
* *Overdenture*: Three or four anterior free-standing implants with retentive prosthetic abutments
* *Overdenture*: Two to four anterior implants joined by bars with or without distal cantilevers (Fig. 12.5)
* *Full-arch fixed prosthesis*: Four to six anterior implants (one- to two-unit distal cantilevers)
* *Full-arch fixed prosthesis*: Six to eight anterior and posterior implants with one, two, or three fixed prostheses

Mandibular implant overdentures have been discussed in Chapter 10. Treatments using two implants have a significant cost–benefit ratio for the patient and offer considerable satisfaction for the patient and clinician. The use of more than two implants is feasible with or without joining bars and cantilever extensions, creating a situation where the denture becomes

virtually implant-borne. Such an overdenture often requires a cast substructure to prevent denture fracture. Accessibility for hygiene and maintenance is a relative advantage over fixed implant bridges. There is some risk of accelerated resorption in the premaxilla of an opposing maxillary denture-bearing arch.

Brånemark pioneered the fixed full-arch prosthesis protocol using five or six implants. It is an excellent treatment utilizing implants in the anterior mandible where bone is dense and aesthetics are less demanding. Implants are visible when the lip is retracted and a space is maintained under the prosthesis for hygiene access. The prosthesis was traditionally fabricated in acrylic resin over a cast gold framework (Carlsson 2009). Other treatment modalities and refinements have evolved for full-arch edentulism utilizing additional implants posterior to the mental canals:

* Computer-aided design and computer-aided manufacturing (CAD/CAM) fabricated bars with anchors supporting an overdenture
* Fixed full-arch segmented metal-ceramic prostheses
* Implant placement with immediate restoration (Fig. 12.6a,b and Fig. 12.7).

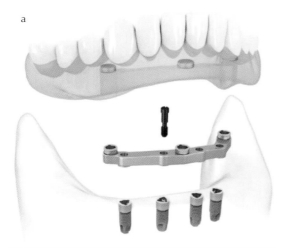

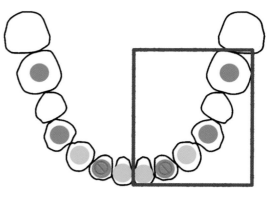

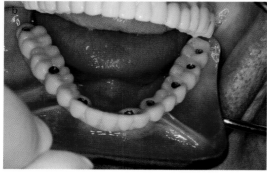

12.6. (a) Depiction of NobelProcera® CAD/CAM bar over-denture with four locator attachments (courtesy of Nobel Biocare). (b) Mandibular full-arch screw-retained FDP supported by eight implants (courtesy of Dr. B. Kim).

12.7. Diagram for implant support of mandibular fixed full-arch bridgework. Green dots depict six-implant support. Eight implants may be used by adding four implants *(yellow dots)* at the expense of two green dots. The blue rectangle is a reminder of splitting the prosthesis to accommodate mandibular flexure. Alternatively, three independent FDPs may be used on six or eight implants (courtesy of H. Byrne).

12.4 Maxillary full-arch implant prostheses

Maxillary edentulous arches pose several problems:

- *Inadequate bone volume and density:* this often necessitates the placement of implants in non-ideal locations where bone is available, usually toward the lingual and at unfavorable angles. A removable prosthesis with a flange may give a better aesthetic result than a fixed bridge when there is significant ridge atrophy.

- *Biomechanical*: Support cannot be evenly distributed when implants cannot be optimally spaced or angled. Maxillary resorption is predominantly from the buccal side, as compared with resorption in the mandible; this leads to lingual placement of implants in the maxilla relative to prosthetic tooth position. For these reasons, the splinting of implants with bars or FDPs is often favored over individual implant loading (e.g., by using locators) in the maxilla.

- *Phonetic*: Ridge resorption may make it difficult to achieve a good anterior palatal shape for phonetics, especially if conventional bridgework is used. A patient may be more satisfied with a removable design that eliminates the spaces that permit airflow during speech.

- *Plaque control*: This is difficult for fixed bridgework and bars, especially if dexterity is compromised, for example, by old age or ill health. It is easier for patients to maintain a removable prosthesis with individual implant supports.

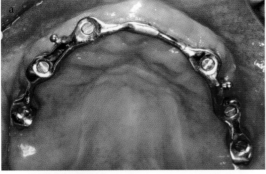

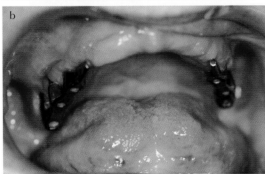

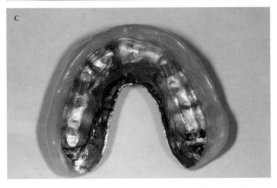

12.8. (a) Maxillary bar with six implants for overdenture (courtesy of Dr. J. Marshall). (b) Maxillary bilateral overdenture bars with three implants each side. (c) Maxillary overdenture with cast base and Hader retentive clips.

Maxillary full arch options

- *Overdenture*: 2 to 6 free standing implants with individual prosthetic abutments
- *Overdenture*: 2 to 6 implants joined by bars with or without cantilevers (Fig. 12.8a–c)

- *Full-arch fixed prosthesis*: 4 to 6 anterior implants (1- or 2-unit cantilevers)
- *Full-arch fixed prosthesis*: 6 to 8 anterior and posterior implants. The prosthesis may be one-piece or segmented (Wismeijer et al. 2010).

Maxillary overdentures

Overdentures with two implants are challenging to execute in the maxilla, due to unfavorable implant angulation and alignment or lingual placement. The lack of vertical space for attachments may also risk fracture of the denture base and compromise appearance. Furthermore, implant failure is higher in low-density maxillary bone (Goodacre et al. 2003).

When more than two implants are in good alignment, it may be possible to use locator or ball abutments on individual implants. However, joining more than two implants with bars has become the more popular method. When implants are joined with bars, complexity increases, forces are more evenly spread over all the implants, and the patient feels that the prosthesis is more like a fixed bridge. Bars allow for the use of shorter implants, for the splinting of misaligned and poorly spaced implants, and for the creation of viable cantilever extension supports (Annibali et al. 2012; Van Assche et al. 2012). Without bars, isolated or misaligned implants may be subjected to excessive and off-axis forces. Sanna et al. (2009) found that interconnected implants had a higher survival rate than individual implants (99.3% versus 87.5%).

Overdenture designs are convenient for the patient in that they facilitate plaque control. A labial flange and partial metal palatal coverage enable good strength, aesthetics, phonetics, and comfort. In many cases, a CoCr framework is recommended for reinforcement of the acrylic denture base and permanent mounting of retentive matrices. This prevents resin base fractures and allows for the elimination of palatal vault coverage.

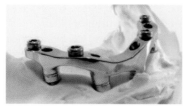
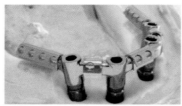
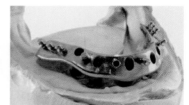

Free Form Milled Bar with Locator® attachments   Dolder® Bar with gold riders   Montreal Bar

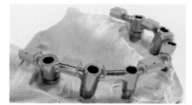
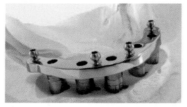
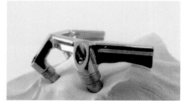

Hader Bar® with clips and housings   Free Form Milled Bar with ball attachments   Possibility to restore severe implant angulations

12.9. Alternative NobelProcera bar designs (courtesy of Nobel Biocare).

A technical overdenture variation uses a milled Ti framework or bar, fabricated by the CAD/CAM method, which is surmounted by locator attachments for retention (Fig. 12.9). Another method uses spark erosion to produce a precisely fitting removable framework over a bar.

Maxillary implant FDP

An implant metal-ceramic FDP is considered by many to be the ultimate treatment for an edentulous arch. However, it is not always possible to achieve a good aesthetic result because of premaxillary resorption, and the resultant need for visible gingiva, and lip support. Pink porcelain is used for these cases. Due to compromise in implant placement, it is often necessary to fabricate a substructure, such as cast telescopic copings, or a CAD/CAM fabricated bar, that is surmounted by a secondary screw-retained or cemented fixed metal-ceramic prosthesis (Fig. 12.10a–c). In FDP cases, oral hygiene procedures will be difficult. Screw-retained

prostheses are often favored by specialists for management of risk.

Occasionally, a fixed prosthesis may be retained by specialized clips which are removable by the patient for oral hygiene procedures. These prostheses are conducive to plaque control, but are technically complex.

12.5 Full-arch fixed rehabilitation approaches

Several approaches are possible for the rehabilitation of full arches. These include:

- *Conventional or traditional approach*: Extractions are followed by an interim removable prosthesis, implant placement and then the definitive restoration.
- *Immediate implant placement approach*: Implants are placed in fresh extraction sites and an interim removable prosthesis is worn until osseointegration is complete. This is followed in 2–6 months by the definitive restoration.

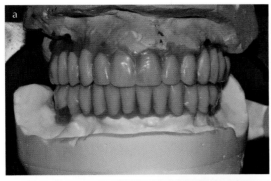

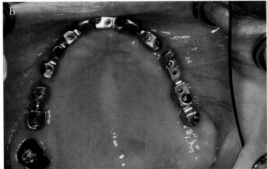

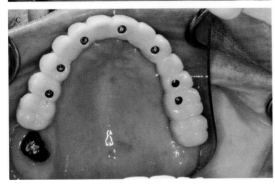

12.10. (a) Diagnostic mock-up for maxillary and mandibular full-arch prostheses (courtesy of Dr. B. Kim). (b) Screw-retained telescopic substructures with retentive screw-holes for superstructure (courtesy of Dr. B. Kim). (c) Final screw-retained FDP (courtesy of Dr. B. Kim).

- *Immediate loading of immediately placed implants*: The prosthesis may be interim or definitive.
- *Staged approach*: Some patients refuse the interim step of a removable prosthesis and wish to go directly to a fixed restoration regardless of the risk. A more conservative *staged approach* may be a better solution for such cases despite the fact that there are many steps and much chairside time. With a staged approach, extractions and implant placements are carried out sequentially, while placing interim fixed or removable prostheses. Cordaro et al. (2007) have described such a staged rehabilitation strategy for full-arch fixed restoration of impending tooth loss (e.g., terminal periodontitis), without the use of removable provisionals. With this approach, some strategic teeth are retained to support provisional cemented bridges, while others are extracted with immediate implant placement. Following integration of the first group of implants, the remaining teeth are extracted, and the already integrated implants support a new provisional prosthesis. After integration of the second group of implants, the definitive fixed prostheses are placed. Although challenging, many clinicians are comfortable with such an approach, as it allows conventional healing times for osseointegration, and is positive from the patient's perspective. It also allows the clinician to work on patient compliance and thus improve outcomes (Fig. 12.11a,b).
- *Immediate loading of immediately placed implants*: This method is becoming popular with the advent of the NobelGuide™, Nobel-Clinician™, and other CT-driven surgical protocols and CAD/CAM technology (see Chapter 11). This option greatly reduces clinical chair time and accelerates treatment. However, there is the potential for significant aesthetic problems even in cases with good implant sites.

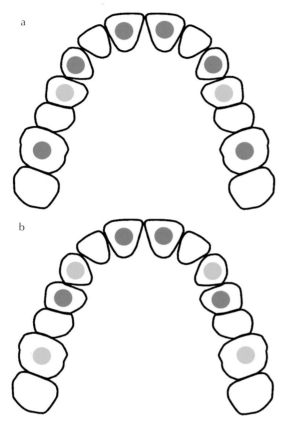

12.11. (a) Diagram of six or eight implant support for an FDP; green dots indicate primary implant locations; yellow dots indicate additional implant locations. (b) Diagram of staged approach; phase I extractions and implants *(green dots)*; phase II extractions and implants *(yellow dots)*; other teeth at nonimplant sites can be extracted at a convenient time (courtesy of H. Byrne).

12.6 Cases with a natural arch opposing an overdenture arch

When these cases are encountered, the primary risk is that of occlusal overload on the implant overdenture with implant abutment, attachment, or denture base wear or fracture. The clinician should pay close attention to any history or evidence of bruxism. It is relatively easy to restore a mandibular arch with an implant prosthesis opposing a complete denture. However, it is more

difficult to predict the consequences of occlusal overload when such a restoration opposes a natural dentition, with or without fixed prostheses or Class III removable prostheses. Notwithstanding the unpredictability of destructive forces on the implants and restorative materials, implant treatment is the only rational treatment in these circumstances, given the consequences of a complete denture in the same situation. Some specialists would favor a fixed implant rehabilitation in these cases.

12.7 Implant-supported removable partial dentures

It is not unusual for clinicians to utilize implants for the support and retention of conventional removable partial dentures. Although this is a clinical usage of implants that has not been well documented, natural tooth roots have served a similar purpose for both complete and partial dentures. From a theoretical viewpoint, it would seem appropriate to use implants for vertical support and retention in distal extension cases (Kennedy Class I and II) and anterior cases with missing canines (Class IV), where fixed implant restoration is not an option.

This situation somewhat mirrors the implant overdenture scenario. The mandibular implant overdenture has become a resounding clinical success, and the implant supported RPD may become similarly so. These cases require thoughtful planning to decide the number and location of implants needed to support function, and the vertical space requirements for attachments. A minimum of between 10.0 and 15.0 mm vertical space is desirable to achieve aesthetic and mechanical success. No formal guidelines are available in the literature thus far. Shahmiri and Atieh (2010) suggest that although implant RPD support may be a convenient treatment modality, the management of Class I RPDs in this way is questionable, given the lack of clinical research data (Fig. 12.12a,b).

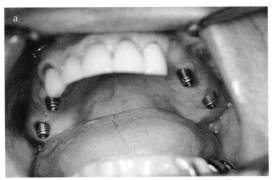

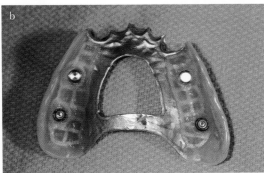

12.12. (a) Locator support for an RPD; abutments are to tall in this example. (b) Locator matrices in RPD base with two retentive inserts placed during delivery.

Treatment planning factors

- Condition of the residual dentition and occlusion
- Compliance in plaque control
- The number of strategic implant supports needed
- Space for implant attachments without compromising denture base strength or aesthetics.

Potential benefits

- Reduced bone resorption under RPD base
- Significant improvement in stability, retention, and function compared to soft tissue supported bases especially Kennedy classes I, II, and IV

- Excellent retention where no innate retention exists.

12.8   Shortened loading protocols

Over the years, a myriad of developments have been introduced aimed at the simplification and concision of implant treatment without negatively influencing outcomes. There is constant pressure to reduce the number of interventions and duration of treatment. The completion of surgical and restorative procedures in one sitting is likely preferred by patients (Szmukler-Moncler et al. 2000; Morton and Ganeles 2007; Moy et al. 2008; Gallucci et al. 2009; Glauser 2009; Wismeijer et al. 2010).

The theory and practice of the orthopedic principle of early stimulation of healing by light loading of bone fractures has found some expression in implant prosthodontics. Light functional loading on a bone fracture site is known to increase vascularization and osteoid formation. Furthermore, the evidence that textured implants (SLA®, TiUnite®, and TiOBlast™) led to earlier osseointegration, compared with smooth surfaces, encouraged the adaptation of early loading strategies (Rocci et al. 2003; Del Fabbro et al. 2006; Schincaglia et al. 2007).

Early loading protocols have been proposed with the goal of shortening treatment times (Attard and Zarb 2005). Henry and Liddelow (2008) suggested a cautious recommendation for immediate loading based on high implant survival rates, but limited scientific evidence. A review by Strub et al. (2012) on immediate loading showed implant survival rates ranging from 95.8–100%. Mandibular implant survival rates ranged from 79% to 100%, and restoration survival rates for both jaws ranged from 96.4% to 100%. They stressed the importance of such factors as patient selection, primary implant stability, splinting of implants and surgical skill for the prognosis of immediately loaded implants. Esposito et al. (2007) recommended careful patient selection and a high degree of primary implant stability (i.e., a high value of insertion torque). They noted that limited data showed no significant difference between early and delayed loading protocols. Atieh et al. (2009) noted a higher risk of implant failure for immediate loading of immediately placed implants. More clinical validation is needed before early loading protocols become mainstream.

Loading protocols

Loading has been classified as follows (Cochran et al. 2004; Moy et al. 2009):

- *Immediate loading*: within 48 hours
- *Early loading*: between 48 hours and 3 months
- *Delayed loading*: after 3 months.

An ITI consensus (Wismeijer et al. 2010) has recommended delayed loading after 2 months. A longer healing period is recommended in certain circumstances:

- Alveolar ridge augmentation
- Sinus floor elevation
- Parafunction
- Maxillary overdentures
- Compromised host status.

Guidelines for immediate loading

- Use careful case selection. Avoid healing issues, smokers, poor plaque control.
- Ensure there is good bone density (Type I and II are best).
- Select a minimum implant length of 10.0 mm.
- Ensure a good initial stability of implants: Torque values of ≥40 Ncm.
- Use screw type tapered implants. These give better initial stability (e.g., NobelActive™).
- Use surface textured implants for more rapid integration (Del Fabbro et al. 2006).

- Splint the implants together with a rigid framework to minimize micro-motion.
- Ensure that there is little or no function or occlusal contact, especially on crowns or FDPs, especially in lateral excursions.
- There should be minimal manipulation of screws and abutments after surgery.
- Plan to have an even distribution of implants in the arch.
- Grafting or site development is not recommended.
- Aesthetics becomes a secondary goal, compared with implant stability and osseointegration.
- A high skill level is required, due to the higher risk of complications for a complex procedure.

Stability-dip

The *early loading* concept is less popular than delayed loading due to the fact that success may be compromised by the *stability-dip* of implants. Stability-dip is seen at 3–6 weeks during bone healing, when old damaged bone is being removed and replaced by fresh callus (Raghavendra et al. 2005). It is possible to get excellent initial stability in Type I or Type II bone; stability then declines but later recovers. Stability-dip is more likely to be a problem with single crowns than splinted multi-unit implant prostheses (FDPs and overdenture bars). Many case reports on immediate loading of single crowns involve temporary crowns placed immediately, but out of occlusion. Cases with complete edentulism, using bars or other rigid frameworks, run a lesser risk of stability-dip because of lower peak occlusal forces on individual implants.

Micro-motion

A threshold of micro-motion in the region of between 50 and 100 μm along the implant bone interface has been suggested as being tolerated while still permitting osseointegration (Brunski 1993). Implant movement in the 200-micron range is likely to cause a fibrous implant interface or failure of osseointegration. Multiple implants must be well spaced and continuously rigidly splinted by the superstructure during the osseointegration period to limit micromotion. Biomechanical stability is enhanced the greater the number of splinted implants.

Full-arch immediate loading

In 1979, Ledermann pioneered immediate loading with overdentures (Uribe et al. 2005). The technique used four splinted implants in the anterior mandible for immediate loading by an overdenture. More recently, four to six implants have been placed in an edentulous arch to support a full-arch fixed restoration (Tarnow et al. 1997). A fixed interim or definitive, screw-retained FDP or bar overdenture is delivered immediately after implant surgery.

Immediate loading has been proven to be successful for single implant crowns (Chiapasco 2004; De Bruyn et al. 2008; Calandriello and Tomatis 2011) and full-arch prostheses, and has been promoted with the NobelGuide and NobelClinician systems for guided surgery and immediate restoration.

According to an ITI consensus statement (Wismeijer et al. 2010) the literature supports loading of textured implants 6–8 weeks after implant placement, with fixed or removable prostheses in the mandible, and for fixed prostheses in the maxilla. There is also some evidence to support immediate or early loading of overdentures in the mandible, and immediate loading of fixed full-arch maxillary and mandibular prostheses.

There is currently insufficient scientific validation for immediate loading with maxillary overdentures, and immediate loading with fixed and removable prostheses in either jaw.

12.9   CAD/CAM prosthetics

Computer-assisted design (CAD) and computer-assisted manufacturing (CAM) can be used to create implant restorations following digital image capture from the oral cavity or from an implant master cast (Jokstad 2009; Koutayas et al. 2009) (Fig. 12.13a,b).

Standard implant connection configurations should not be a problem when compared to the complexity of natural tooth preparations, when acquiring clinical digital images. Much CAD/CAM work is currently done by scanning the master implant cast, and designing and milling the prosthesis in ceramic (Zirconia or Alumina) or Ti. Single or multi-unit substructures and bars can be fabricated in this manner. Aesthetic porcelains, if necessary, are then applied to the milled restorations by hand at the dental laboratory. It is increasingly possible to obtain digital optical impressions and to design and fabricate restorations using CAD/CAM. This method is likely to become routine as digital scanning and other technologies advance.

CAD/CAM enables a laboratory to minimize abutment inventory, reduce manual technical procedures, and assure quality and machine-fit of final implant restorations. CAM is usually done at a remote central location and the restoration returned to a local laboratory for final customization. Several comprehensive systems are available, for example, Procera® by Nobel-Biocare, CARES® by Straumann, and Compartis® by Dentsply. Drago (2007) discusses a Biomet-3i™ system that uses coded (Encode®) healing abutments, which facilitate CAD/CAM procedures.

It is impossible to totally eliminate accuracy errors with impressions, laboratory master casts, and lost-wax casting techniques. In the future, it will be possible to create the most accurate results through digital impressions, virtual design, and computer-aided manufacturing. It is already feasible, though uncommon, to combine virtual design, guided surgery,

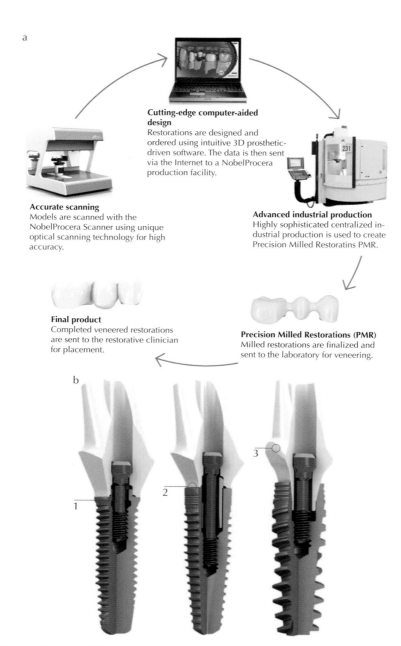

Cutting-edge computer-aided design
Restorations are designed and ordered using intuitive 3D prosthetic-driven software. The data is then sent via the Internet to a NobelProcera production facility.

Accurate scanning
Models are scanned with the NobelProcera Scanner using unique optical scanning technology for high accuracy.

Advanced industrial production
Highly sophisticated centralized industrial production is used to create Precision Milled Restoratins PMR.

Final product
Completed veneered restorations are sent to the restorative clinician for placement.

Precision Milled Restorations (PMR)
Milled restorations are finalized and sent to the laboratory for veneering.

12.13. (a) NobelProcera design and fabrication process (courtesy of Nobel Biocare). (b) Nobel Procera custom zirconia abutments on (1) external hex, (2) trichannel, and (3) internal hex (platform-switching) connections (courtesy of Nobel Biocare).

and computerized fabrication of final restorations for delivery at the time of surgery.

Advantages of CAD/CAM

- Reduced dependence on conventional laboratory technology
- Improved quality control
- Improved efficiency.

Disadvantages of CAD/CAM

- Cost: setup cost, ongoing training cost, software update cost
- There may be a steep learning curve
- Possible rapid obsolescence of software and systems.

References

Annibali S, Cristalli MP, Dell'Aquila D, Bignozzi I, La Monaca G, Pilloni A. (2012) Short dental implants: a systematic review. *J Dent Res.* 91(1): 25–32.

Atieh MA, Payne AG, Duncan WJ, Cullinan MP. (2009) Immediate restoration/loading of immediately placed single implants: is it an effective bimodal approach? *Clin Oral Implants Res.* 20(7): 645–59.

Attard NJ, Zarb GA. (2005) Immediate and early implant loading protocols: a literature review of clinical studies. *J Prosthet Dent.* 94(3):242–58.

Brunski JB. (1993) Avoid pitfalls of overloading and micro-motion of intraosseous implants. *Dent Implantol Update.* 4(10):77–81.

Calandriello R, Tomatis M. (2011) Immediate occlusal loading of single lower molars using Brånemark System® Wide Platform TiUnite™ implants: a 5-year follow-up report of a prospective clinical multicenter study. *Clin Implant Dent Relat Res.* 13(4):311–18.

Carlsson GE. (2009) Dental occlusion: modern concepts and their application in implant prosthodontics. *Odontology.* 97(1):8–17.

Chiapasco M. (2004) Early and immediate restoration and loading of implants in completely edentulous patients. *Int J Oral Maxillofac Implants.* 19 Suppl: 76–91.

Cochran DL, Morton D, Weber HP. (2004) Consensus statements and recommended clinical procedures regarding loadingprotocols for endosseous dental implants. *Int J Oral Maxillofac Implants.* 19 Suppl:109–13.

Cordaro L, Torsello F, Ercoli C, Gallucci G. (2007) Transition from failing dentition to a fixed implant-supported restoration: a staged approach. *Int J Periodontics Restorative Dent.* 27(5):481–7.

Dawson A, Chen S. (eds.) (2009) *The SAC Classification in Implant Dentistry.* Quintessence, Berlin.

De Bruyn H, Van de Velde T, Collaert B. (2008) Immediate functional loading of TiOblast dental implants in full-arch edentulous mandibles: a 3-year prospective study. *Clin Oral Implants Res.* 19(7):717–23.

Del Fabbro M, Testori T, Francetti L, Taschieri S, Weinstein R. (2006) Systematic review of survival rates for immediately loaded dental implants. *Int J Periodontics Restorative Dent.* 26(3):249–63.

Drago C. (2007) *Implant Restorations: A Step-by-Step Guide,* 2nd ed. Blackwell-Munksgaard, Ames.

Esposito M, Grusovin MG, Willings M, Coulthard P, Worthington HV. (2007) Interventions for replacing missing teeth: different times for loading dental implants. *Cochrane Database Syst Rev.* (2):CD003878.

Gallucci GO, Morton D, Weber HP. (2009) Loading protocols for dental implants in edentulous patients. *Int J Oral Maxillofac Implants.* 24 Suppl: 132–46.

Glauser R. (2009) Shortened clinical protocols: the (r)evolution is still ongoing. In: A Jokstad (ed.), *Osseointegration and Dental Implants.* Wiley-Blackwell, Ames, pp. 273–8.

Goodacre CJ, Bernal G, Rungcharassaeng K, Kan JY. (2003) Clinical complications with implants and implant prostheses. *J Prosthet Dent.* 90(2):121–32.

Henry PJ, Liddelow GJ. (2008) Immediate loading of dental implants. *Aust Dent J.* 53 Suppl 1:S69–81.

Jokstad A. (2009) *Osseointegration and Dental Implants.* Wiley-Blackwell, Ames.

Koutayas SO, Vagkopoulou T, Pelekanos S, Koidis P, Strub JR. (2009) Zirconia in dentistry: part 2. Evidence-based clinical breakthrough. *Eur J Esthet Dent.* 4(4):348–80.

Morton D, Ganeles J. (2007) In: D Wismeijer, D Buser, U Belser (eds.), *ITI Treatment Guide. Volume 2. Loading Protocols in Implant Dentistry: Partially Dentate Patients.* Quintessence, Berlin.

Moy P, Palacci P, Ericsson I. (eds.) (2008) *Immediate Function and Esthetics in Implant Dentistry.* Quintessence, London.

Moy PK, Romanos GE, Roccuzzo M. (2009) Loading protocols and biological response. In: A Jokstad (ed.), *Osseointegration and Dental Implants*. Wiley-Blackwell, Ames, pp. 239–53.

Raghavendra S, Wood MC, Taylor TD. (2005) Early wound healing around endosseous implants: a review of the literature. *Int J Oral Maxillofac Implants*. 20(3):425–31.

Rocci A, Martignoni M, Burgos PM, Gottlow J, Sennerby L. (2003) Histology of retrieved immediately and early loaded oxidized implants: light microscopic observations after 5 to 9 months of loading in the posterior mandible. *Clin Implant Dent Relat Res*. 5 Suppl 1:88–98.

Sanna A, Nuytens P, Naert I, Quirynen M. (2009) Successful outcome of splinted implants supporting a "planned" maxillary overdenture: a retrospective evaluation and comparison with fixed full dental prostheses. *Clin Oral Implants Res*. 20(4): 406–13.

Schincaglia GP, Marzola R, Scapoli C, Scotti R. (2007) Immediate loading of dental implants supporting fixed partial dentures in the posterior mandible: a randomized controlled split-mouth study– machined versus titanium oxide implant surface. *Int J Oral Maxillofac Implants*. 22(1):35–46.

Shahmiri RA, Atieh MA. (2010) Mandibular Kennedy Class I implant-tooth-borne removable partial denture: a systematic review. *J Oral Rehabil*. 37(3): 225–34.

Strub JR, Jurdzik BA, Tuna T. (2012) Prognosis of immediately loaded implants and their restorations: a systematic literature review. *J Oral Rehabil*. 39(9):704–17.

Szmukler-Moncler S, Piattelli A, Favero GA, Dubruille JH. (2000) Considerations preliminary to the application of early and immediate loading protocols in dental implantology. *Clin Oral Implants Res*. 11(1):12–25.

Tarnow DP, Emtiaz S, Classi A. (1997) Immediate loading of threaded implants at stage 1 surgery in edentulous arches: ten consecutive case reports with 1- to 5-year data. *Int J Oral Maxillofac Implants*. 12(3):319–24.

Tarnow DP, Cho S-C, Froum SJ. (2010) Esthetic complications with adjacent implant restorations. In: SJ Froum (ed.), *Dental Implant Complications. Etiology, Prevention, and Treatment*. Wiley-Blackwell, Ames, pp. 216–26.

Uribe R, Peñarrocha M, Balaguer J, Fulgueiras N. (2005) [Immediate loading in oral implants. Present situation]. [Article in English, Spanish] *Med Oral Patol Oral Cir Bucal*. 10 Suppl 2:E143–53.

Van Assche N, Michels S, Quirynen M, Naert I. (2012) Extra short dental implants supporting an overdenture in the edentulous maxilla: a proof of concept. *Clin Oral Implants Res*. 23(5): 567–76.

Wismeijer D, Casentini P, Gallucci GO, Chiapasco M. (2010) In: D Wismeijer, D Buser, U Belser (eds.), *ITI Treatment Guide: Volume 4: Loading Protocols in Implant Dentistry: Edentulous Patients*. Quintessence, Berlin.

Wittneben JG, Webber HP. (2013) In: D Wismeijer, S Chen, D Buser (eds.), *ITI Treatment Guide: Volume 6: Extended Edentulous Spaces in the Esthetic Zone*. Quintessence, Berlin.

13

Complications

13.1   Introduction

Implant complication rates increase with the increasing complexity of clinical situations in which they are used. Many failures can be attributed to the steep learning curve of implant surgery and oversights during treatment planning. The level of implant training within the profession and the quality of treatment are improving with the introduction of implant programs to dental school curricula and the American Dental Association (ADA) accreditation requirement for implant competency.

Implant complications may relate to problems during surgical placement, healing or during function (Froum 2010). There may be problems with the implant itself, or the prosthetic reconstruction. Some complications are severe due to the loss or impending loss of the implant followed by the loss of the restoration. Other complications are mild in that the problem can be tolerated, for example, aesthetics, or be remedied by, for example, screw tightening or modification of the prosthesis. Remedies may be expensive and not necessarily completely successful. Some complications will recur, as with clip renewal for overdentures.

There is a tendency in research to discuss implant success in terms of predicted implant survival and prosthesis survival, while placing less emphasis on technical and aesthetic complications. An implant that is poorly positioned creates several problems that may affect the outcome: aesthetic, biomechanical (e.g., overload), and biological (e.g., plaque control). Furthermore, these complications may be cumulative, such as when functional overload

Fundamentals of Implant Dentistry, First Edition. Gerard Byrne.
© 2014 John Wiley & Sons, Inc. Published 2014 by John Wiley & Sons, Inc.
Companion website: www.wiley.com/go/byrne/implants

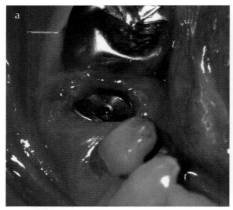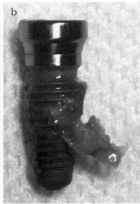

13.1. (a) Implant failure due to infection 1 month after placement. (b) Implant removed (courtesy of Dr. C. Goodacre).

leads to bone loss accompanied by screw-loosening and fracture or porcelain fracture. A recent report showed that only 66.4% of implant patients were completely free from any type of reported complications (Albrektsson and Donos 2012) (Fig. 13.1a,b).

13.2 Implant treatment outcomes and complications

High survival rates of implant-supported prostheses have validated the use of implant restorations for oral rehabilitation (Adell et al. 1981, 1990; Lindquist et al. 1996; Buser et al. 1997) The reader is reminded of *implant success criteria* listed in Chapter 6, while realizing that the criteria that determine success or failure of implant prostheses are less clearly defined. Implant studies commonly use implant survival, radiographic bone loss, or prosthesis survival as outcome measures. Implant failure is usually reported, whereas progressive bone loss or prosthesis complications may not be reported. Although some implants may fail, a prosthesis may continue to function adequately after repair, or with fewer implants. This was seen in some of the original Brånemark full-arch cases

(Brånemark 2005). Similarly, a prosthesis will continue to function satisfactorily despite poor aesthetics, or even in the presence of infection or progressive bone loss. To call such a case successful is disingenuous, just as the presence of abutment caries would not make a traditional tooth-borne FDP successful.

Berglundh et al. (2002), in a systematic review, noted that implant loss was most frequently reported, whereas biological complications were considered in only 40–60% of studies, and technical complications in 60–80% of studies. This observation indicates that data on the incidence of biological and technical complications may be underestimated and should be interpreted with caution.

The definition of implant treatment success must take into account not only the quality and durability of implant osseointegration, but also the quality of aesthetics and trouble-free functionality of the prosthesis. Thus, the implant may fail or be in the process of failing *(survival)*, or *the prosthesis* may fail or develop complications. The implant may fail to integrate *(early failure)*, or may lose integration *(late failure)* when placed in function. The profession needs more information on aesthetic outcomes and rates of implant loss through either

Table 13.1 Summary of 10-year FDP survival estimates

Type of reconstruction	No. of reconstructions	10-year survival summary estimate (95%CI)
Conventional FDP	1218	89.2% (76.1–95.3%)
Cantilever FDP	239	80.3% (75.2–84.4)
Resin-bonded FDP	51	65% (51.4–76.9)
Implant FDP	219	86.7% (82.8–89.8)
Combined implant/tooth FDP	72	77.8 (66.4–85.7)
Implant single crown	69	89.4 (79.3–95.60

CI, confidence interval.
Source: Adapted from Jokstad (2009).

peri-implantitis or overload. Berglundh et al. (2002) further reported that 2.5% of all implants failed before loading and 2–3% failed during function; failure rates are higher in grafting sites. Esposito et al. (1998) reported that 40% of implant failures were early and 60% were late. Rosenberg and Torosian (1998) reported an overall implant failure rate of 7.5%. Eckert et al. (2005) reported a 5-year survival rate of six implant systems of 96%.

From a prosthetic perspective, Pjetursson et al. (2004a, 2004b) and Lang et al. (2004) have reviewed implant survival rates and fixed prosthesis complication rates, and these are shown in Table 13.1 and Table 13.2. This information has been further reviewed by Pjetursson et al. (2012), Jung et al. (2012), and by Romeo and Storelli (2012). Goodacre et al. (2003) has also reported on general prosthetic complication rates.

Complications may be classified as follows:

- *Surgical*, that is, prior to function (Fig. 13.1a,b)
- *Prosthetic*, that is, functional
- *Minor*, easily correctible
- *Major*, not easily correctible
- *Repetitive*, for example, repeated screw loosening or overdenture fracture or clip failure
- *Cumulative*, a combination of problems with the same case over time

- *Loss of an implant*, but restoration continues to function as with multi-unit FDPs
- Loss of implant and restoration.

The likelihood of complications is related to the following practice trends:

- The total number of restorations has increased dramatically in the past 20 years, with double digit inflation in implant industry.
- More inexperienced general dentists, with minimal implant education or training, rather than specialists are placing and restoring implants.
- More compromised implant sites are being treated, and more aggressive protocols such as immediate placement and immediate loading are being used.
- Proven implant designs are being replaced by designs with different connections and surfaces that have no long-term data.

Other complications not directly related to surgery or restoration:

- *Swallowing or inhalation* of surgical or prosthetic components. When working with small unfamiliar components intraorally, it is paramount to exercise precaution in order

Table 13.2 Summary of complications with implant supported reconstructions (CI = confidence interval)

Types of complication	Implant supported FDPs		Combined implant tooth supported FDPs		Implant supported single crowns	
	No. of reconstructions	Cumulative 5-year complication rates (95% CI)	No. of reconstructions	Cumulative 5-year complication rates (95% CI)	No. of reconstructions	Cumulative 5-year complication rates (95% CI)
Soft tissue problems	751	8.6% (5.1–14.1)	184	7.0% (1.7–25.8%)	267	9.7% (5.1–17.9%)
Bone loss >2.0 mm					509	6.3% (3.0–13.0%)
Aesthetic problems					418	8.7% (3.2–22.6%)
Implant fracture	2559	0.5% (0.3–1.1%)	530	0.8% (0.4–1.7%)	1312	0.14% (0.03–0.64%)
Screw fracture	2590	1.5% (0.8–2.8%)	511	0.6% (0.3–1.1%)	510	0.35% (0.09–1.4%)
Abutment or screw loose	2453	5.6% (3.7–8.3%)	296	6.9% (4.7–10.3%)	752	12.7% (5.7–27.0%)
Loss of retention	93	5.7% (3.0–11.0%)	286	7.3% (5.3–10.1%)	374	5.5% (2.2–13.5%)
Veneer fracture	948	11.9% (7.7–18.2%)	125	7.2% (4.8–10.9%)	508	4.5% (2.4–8.4%)
Ceramic fracture	521	8.8% (5.0–15.1%)	125	7.2% (4.8–10.9%)	402	3.5% (1.7–7.0%)

Source: Adapted from Jokstad (2009).

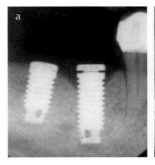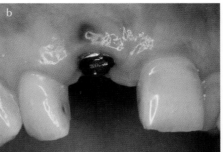

13.2. (a) Incompletely seated cover screw at time of surgery with resultant bone loss (courtesy of Dr. C. Goodacre). (b) Fistula associated with a loose cover screw (courtesy of Dr. C. Goodacre).

to avoid the risk of swallowing or inhalation. This risk is not unique to implant treatment, but can be prevented by using floss ties on components (when possible) and always using gauze squares as a safety net. Abutments and small screws require particular attention. It is usually wise to carry screws into the mouth within a larger component, as for example, by holding an abutment screw within an abutment.

- Problems *identifying implants* and restoration designs provided by other clinicians.

13.3 Complications during the surgical and healing phases, early failure

Implant surgery, as with any minor oral surgery procedure, will have its share of complications ranging from intraoperative to postoperative problems (see Chapter 7).

Failure of an implant to integrate is likely when the implant is not a precise and stable fit in the prepared site, or when there is excessive bone damage from heat generated during drilling (Fig. 13.1a,b). Lack of integration may be discovered early due to infection, at second-stage surgery, or later when impression copings are placed.

When an implant has failed to integrate, it must be removed (backed out), and the site

debrided and grafted, thus restoring a healthy status of the site for follow-up implantation 6 months later. Lack of integration may be absolute or relative. Poor quality integration or incomplete integration is not readily detectable clinically, and may be a prelude to bone loss in function, perhaps soon after restoration. Radiographs are generally of insufficient resolution to diagnose fine fibrous encapsulation of implants (Fig. 13.2a,b).

General complications related to surgery and healing

- Infection, hemorrhage, edema, and bruising
- Life-threatening problems during anesthesia and surgery, for example, arterial damage
- Peri-implant infection with early implant loss
- Damage to vital anatomic structures necessitating implant removal. Early diagnosis and corrective action is essential, for example, perforation of cortical plates, sinus lining, nasal floor
- Sinus infection
- Osteonecrosis
- Neural damage with sensory problems (Palma-Carrió et al. 2011) (Fig. 13.3)
- Dehiscence and fenestration of cortical plates
- Implant malposition
- Implant fracture.

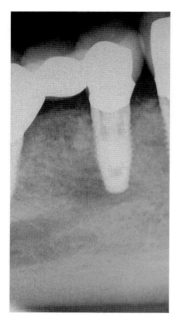

13.3. Neurosensory problem with impingement on mental canal (courtesy of Dr. C. Goodacre).

Etiology of complications

- Poor infection control
- Traumatic surgery, for example, overheating of bone
- Lack of primary implant stability (e.g., poorly prepared osteotomy)
- Inadequate quantity or density of bone
- Impaired healing ability of bone (e.g., smoker, diabetes mellitus, irradiation)
- Disruption of implant-bone interface (e.g., accidental loading)
- Early loading, which disrupts osseointegration (i.e., poor case selection for early loading).

Patient risk factors

- Age: there are increased complication rates with increasing age due to health issues
- Uncontrolled systemic diseases that affect healing, for example, diabetes, immunodeficiency
- Certain medications, for example, bone antiresorptive therapy
- Smoking or poor oral hygiene (Fig. 13.4a,b)
- Prior oncologic irradiation to the implant site.

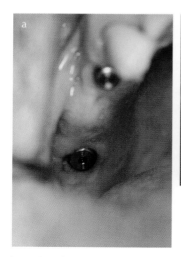
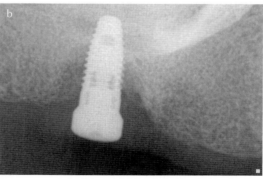

13.4. (a) Early implant failure with purulent discharge and 7.0 mm pocketing. (b) Radiograph of bone loss.

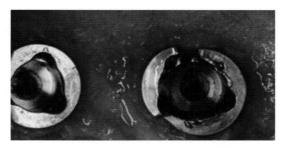

13.5. Implant fracture (courtesy of Dr. E. Kim).

Operator risk factors

- Inadequate diagnosis and planning, for example, bone volume
- Damage to flap or bone blood supply
- Traumatic surgery, for example, overheating bone
- Improper size of osteotomy with lack of primary stability.

13.4   Implant fracture

Implant damage or fracture is relatively rare and has been estimated as 0.6% of all cases and 1.5% of partially edentulous cases (Eckert et al. 2000) (Table 13.2). Mishandling of implants during surgical insertion may cause damage or fracture (Fig. 13.5). Damage may also occur when torquing incorrectly aligned abutments in the prosthetic phase. Functional overloading is associated with complications such as screw loosening, screw fractures, and prosthesis and implant fractures. Bruxism and off-axis forces are implicated in implant overload. Empirical solutions based on satisfactory outcomes with tooth-borne prostheses and dentures are applied. To date, there is no research evidence from long-term studies that suggests specifying a particular occlusal design for implant restorations.

Metal components undergo cyclic bending and may ultimately undergo fatigue failure in certain conditions where metal is thin and where stress is concentrated. Implant fracture is most likely in molar areas where biting force is the greatest (between 600 and 800 N), where a moment force is introduced by a cantilever, or where there is bruxism.

There may be more risk of fracture of the implant collar with a precisely fitting internal connection, than one with an external hex connection. Conversely, external connections are more likely to have abutment screw failure. Internal connections can produce *hoop* stresses on the thinnest section of the implant with a risk of *flowering* cracks. The phenomenon of hoop fracture may increase with the prevalence of these newer internal connection designs and may make a case for the use of stronger Ti implant alloys. Implants with external hex connections tend to fracture within the implant body where the abutment screw terminates, leading to bone loss. Marginal bone loss or implant loss may also be the result of excessive loading (Quirynen et al. 1992; Isidor 1997; van Steenberghe et al. 1999). A screw fracture may be retrieved, but an implant fracture cannot be. A fractured implant must be removed with a correctly sized trephine drill when it poses an infection risk, or needs to be replaced by a new wider diameter implant.

Causes of implant damage may be summarized as follows:

- Attempts to self-thread an implant into dense cortical bone without tapping
- Damage to an implant by using incorrect components or drivers
- Functional overload of an implant, for example, cantilevers, bruxism, and inadequate number and diameter of implants
- A poorly fitting prosthesis that causes resting strain at the implant–abutment connection
- An implant design that incorporates mechanical weak points, for example, deep slots or thin collar dimensions.

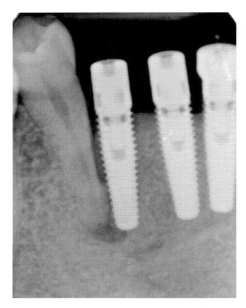

13.6. Implant placed too close to adjacent tooth resulting in direct tooth damage and loss of both tooth and implant (courtesy of Dr. C. Goodacre).

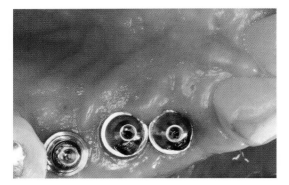

13.7. Implants placed too close together, risking aesthetic, bone loss and plaque control problems, and technical issues (courtesy of Dr. E. Kim).

13.5   Implant malposition and problems with treatment planning

Implant malposition (or poor angulation: m–d, b–l) has implications for the aesthetics, biology and biomechanics of an implant prosthesis (Froum 2010) (Fig. 13.6). It is easy to understand the aesthetic component, as for example, when placing implants in embrasure spaces rather than tooth spaces. However, the biomechanical and biological aspects are also very important. Placement of implants at an adverse angle can create moment forces on the implant restoration. These moment forces may lead to overload that contributes to bone loss and/or mechanical failure of components. Implants that are placed too close together or too close to an adjacent tooth can cause aesthetic, hygiene, and bone loss problems. In some extreme cases, the implants may not be restorable due to position or space restrictions. Vertical malposition leads to bone loss when the implant is placed too deep relative to the bone crest, or an aesthetic problem when the implant protrudes too far from the ridge crest.

Malposition may occur due to uncorrected bone volume issues, or as a consequence of poor planning or execution. There are very limited data on aesthetic success, or patient-centered outcomes.

Avoidance of malposition

* Referral (as per SAC guidelines: see Chapters 5 and 11)
* Comprehensive assessment and diagnosis
* Prosthetic driven treatment planning
* CBCT scans, radiographic and surgical guides
* Plan ridge augmentation as needed (Fig. 13.7 and Fig. 13.8).

13.6   Complications during function

Prosthetic phase or functional complications are technical, biological and aesthetic, and

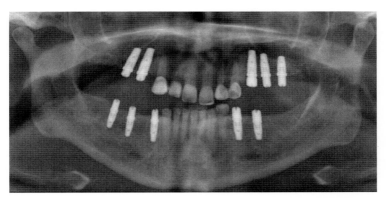

13.8. Planning problem: implants placed posteriorly, but anterior teeth failing due to caries and bruxism habit.

related to poor implant position, poor management of forces, or poor plaque control (Goodacre et al. 1999; Berglundh et al. 2002; Andreiotelli et al. 2010). Poorly placed implants may be unrestorable. Pjetursson et al. (2004a, 2004b) and Lang et al. (2004) presented valuable and comprehensive information on complication rates for conventional FDPs, implant FDPs, combination FDPs, and implant single crowns in four systematic reviews. The pooled data on biological and technical complications is presented in Jokstad (2009). Selected data are presented in Table 13.1 and Table 13.2. Compiled data showed that 50% of implant fixed prostheses had some complications within a 10-year period and 39% had some complications within a 5-year period. According to a review by Goodacre et al. (2003), the most common prosthetic complications are: loosening of the overdenture retentive mechanism (33%), resin veneer fracture with fixed partial dentures (22%), overdentures needing to be relined (19%), and overdenture attachment fracture (16%). Some cases may have a combination of complications, that is, soft tissue, bone (peri-implantitis), prosthetic (screw fractures etc.), and aesthetic complications. Complications cause added cost and inconvenience

over the lifetime of an implant prosthesis (Papaspyridakos et al. 2012).

Avoidance of prosthetic phase complications

- Identify risk factors at diagnosis and treatment planning phase
- Do not compromise on implant support
- Have a treatment plan with clear, definable goals
- Define realistic expectations for patient outcomes.

13.7   Aesthetic complications

The gingiva frames the teeth and creates aesthetic balance. When this balance is pleasing, it must be maintained. When the balance is asymmetric, then this must be demonstrated to the patient in advance of treatment, and a suitable compromise worked out. Photographs, study models and interim restorations study models, and interim restorations are invaluable for patient education and treatment planning. Aesthetic compromise can be the result of

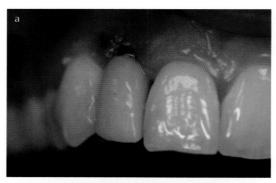

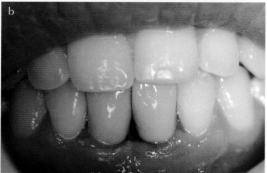

13.9. Aesthetic problems: (a) Implant collar exposure #7. (b) Adjacent incisor implants and single crowns with no interdental papilla (courtesy of Dr. E. Kim).

planning, surgical, prosthetic, or maintenance mistakes (Fig. 13.9a,b). *Aesthetic problems usually arise from incorrect implant placement apico-coronally, facio-lingualiy, or mesio-distally.* Implant placement must be *prosthetically driven*. When there is labial or vertical bone deficiency, there must be a diagnostic mock-up of the prosthesis in order to determine what is required for an aesthetic result. Even when the bone and soft tissue are adequate, the implant may still be positioned incorrectly or the tissues may recede. Soft tissue biotype plays an important role in determining aesthetic outcomes.

When two or more adjacent incisors are missing and replaced with implants, there is a likelihood that the interproximal papilla will be missing, which is unaesthetic. When possible, avoid placement of two adjacent implants in asymmetric positions, that is, canine : lateral, and central : lateral. Instead, consider replacing the lateral incisor with a single implant in the central or cuspid site, using a cantilevered ovate pontics.

Notes on implant placement in the aesthetic zone

Aesthetic problems are related to implant mal-position and soft tissue deficiency, are intractable and therefore should be avoided and preempted at diagnosis and treatment planning (Chen and Buser 2010). When an implant is well positioned, there are generally enough prosthetic components available to enable a good aesthetic result.

Dawson and Chen (2009) refer to *comfort and danger zones* for implant placement in order to sensitize practitioners to the perils of misplacement.

The optimum result may be achievable with immediate placement in a healthy extraction socket, with autograft in-fill around the implant. Immediate placement may offer a good solution for bone and soft tissue height preservation. Platform-switching may also help to preserve bone and soft tissue in the aesthetic zone. One-stage implants with integral transmucosal extensions (as per Straumann) are not as flexible prosthetically and hence aesthetically, as implants that are designed to be placed at the level of the bony crest. When an implant is well positioned, there are generally enough prosthetic components available to enable a good aesthetic result.

Mesio-distal placement is also very critical for aesthetics. If the implant is too close to, or is angled towards an adjacent tooth, or if the implant is positioned in an embrasure space, there will be an aesthetic problem.

Common placement problems with aesthetic implications

- Implant placement too far labially may lead to bone dehiscence, fenestration, soft tissue recession, or metal showing through the mucosa. This happens more often with immediate placement when the socket is allowed to guide the surgical drills.
- Implant placement too far lingually causes the emergence profile to be deficient or results in the need for a tissue lap pontic; this has aesthetic and hygiene implications.
- Implant placement too far apically leads to bone and possibly gingival recession and an asymmetric gingival line.
- Implant placement too far coronally risks a visible implant collar.
- Implant placement too close to another implant or to one side of a space causes the dental papillae to be deficient and creates a higher risk of bone loss.
- Poor implant angulation mimics malposition.

Avoidance of implant malposition

- If doubts about bone volume arise, use CT imaging for diagnosis.
- Choose the correct implant diameter and shape for the clinical situation.
- Plan to leave between 1.0 and 2.0 mm bone labially, or augment the ridge in advance.
- Use a surgical guide that shows the labial outline of the future tooth or teeth.
- Do not take intraoperative risks when bone volume is inadequate, instead abort surgery.
- Do not risk damage to the labial bony plate.

Soft tissue management for aesthetics

- Be familiar with soft tissue biotypes and aesthetic limitations.

- Maintain papillae by leaving adequate space next to the natural tooth: 2.0 mm.
- Preserve marginal bone and soft tissue height.
- Perform mucogingival surgery to build up deficient soft tissue or to increase the band of attached mucosa.
- Perform bone augmentation to build bone volume.
- Create an optimum soft tissue profile with provisional crowns.

13.8   Mechanical complications

Mechanical complications relate to planning and execution problems, and adverse functional forces or overload (Brägger et al. 2001; Goodacre et al. 2003; Froum 2010) (Fig. 13.10, Fig. 13.11, Fig. 13.12, and Fig. 13.13). Examples include:

- Incomplete seating of abutments
- Screw loosening: either an abutment or prosthetic screw
- Screw fracture (Fig. 13.10)
- Implant fracture
- Ceramic abutment fracture
- Fracture of veneering porcelain or resin

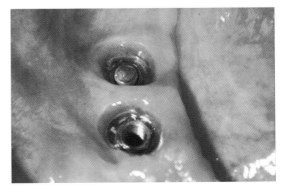

13.10. Mechanical problem: abutment screw fracture with external hex implant (courtesy of Dr. C. Goodacre).

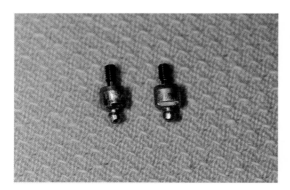

13.11. Mechanical problem: ball abutment wear.

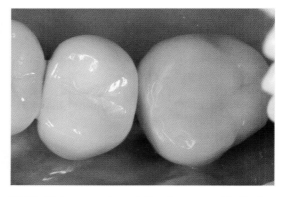

13.13. Molar crown has rotational movement indicating abutment screw loosening (courtesy of Dr. C. Goodacre).

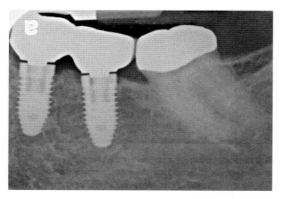

13.12. Incomplete seating of a two-unit FDP (courtesy of Dr. C. Goodacre).

- An uncementing problem with short or small abutments
- Loss of resin plugs from screw access holes
- Overdenture attachment component wear, or fracture of denture base (Fig. 13.11)
- Fixed (hybrid) prosthesis problems, for example, cantilever fracture and resin fracture (Fig. 13.12 and Fig. 13.13).

The region of osseointegration of implants seems to be extremely resistant to occlusal overload. Current evidence does not point to occlusal forces as being a substantial risk factor for bone loss or loss of osseointegration. However, Isidor (1997) has shown a positive relationship between bone loss and overload in an animal study.

Parafunction is outside the clinician's control. Parafunction imparts potential risks for screw loosening and fracture, bone loss, and restoration fractures. Forces may be mitigated by providing an occlusal device that equalizes forces during periods of parafunction. Compliance cannot be guaranteed, and there are financial implications for the patient regarding remakes and repairs. Patients must be made aware of this prior to implant treatment.

13.9 Peri-implant soft tissue complications

There are several common peri-implant complications as follows:

- *Peri-implant mucositis* is a term used to describe reversible inflammatory reactions in the mucosa adjacent to an implant. It has been shown experimentally that there is a cause-and-effect relationship between bacterial plaque and the developing mucositis (Pontoriero et al. 1994). Mucositis may progress to peri-implantitis. This is analogous to the progress of gingivitis to periodontitis.
- *Hyperplasia* is a sequela of uncontrolled mucositis and is often seen in cases with

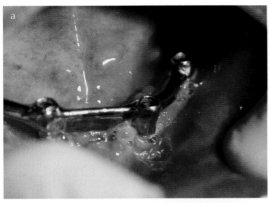

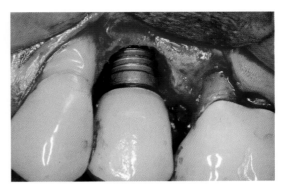

13.15. Surgically exposed peri-implant bone loss after 2 months, resulting from cement remaining subgingivally (courtesy of Dr. C. Goodacre).

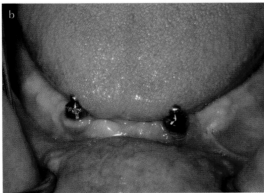

13.14. (a) Inflammatory hyperplasia next to an overdenture implant bar. (b) Gingival inflammation and recession in case with an inadequate band of keratinized gingiva (courtesy of Dr. E Kim).

poor oral hygiene or restricted access for hygiene, such as may occur with FDPs and bar overdentures (Fig. 13.14a,b).

*   *Peri-implantitis* is an inflammatory process affecting the tissues around an osseointegrated implant resulting in loss of supporting bone (Lang and Berglundh 2011). Untreated peri-implantitis will lead to progressive bone loss with loss of the implant, and may jeopardize the implant-supported prosthesis. The effect of inadequate plaque control may be potentiated by local factors tissue, poor fit of the prosthesis, or such as untreated adjacent periodontitis, smoking, implant overloading, the absence

of keratinized tissue, poor fit of the prosthesis, cement residue left in the implant sulcus (Fig. 13.15), or systemic health issues.

*   *Gingival recession* is caused by underlying bone recession or dehiscence. This may occur when the remaining cortical plates are too thin, or are damaged during surgery. This aesthetic problem is very difficult to resolve.

*   *Fistula* formation may be caused by incomplete seating of cover screws or abutments (Fig. 13.2b). The source of the problem must be investigated by removing and retightening the offending component.

Complications must be carefully assessed, monitored, and treated to avoid more serious protracted peri-implant problems (see Chapter 6). A consistent recall strategy is the basis for good preventive care. Patients with removable prostheses often neglect recall unless problems arise. Early diagnosis and intervention are recommended for peri-implantitis (Roos-Jansåker et al. 2003).

13.10   Peri-implant bone loss

The role of overload and peri-implantitis in implant bone loss is controversial (Fig. 13.16). Bone loss has been shown to occur due to

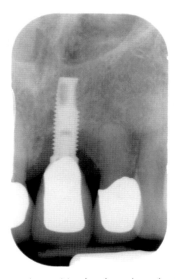

13.16. Progressive peri-implant bone loss after 8 years in a patient who is a smoker. There was no evidence of adverse occlusal forces.

occlusal overload around short implants and in soft bone (De Smet et al. 2001; Isidor 2006). Peri-implant bone loss has also been produced experimentally by bacterial plaque in the same manner as periodontitis (Schou et al. 1993). Smoking is a significant risk factor. Weber and Cochran (1998) have noted the conundrum of peri-implantitis bone loss in terms of the relative importance of etiologic factors such as: inadequate plaque removal, inadequate bone healing, unfavorable quality and quantity of bone, or biomechanical problems. The clinician must manage plaque control as for normal teeth, and also plan and manage occlusal loading (Klinge et al. 2005). Bone loss is best diagnosed and monitored with radiographs.

Functional bone loss around an implant may occur for several reasons

- When an abutment is connected to an implant at second-stage surgery, crestal bone recedes 1.0–2.0 mm from the implant–abutment junction (IAJ). This is considered to be due to microflora at the IAJ and the periodontal concept of *biologic width*.
- When the cortical bone is thin or loses its blood supply after osteotomy, it may resorb causing dehiscence or fenestration.
- Poor plaque control may lead to peri-implantitis bone loss. Smoking is a compounding risk factor.
- Bone may be lost through functional overload. Adverse forces may lead to bone damage, inflammation, resorption and replacement with fibrous tissue, usually at the collar of the implant. *Stress shielding* with smooth implant collars has been implicated in cervical bone loss (see Chapter 3). The stress-shielding phenomenon may be related to the quality of integration at the time of loading.
- Implant fracture leads to adjacent bone loss at the fracture line.

Peri-Implantitis

The initial inflammatory reaction (Lang and Tonetti 2010) to bacterial plaque (mucositis) can progress to peri-implantitis (Esposito et al. 2012a, 2012b) (see Chapter 6). Peri-implantitis is an inflammatory reaction with bone loss. It may be complicated by the exposure of implant threads or textured surfaces to plaque and calculus. Peri-implantitis is one of the most significant risk factors associated with implant failure. The microbiota found in mucositis and peri-implantitis have been found to resemble those isolated from individuals with gingivitis and periodontitis (Rosenberg et al. 2004) The pathogenesis of peri-implantitis is different from periodontitis in that inflammatory lesions spread into the marrow spaces rather than being confined to the soft tissues (Froum 2010; Schwarz and Becker 2010)

Symptoms of peri-implantitis may include bleeding on probing, increased probing pocket depth, suppuration, pain, and finally mobility. The incidence of peri-implantitis has been

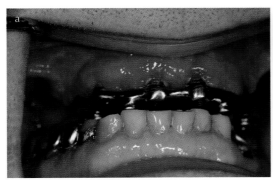
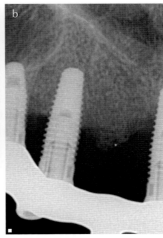

13.17. (a) Peri-implantitis with implant exposure in a maxillary overdenture case. (b) Radiograph showing advanced peri-implant bone loss in the same case.

reported to be in the range of 12–40% by Lindhe and Meyle (2008), and 9.6% by Atieh et al. (2012). It is accepted that patients with chronic periodontitis have a higher incidence of peri-implantitis, perhaps from the same underlying etiology (Karoussis et al. 2007). Smokers also have an increased risk of peri-implantitis implant failure, 16.6% incidence compared with non-smokers having an incidence of 6.9% (Wallace 2000; Baig and Rajan 2007) (Fig. 13.17a,b).

Avoidance of peri-implantitis

- Educate the patient about plaque control and the risk factors for peri-implantitis.
- Explain the possible outcomes of peri-implantitis before treatment.
- Eliminate periodontal disease prior to implant treatment.
- Explain smoking as a risk factor in peri-implantitis and institute smoking cessation.
- Be cognizant of metabolic diseases that affect bone healing capacity.
- Patient should demonstrate excellent plaque control measures.

- There should be a minimum of one yearly evaluation of plaque index, bleeding on probing (BoP), and probing depth.
- A radiograph is indicated if a peri-implant pocket is >6.0 mm.
- Institute cumulative interceptive supportive therapy (CIST) when soft/hard tissue problems arise (see Chapter 6).

13.11 Avoidance of implant complications

There is an expression that the "key to diagnosis is awareness." It follows that the key to successful diagnosis and treatment is thorough data collection and patient assessment. Data must be carefully compiled and diagnoses made before formulating and carrying out elective treatment. Assessment is ongoing during treatment. A good maintenance system allows early diagnosis and intervention.

Immediate postsurgical assessment

If primary stability was not achieved at implant surgery there is a high likelihood of early implant failure. Lack of stability and infection may become apparent within 2 weeks after placement of the implant. There may be other signs and symptoms such as pain or purulent discharge. This infection should be treated quickly by removing the implant, thereby limiting the infection and potential bone damage. Once infection has been controlled, a decision can be made as to whether to debride and graft (GBR) or to place a new wider-diameter implant.

Stage-two surgery and preprosthetic assessment

A clinical and radiographic assessment helps confirm or deny osseointegration. Pain or mobility during cover screw removal or abutment insertion may be indicative of a problem. The implant should produce a ringing sound when percussed with a metal instrument, indicating ankylosis. Neither test confirms that implant integration is mature or complete. Stability testing devices may have a role to play in the future (e.g., Osstell™ and Periotest®). If there is doubt about integration, then it is best to delay prosthetic restoration.

Routine maintenance and implant assessment

Routine follow-up checks must be done to evaluate plaque control, peri-implant soft tissue health, bone levels, and prosthetic stability. When problems are noted, steps can be taken to limit more serious long-term damage.

13.12 Diagnosing and treating other clinicians' implant cases

We live in a relatively mobile society; people move for many reasons, and dentists retire. While traditional prosthetic procedures were universally understood and recognizable,

implant dentistry is considerably more varied, complex, and challenging. As implant dentistry becomes more popular, the clinician must anticipate implant cases from other dentists presenting for routine maintenance and with problems. The clinician must examine such cases carefully and determine whether the patient should seek specialist follow-up care or whether routine maintenance would be a satisfactory option. In all such cases, one should connect with the clinician of record, when possible, for the implant dental record and radiographs. In circumstances when this information is no longer available, it may be necessary to do some detective work online or with your laboratory technician in order to determine the kind of implant that was used, of which generation, and how the restoration was attached. Some websites use radiographic images for implant recognition (Implant Identification websites 2013). Such clinical scenarios are a reminder of the importance of accurate record keeping, and good communication.

References

Adell R, Lekholm U, Rockler B, Brånemark P-I. (1981) A 15-year study of osseointegrated implants in the treatment of the edentulous jaw. *Int J Oral Surg.* 10(6):387–416.

Adell R, Eriksson B, Lekholm U, Brånemark P-I, Jemt T. (1990) Long-term follow-up study of osseointegrated implants in the treatment of totally edentulous jaws. *Int J Oral Maxillofac Implants.* 5(4):347–59.

Andreiotelli M, Att W, Strub JR. (2010) Prosthodontic complications with implant overdentures: a systematic literature review. *Int J Prosthodont.* 23(3): 195–203.

Albrektsson T, Donos N. (2012) Implant survival and complications. The Third EAO consensus conference 2012. Working Group 1. *Clin Oral Implants Res.* Suppl 6:63–5.

Atieh MA, Alsabeeha NH, Faggion CM Jr, Duncan WJ. (2012, 2012) The frequency of peri-implant diseases: a systematic review and meta-analysis. *J Periodontol.* 84(11):1586-98.

Baig MR, Rajan M. (2007) Effects of smoking on the outcome of implant treatment: a literature review. *Indian J Dent Res.* 18(4):190–5.

Berglundh T, Persson L, Klinge B. (2002) A systematic review of the incidence of biological and technical complications in implant dentistry reported in prospective longitudinal studies of at least 5 years. *J Clin Periodontol.* 29 Suppl 3:197–212; discussion 232–3.

Brånemark P-I. (2005) *The Osseointegration Book:From Calvarium to Calcaneus.* Quintessence, Chicago.

Brägger U, Aeschlimann S, Bürgin W, Hämmerle CH, Lang NP. (2001) Biological and technical complications and failures with fixed partial dentures (FPDs) on implants and teeth after four to five years of function. *Clin Oral Implants Res.* 12(1): 26–34.

Buser D, Mericske-Stern R, Bernard JP, Behneke A, Behneke N, Hirt HP, Belser UC, Lang NP. (1997) Long-term evaluation of non-submerged ITI implants. Part 1: 8-year life table analysis of a prospective multi-center study with 2359 implants. A systematic review of the incidence of biological and technical complications in implant dentistry reported in prospective longitudinal studies of at least 5 years. *Clin Oral Implants Res.* 8(3): 161–72.

Chen ST, Buser D. (2010) Esthetic complications due to implant malpositions: etiology, prevention, and treatment. In: S Froum (ed.), *Dental Implant Complications: Etiology, Prevention and Treatment.* Wiley-Blackwell, Ames, pp. 134–55.

Dawson A, Chen S. (eds.) (2009) *The SAC Classification in Implant Dentistry.* Quintessence, Berlin.

De Smet E, van Steenberghe D, Quirynen M, Naert I. (2001) The influence of plaque and/or excessive loading on marginal soft and hard tissue reactions around Brånemark implants: a review of literature and experience. *Int J Periodontics Restorative Dent.* 21(4):381–93.

Eckert SE, Meraw SJ, Cal E, Ow RK. (2000) Analysis of incidence and associated factors with fractured implants: a retrospective study. *Int J Oral Maxillofac Implants.* 15(5):662–7.

Eckert SE, Choi YG, Sánchez AR, Koka S. (2005) Comparison of dental implant systems: quality of clinical evidence and prediction of 5-year survival. *Int J Oral Maxillofac Implants.* 20(3):406–15.

Esposito M, Hirsch JM, Lekholm U, Thomsen P. (1998) Biological factors contributing to failures of osseointegrated oral implants. (I). Success criteria and epidemiology. *Eur J Oral Sci.* 106(1):527–51.

Esposito M, Grusovin MG, Worthington HV. (2012a) Interventions for replacing missing teeth: treatment of peri-implantitis. *Cochrane Database Syst Rev.* (1):CD004970.

Esposito M, Klinge B, Meyle J, Mombelli A, Rompen E, van Steenberghe D, Van Dyke T, Wang HL, van Winkelhoff AJ. (2012b) Working Group on the Treatment Options for the Maintenance of Marginal Bone Around Endosseous Oral Implants, Stockholm, Sweden, 8 and 9 September 2011. Consensus statements. *Eur J Oral Implantol.* 5 Suppl:S105–6.

Froum S. (ed.) (2010) *Dental Implant Complications: Etiology, Prevention and Treatment.* Wiley-Blackwell, Ames.

Goodacre CJ, Kan JY, Rungcharassaeng K. (1999) Clinical complications of osseointegrated implants. *J Prosthet Dent.* 81(5):537–52.

Goodacre CJ, Bernal G, Rungcharassaeng K, Kan JY. (2003) Clinical complications with implants and implant prostheses. *J Prosthet Dent.* 90(2): 121–32.

Implant Identification websites (2013) http://whatimplantisthat.com/; http://osseosource.com/dental-implants/; http://www.whichimplant.com/

Isidor F. (1997) Histological evaluation of peri-implant bone at implants subjected to occlusal overload or plaque accumulation. *Clin Oral Implants Res.* 8(1):1–9.

Isidor F. (2006) Influence of forces on peri-implant bone. *Clin Oral Implants Res.* 17 Suppl 2: 8–18.

Jokstad A. (2009) *Osseointegration and Dental Implants.* Wiley-Blackwell, Ames.

Jung RE, Zembic A, Pjetursson BE, Zwahlen M, Thoma DS. (2012) Systematic review of the survival rate and the incidence of biological, technical, and aesthetic complications of single crowns on implants reported in longitudinal studies with a mean follow-up of 5 years. *Clin Oral Implants Res.* 23 Suppl 6:2–21.

Karoussis IK, Kotsovilis S, Fourmousis I. (2007) A comprehensive and critical review of dental implant prognosis in periodontally compromised partially edentulous patients. *Clin Oral Implants Res.* 18(6):669–79.

Klinge B, Hultin M, Berglundh T. (2005) Peri-implantitis. *Dent Clin North Am.* 49(3):661–76.

Lang NP, Tonetti MS. (2010) Peri-implantitis: etiology, pathogenesis, prevention, and therapy. In: S Froum (ed.), *Dental Implant Complications: Etiology,*

Prevention and Treatment. Wiley-Blackwell, Ames, pp. 119–33.

Lang NP, Pjetursson BE, Tan K, Brägger U, Egger M, Zwahlen M. (2004) A systematic review of the survival and complication rates of fixed partial dentures (FPDs) after an observation period of at least 5 years. II. Combined tooth—implant-supported FPDs. *Clin Oral Implants Res.* 15(6):643–53.

Lang NP Berglundh T; Working Group 4 of Seventh European Workshop on Periodontology. (2011) Periimplant diseases: where are we now?—Consensus of the Seventh European Workshop on Periodontology. *J Clin Periodontol.* 38 Suppl 11: 178–81.

Lindhe J Meyle J; Group D of European Workshop on Periodontology. (2008) Peri-implant diseases: Consensus Report of the Sixth European Workshop on Periodontology. *J Clin Periodontol.* 35 (8 Suppl):282–5.

Lindquist LW, Carlsson GE, Jemt T. (1996) A prospective 15-year follow-up study of mandibular fixed prostheses supported by osseointegrated implants. Clinical results and marginal bone loss. *Clin Oral Implants Res.* 7(4):329–36.

Palma-Carrió C, Balaguer-Martínez J, Peñarrocha-Oltra D, Peñarrocha-Diago M. (2011) Irritative and sensory disturbances in oral implantology. Literature review. *Med Oral Patol Oral Cir Bucal.* 16(7): e1043–6.

Papaspyridakos P, Chen CJ, Chuang SK, Weber HP, Gallucci GO. (2012) A systematic review of biologic and technical complications with fixed implant rehabilitations for edentulous patients. *Int J Oral Maxillofac Implants.* 27(1):102–10.

Pjetursson BE, Tan K, Lang NP, Brägger U, Egger M, Zwahlen M. (2004a) A systematic review of the survival and complication rates of fixed partial dentures (FPDs) after an observation period of at least 5 years. I: implant supported FPDs. *Clin Oral Implants Res.* 15(6):625–42.

Pjetursson BE, Tan K, Lang NP, Brägger U, Egger M, Zwahlen M. (2004b) A systematic review of the survival and complication rates of fixed partial dentures (FPDs) after an observation period of at least 5 years. IV: cantilever FPDs. *Clin Oral Implants Res.* 15(6):667–76.

Pjetursson BE, Thoma D, Jung R, Zwahlen M, Zembic A. (2012) A systematic review of the survival and complication rates of implant-supported fixed dental prostheses (FDPs) after a mean observation period of at least 5 years. *Clin Oral Implants Res.* 23 Suppl 6:22–38.

Pontoriero R, Tonelli MP, Carnevale G, Mombelli A, Nyman SR, Lang NP. (1994) Experimentally induced peri-implant mucositis. A clinical study in humans. *Clin Oral Implants Res.* 5(4):254–9.

Quirynen M, Naert I, van Steenberghe D. (1992) Fixture design and overload influence marginal bone loss and fixture success in the Brånemark system. *Clin Oral Implants Res.* 3(3):104–11.

Romeo E, Storelli S. (2012) Systematic review of the survival rate and the biological, technical, and aesthetic complications of fixed dental prostheses with cantilevers on implants reported in longitudinal studies with a mean of 5 years follow-up. *Clin Oral Implants Res.* 23 Suppl 6:39–49.

Roos-Jansåker AM, Renvert S, Egelberg J. (2003) Treatment of peri-implant infections: a literature review. *J Clin Periodontol.* 30(6):467–85.

Rosenberg ES, Torosian J. (1998) An evaluation of differences and similarities observed in fixture failure of five distinct implant systems. *Pract Periodontics Aesthet Dent.* 10(6):687–98.

Rosenberg ES, Cho SC, Elian N, Jalbout ZN, Froum S, Evian CI. (2004) A comparison of characteristics of implant failure and survival in periodontally compromised and periodontally healthy patients: a clinical report. *Int J Oral Maxillofac Implants.* 19(6):873–9.

Schou S, Holmstrup P, Stoltze K, Hjørting-Hansen E, Kornman KS. (1993) Ligature-induced marginal inflammation around osseointegrated implants and ankylosed teeth. *Clin Oral Implants Res.* 4(1): 12–22.

Schwarz F, Becker J. (2010) *Peri-implant Infection: Etiology, Diagnosis and Treatment.* Quintessence, London.

van Steenberghe D, Naert I, Jacobs R, Quirynen M. (1999) Influence of inflammatory reactions vs. occlusal loading on peri-implant marginal bone level. *Adv Dent Res.* 13:130–5.

Wallace RH. (2000) The relationship between cigarette smoking and dental implant failure. *Eur J Prosthodont Restor Dent.* 8(3):103–6.

Weber HP, Cochran DL. (1998) The soft tissue response to osseointegrated dental implants. *J Prosthet Dent.* 79(1):79–89.

Appendix A

Fundamentals of Implant Dentistry, First Edition. Gerard Byrne.
© 2014 John Wiley & Sons, Inc. Published 2014 by John Wiley & Sons, Inc.
Companion website: www.wiley.com/go/byrne/implants

IMPLANT AND PATIENT INFORMATION AND CONSENT FORM

Patient Name _____

1. I understand that dental implant procedures involve a surgical phase (inserting the implants) and a prosthodontic phase (replacing teeth) and that a separate fee is charged for each phase.

2. I understand that after the surgical phase is completed, the completion of my treatment may range from 4–10 months and that additional procedures may extend completion time.

3. I have been informed and I understand the purpose and the nature of the implant surgery procedure. I understand there will be two planned surgical procedures: 1) opening the gum tissue followed by a precision drilling of small openings into the underlying jaw bone, and then the filling of these openings with dental implants similar in size to a small single tooth root. The gum tissue will be closed over the implants with sutures (stitches) which will be removed in 7–14 days. I understand that I cannot wear any denture over the healing implants for at least two weeks and that my present denture must be adjusted and/or lined with soft lining before it can be worn. 2) I understand a second surgical procedure, 3–6 months after the first procedure, will be necessary to place implant abutments through the gum. I also understand that the healing of the gum following the second surgical procedure may result in irregularities that may require other surgical corrections that may incur an additional fee (e.g. gum or bone grafts).

3a. I hereby authorize the following Drs. _____ and such assistants as may be selected by them, to treat the condition(s) described as follows:

Surgical:

Restorative:

4. Alternatives to this treatment have been explained to me which may include but are not limited to: 1) Continuing with my present denture or not replacing missing teeth; 2) Constructing a new denture without surgical correction or placement of a fixed (non-removable) bridge if adequate teeth are available; 3) Constructing a new denture with surgical procedures which may include but are not limited to: moving muscle attachments, nerves, bone, or soft tissue grafting. I understand and have considered these alternatives, but I want dental implants to help secure the replacement tooth or teeth.

5. I understand there are possible risks and side effects involved with surgery, drugs, and anesthesia. Such complications may include pain, swelling, infection, discoloration, numbness of the lip, tongue, chin, cheek, or teeth may occur. The exact duration of complications may not be determinable and may be irreversible. Also possible are inflammation of a vein, injury to teeth present, bone fractures, sinus penetration, delayed healing, allergic reactions or side effects to drugs or medications used.

6. If you are taking a bisphosphonate, a drug most often prescribed for osteoporosis, you may be at risk for developing osteonecrosis of the jaw. Common names of this class of drug include Fosamax, Actonel, and Boniva. Please ask your provider if you have any questions relative to the risks of these drugs and your procedure.

7. I understand that if no implants are done, any of the following could occur: loss of bone, gum tissue inflammation, infection, tooth or gum sensitivity, looseness and/or drifting of teeth, looseness of dentures/bridges and the necessity of tooth extraction. Also possible are temporomandibular joint (jaw) problems, headaches, referred pains to the back of the neck and facial muscles, and tired muscles when chewing.

8. It has been explained to me that there is no method to accurately predict gum and bone healing capabilities in each patient following the placement of the implant and that in some instances implants fail and must be removed. I have been informed and understand that the practice of dentistry is not an exact science; no guarantees or assurances as to the outcome of results of treatment or surgery can be made.

A.1 Implant consent form.

9   If an implant fails to integrate to the bone at or before the second stage procedure (abutment connection), I understand I have the fellowing options: 1) Removal of the implant and replacement of a new implant at the proper time. There will be no surgical fee for this replacement but I will be responsible for any additional procedures necessary to improve chances of success; 2) Removal of the implant and no replacement. Again, no there will be no surgical fee for the removal of the implant but there may be additional costs for modifications in the planned prosthesis.

10.   I understand that smoking, alcohol, or improper diet affect gum healing and may limit the success of the implant(s). I agree to follow the doctor's hygiene and diet instructions. I agree to report to my doctor for regular examinations as instructed.

11.   I agree to conscious sedation/anesthesia if necessary, depending on the choice of the doctor. If conscious sedation is indicated, I understand that drowsiness may occur and that I will not drink alcohol or take any medicines other than those prescribed or recommended by my doctor for the implant procedure. I have reported all medications prescribed by other doctors or that I take non-prescribed. I will follow doctor's presedation instructions, including not eating or drinking eight (8) hours prior to sedation and arrange a driver to take me home. I agree not to operate a motor vehicle or hazardous equipment or devices for at least 24 hours or more until fully recovered from the effects of the anesthesia or drugs given for my care.

12.   I have been given an accurate report of my physical and mental health history. I have also reported any prior allergic or unusual reactions to drugs, food, insect bites, anesthetics, pollens, or dust.

13.   I consent to photography, filming, and recording of the procedure to be performed for the advancement of implant dentistry, provided my identity is not revealed.

14.   It has been explained to me that after the completion of healing from the surgical phase (integration of the implants and placement of the abutments) that the prosthodontic phase (replacement of teeth) must be completed.

15.   I understand that the prosthodontic phase will likely be completed by another (my general dentist, a dental student or other dentist recommended) and that the fee for the prosthodontic phase is separate and in addition to the surgical phase.

16.   I have been informed and understand that:

(a)   the design or type of prosthesis (tooth, bridge or denture) may require modification due to the number or final position of the implants

(b)   the prosthesis that attaches to the implants may not look, feel or chew as well as natural teeth

(c)   cleaning the implants and prosthesis may be more difficult than natural teeth

17.   I understand that I must thoroughly clean my implants and prosthesis as prescribed and that I must have periodic professional cleanings and prosthesis evaluations. Just as can occur with conventional dental work, repairs or replacements may generate additional fees and would be handled on a case-by-case basis.

18.   I understand there are two estimated fees for my treatment:

1)   Surgical phase $ _____   2)   Prosthodontic phase $ _____

19.   I request and authorize medical/dental services for me, including implants and other surgery. I fully understand that during, and following the contemplated procedure, surgery, or treatment, conditions may become apparent which warrant, in the judgement of the doctor, additional or alternative treatment pertinent to the success of comprehensive treatment. I also approve any modification in design, materials, or care, if it is felt this is for my best interest.

I CERTIFY THAT I READ AND WRITE ENGLISH AND HAVE READ AND FULLY UNDERSTAND THE ABOVE AUTHORIZATION AND INFORMED CONSENT FOR IMPLANT SURGERY AND PROSTHESIS AND THAT ALL MY QUESTIONS HAVE BEEN FULLY ANSWERED.

SIGNATURE OF PATIENT OR RESPONSIBLE PERSON (AGE 19 OR OLDER)	DATE SIGNED (M/D/Y)
WITNESS (professional staff member)	DATE SIGNED (M/D/Y)
FACULTY MEMBER & STUDENT	DATE SIGNED (M/D/Y)

A.1 *Continued*

Appendix B

General reference books

Block MS. (2011) *Color Atlas of Dental Implant Surgery*, 3rd ed. Saunders, St. Louis.

Brånemark P-I. (2006) *The Osseointegration Book: From Calvarium to Calcaneus*. Quintessence, Chicago.

Brånemark P-I, Zarb G, Albrektsson T. (1985) *Tissue-Integrated Prostheses: Osseointegration in Clinical Dentistry*. Quintessence, Chicago.

Dibart S, Dibart J-P. (2011) *Practical Osseous Surgery in Periodontics and Implant Dentistry*. Wiley-Blackwell, Ames.

Drago C, Peterson T. (2007) *Implant Restorations: A Step-by-Step Guide*, 2nd ed. Wiley-Blackwell, Ames.

Froum SJ. (ed.) (2010) *Dental Implant Complications: Etiology, Prevention, and Treatment*. Wiley-Blackwell, Ames.

Jokstad A. (ed.) (2009) *Osseointegration and Dental Implants*. Wiley-Blackwell, Ames.

Misch CE. (2005) *Dental Implant Prosthetics*. Elsevier Mosby, St. Louis.

Misch CE. (2007) *Contemporary Implant Dentistry*, 3rd ed. Mosby, St. Louis.

Schroeder A, Sutter F, Krekeler G. (1991) *Oral Implantology: Basics—ITI Hollow Cylinder*. Thieme, New York.

Schroeder A, Sutter F, Buser D, Krekeler G. (1996) *Oral Implantology: Basics—ITI Hollow Cylinder*. Thieme, New York.

Spiekermann H. (1995) *Color Atlas of Dental Medicine: Implantology*. Thieme, Stuttgart.

ITI treatment guides

Belser U, Martin W, Jung R, Hämmerle C, Schmid B, Morton D, Buser D. (2007) In: D Buser, U Belser, D Wismeijer (eds.), *ITI Treatment Guide: Volume 1: Implant Therapy in the Esthetic Zone: Single-Tooth Replacements*. Quintessence, Berlin.

Chen S, Buser D. (2008) In: D Buser, D Wismeijer, U Belser (eds.), *ITI Treatment Guide: Volume 3: Implant Placement in Post-Extraction Sites: Treatment Options*. Quintessence, Berlin.

Cordaro L, Terheyden H. (2014) In: S Chen, D Buser, D Wismeijer (eds.), *ITI Treatment Guide: Volume 7: Ridge Augmentation Procedures in Implant Patients: A Staged Approach*. Quintessence, Berlin.

Dawson A, Chen S. (eds.) (2009) *The SAC Classification in Implant Dentistry*. Quintessence, Berlin.

Jensen S, Katsuyama H. (2011) In: S Chen, D Buser, D Wismeijer (eds.), *ITI Treatment Guide: Volume 5. Sinus Floor Elevation Procedures*. Quintessence, Berlin.

Morton D, Ganeles J. (2007) In: D Wismeijer, D Buser, U Belser (eds.), *ITI Treatment Guide: Volume 2. Loading Protocols in Implant Dentistry: Partially Dentate Patients*. Quintessence, Berlin.

Wismeijer D, Casentini P, Gallucci GO, Chiapasco M. (2010) In: D Wismeijer, D Buser, U Belser (eds.), *ITI Treatment Guide: Volume 4: Loading Protocols in Implant Dentistry: Edentulous Patients*. Quintessence, Berlin.

Wittneben JG, Webber HP. (2013) In: D Wismeijer, S Chen, D Buser (eds.), *ITI Treatment Guide: Volume 6: Extended Edentulous Spaces in the Esthetic Zone*. Quintessence, Berlin.

Fundamentals of Implant Dentistry, First Edition. Gerard Byrne.
© 2014 John Wiley & Sons, Inc. Published 2014 by John Wiley & Sons, Inc.
Companion website: www.wiley.com/go/byrne/implants

Index

Abutment
 CAD/CAM, 76, 154, 216, 222
 ceramic, 66, 156
 custom, 74, 153, 154
 healing, 73, 105, 134, 140, 182, 183, 221
 locating jig, 154, 170
 overdenture, 76, 78
 prefabricated, 66, 75, 153, 168
 standard, 76
 temporary, 75, 140, 151, 166
 transmucosal, 8, 106, 234
 UCLA, 65, 73, 168
Age, of patient, 84
Allograft, 138, 196
Alloplast, 138, 196, 201
Aluminum oxide, 10, 24, 66
Analgesia, 131
Antibiotic prophylaxis, 122, 131
Anticoagulant, 83, 121
Anti-rotation, 8, 71, 157
Attachments for overdenture, 77, 114, 174, 184, 216
Augmentation, *see also* Sinus lift
 ridge, 192–202
 socket, 137
Autogenous graft, 196, 199, 201

BAM (Bio-absorbable membrane),
 see Membranes
Bar, for overdenture, 213–216, 221
BIC, 45, 49, 57, 60, 65
Biofilms, 113
Biologic width, 31, 238
Biomechanics, 43–60
Bisphosphonates, 122
Bleeding on probing (BOP), 15, 35, 113, 238
Block graft, 138, 199, 200
Bone
 graft, 91, 137, 196, 200
 loss, 4, 12, 13, 15, 28, 34, 44, 110, 123, 228, 230, 237–239
 morphogenetic protein, 26, 197
 quality, 110, 127–128, 133, 139, 140
 volume, 125, 137, 147, 166, 176, 194–202
BOP, *see* Bleeding on probing
Brånemark, 1, 3, 10, 23, 25, 72, 103

CAD/CAM, 66
Cantilever, 45, 52, 57–59, 165, 170, 215, 231
Caries, 86, 98
CBCT, *see* Cone beam computed tomography
Cementation, 109, 154, 154, 158, 168
Ceramic implants, 10

Fundamentals of Implant Dentistry, First Edition. Gerard Byrne.
© 2014 John Wiley & Sons, Inc. Published 2014 by John Wiley & Sons, Inc.
Companion website: www.wiley.com/go/byrne/implants